The Anthropology of Welfare

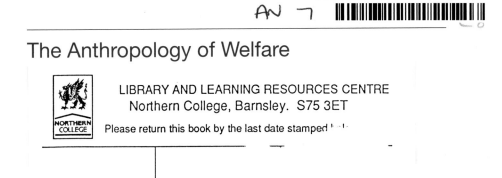
The Anthropology of Welfare provides an overview of what anthropology has to offer welfare studies and vice versa. Case studies from anthropologists in the field examine different branches of welfare and community care, for example:

- Maternity services
- Children with learning difficulties
- Children's homes
- Mothers' centres
- People with HIV
- Mental health centres
- Housing
- Care and provision for the elderly

Examples are taken from urban and rural areas of the UK, USA, Sweden, Germany, Portugal and New Zealand. In each case the theoretical and methodological appropriateness of social anthropology for the study of welfare, and the insights gained by bringing anthropology and welfare together, are examined.

The Anthropology of Welfare will be essential reading for those studying anthropology, social work and social policy and will be of interest to teachers, practitioners and researchers in applied social welfare fields.

Iain R. Edgar and **Andrew Russell** are both Lecturers in Anthropology at the University of Durham.

The Anthropology of Welfare

Edited by Iain R. Edgar and Andrew Russell

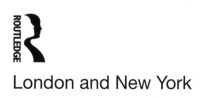

London and New York

First published 1998 by Routledge
11 New Fetter Lane, London EC4P 4EE

Simultaneously published in the USA and Canada
by Routledge
29 West 35th Street, New York, NY 10001

Typeset in Baskerville by Routledge

Printed and bound in Great Britain by T. J. International Ltd, Padstow,
Cornwall

British Library Cataloguing in Publication Data
A catalogue record for this book is available from the British Library

Library of Congress Cataloguing in Publication Data
The anthropology of welfare/edited by Iain Edgar and Andrew Russell.
p. cm.
Includes bibliographical references and index.
1. Public welfare. 2. Social service. 3. Ethnology.
4. Community organization. 5. Social policy.
I. Edgar, Iain R., 1948–. II. Russell, Andrew, 1958–.
HV40.A786 1998
361.8–dc21
97-49568
CIP

ISBN 0-415-16964-X (hbk)
ISBN 0-415-16965-8 (pbk)

Contents

Notes on contributors   vii
Acknowledgements   xi

1 **Research and practice in the anthropology of welfare**   1
Andrew Russell and Iain R. Edgar

2 **'You just get on with it': questioning models of welfare**   16
dependency in a rural community
Pia Christensen, Jenny Hockey and Allison James

3 **Concepts of community in changing health care:**   33
a study of change in midwifery practice
Christine McCourt

4 **The child welfare debate in Portugal:**   57
a case study of a children's home
Karen Aarre

5 **'Equal, but different'? Welfare, gender ideology**   73
and a 'mothers' centre' in southern Germany
Lisa Hoecklin

6 **The co-operation concept in a team of Swedish social**   97
workers: applying grid and group to studies of
community care
Steve Trevillion and David Green

7 **Caring communities or effective networks?**   120
Community care and people with learning
difficulties in South Wales
Charlotte Aull Davies

8 **Staff models and practice: managing 'trouble' in a**   137
community-based programme for chronically
mentally ill adults in the USA
Dana M. Baldwin

 9 **A local anthropology of exclusion**   161
    John Given

10 **Considering the culture of community care:**   183
    anthropological accounts of the experiences of
    frontline carers, older people and a researcher
    Lorna Warren

11 **Treasures on Earth: housing assets, public policy and**   209
    older people in New Zealand
    Sally Keeling

12 **Residents' participation in the management of**   228
    retirement housing in the UK
    Peter Lloyd

13 **Using experiential research methods:**   246
    the potential contribution of humanistic groupwork
    methods to anthropology and welfare research
    Iain R. Edgar

    Index   262

Contributors

Karen Aarre graduated in social anthropology and development studies at the School of Oriental and African Studies, University of London, in 1994. The thesis for her MPhil degree in social anthropology at Oxford was about 'the child' in Portugal, based on fieldwork in a Portuguese children's home. She is currently on an ESRC Research Studentship doing fieldwork in another Portuguese children's home for her DPhil dissertation, also at Oxford.

Dana M. Baldwin is a researcher in the UCLA Neuropsychiatric Institute Drug Abuse Research Center. She received her PhD in anthropology from the University of California at Los Angeles, and has served as a consultant at the RAND Corporation and as a researcher in the Organizational Research Department of the Kaiser Permanente Medical Care Program in California. Her research interests include medical anthropology, qualitative research methods, mental health, and substance abuse.

Pia Christensen is a social anthropologist with research interests in the sociology and anthropology of childhood. Author of a number of publications on the cultural performance of children's sickness, she is currently carrying out research into the social organization of children's time at the University of Hull.

Charlotte Aull Davies is lecturer in the Department of Sociology and Anthropology, University of Wales Swansea. Her research interests include learning disabilities, gender and ethnic identities, nationalism and migration. She is the author of *Welsh Nationalism in the Twentieth Century: The Ethnic Option and the Modern State* (Praeger 1989).

Iain R. Edgar is a lecturer in Social Anthropology at the University of Durham. Previously he practised as a qualified social worker and then taught social work at the University of Northumbria. During this later period, he studied first therapeutic communities and then dreamwork groups to gain a PhD in Social Anthropology from the University of Keele.

John Given is a senior lecturer at the University of Northumbria at Newcastle-upon-Tyne, who established and ran an applied social research centre focusing upon urban issues. He is currently teaching and researching in narrative method.

David Green is a researcher at Brunel University. For the past three years he has been working with Steve Trevillion on the development of new social network and comparative approaches to the study of community care.

Jenny Hockey is a social anthropologist teaching health studies at Hull University. Her publications include *Experiences of Death* (Edinburgh University Press) and *Growing Up and Growing Old* (Sage 1993, with A. James). She co-edits the *Journal of Gender Studies*.

Lisa Hoecklin is completing a DPhil in social anthropology at Oxford. She has an MBA from Washington University and worked for five years in management consulting in the United States and England. In 1992, she conducted a major research project commissioned by the Economist Intelligence Unit into the assumptions and strategies with which multinational organizations manage cultural differences. Her interests in social anthropology are on issues of gender, social policy and organizational management.

Allison James is a social anthropologist at Hull University whose research interests centre on the new social studies of childhood and the life course. Her publications include *After Writing Culture* (Routledge 1997, co-edited with J. Hockey and A. Dawson) and *Theorising Childhood* (Polity Press 1997, with C. Jenks and A. Prout).

Sally Keeling completed an honours degree in social anthropology at the University of Otago, Dunedin, New Zealand in the early 1970s. Since then she has worked in social and educational service management throughout New Zealand. Following a period managing community and residential aged care services, she returned to university to undertake doctoral studies.

Peter Lloyd is emeritus professor of Social Anthropology at the University of Sussex. Since his virtual retirement from teaching he has been involved in many projects relating to the welfare of older people. He was founder of Social Anthropology, Social and Community Work (SASCW), which merged in 1988 to form the British Association of Social Anthropology in Policy and Practice (BASAPP), now Anthropology in Action (A-in-A). He is also Volunteer Community Care Policy Advisor to the Sussex Rural Community Council.

Christine McCourt is a senior lecturer in Health Services Research at the Wolfson Institute, Thames Valley University. She trained in anthropology at the London School of Economics and completed a doctorate in social anthropology and social policy there in 1990. Her research interests are in psychiatry, childbirth and the analysis of institutional change, particularly from the perspectives of people using such services.

Andrew Russell is a lecturer in the Department of Anthropology at the University of Durham. His specializations are in medical anthropology and applied/development anthropology. His DPhil research in social anthropology was carried out amongst the Yakha in the middle hills of East Nepal. He is convenor of the Centre for the Study of Contraceptive Issues at Durham and University College Stockton.

Steve Trevillion is reader in Social Work and Social Policy at Brunel University. He is associated with the development of networking and collaboration. For the past three years he has been working with David Green on the development of new social network and comparative approaches to the study of community care.

Lorna Warren is a lecturer in the Department of Sociological Studies at the University of Sheffield. She has been working on studies of community care since 1983. Her publications include *Changing Services for Older People* (1996).

Acknowledgements

Many human threads are temporally and creatively woven into the outcome of this book. It probably began, unbeknown, with the first meeting of the group Social Anthropology, Social and Community Work (SASCW), which Iain Edgar attended in 1985. SASCW was initiated by Peter Lloyd, following the Grillo report into vocational prospects for anthropology graduates, and it was initially supported by the Wenner-Gren foundation. SASCW progressively brought together social anthropologists working full-time in welfare work as practitioners or researchers, and academic anthropologists with professional interests in this branch of 'anthropology at home'. At the first meeting of SASCW Rosemary Lamb, now deceased, movingly spoke about how she used her anthropological training in her welfare work in rural Northumberland. Ears pricked up; something original and exciting was on the move.

SASCW became the British Association for the Study of Anthropology in Policy and Practice in 1989 with the merger of SASCW with GAPP (Group for Anthropology in Policy and Practice) and ATE (Anthropology in Teaching and Education). As happens, BASAPP later begat Anthropology in Action (A-in-A).

The actual beginning of the book happened at a memorial seminar for David Brooks in Durham in 1994. David, an anthropology lecturer at Durham University, had been a formidable influence on the creative thinking of a generation of social anthropology graduates there, and the gathering was an opportunity for his academic friends and ex-students to meet and honour his memory. Several future contributors to this volume were there. At the meeting, Sue Wright suggested the idea for the book to the editors, who then developed a workshop on the theme of 'Poor Culture, Good Economy? The Anthropology of Community Care' at the 1996 European Association of Social Anthropology (EASA) bi-annual conference in Barcelona. The book rapidly developed thereafter with the excellent support of Heather Gibson and Fiona Bailey, in particular, at Routledge.

Further thanks are due the University of Durham and the British Academy for their financial support for the development of the workshop at the EASA conference. In the final stages, several people supported our (and the book's) welfare in adversity. Todd Rae provided advice on converting computer files and dealing with their viruses, and Malia Fullerton dealt with the vagaries of the Internet. Sally Keeling's input as proofreader for a number of final chapter drafts was also much appreciated. Finally we would like to thank our families for all the care, community and perspective they have provided as this work has progressed.

Chapter 1

Research and practice in the anthropology of welfare

Andrew Russell and Iain R. Edgar

INTRODUCTION

This is a book about human welfare, defined in the broadest sense as the process of normalizing or optimizing the well-being of dependent individuals, organizations and societies. We look at the people who receive welfare, and those who give it, and the social institutions, organizations and networks that are involved in the process. This is also a book about anthropology, in many ways the most far-reaching and inclusive of the social science disciplines, and what it has to say about welfare, its provision and distribution. The book champions the relevance of social anthropology to welfare research and practice, and the value of welfare as a research topic in anthropology. It also looks at methods in welfare practice and how these can be incorporated into social anthropological enquiry.

Various new and 'applied' fields of anthropology have formed in the past fifty years or so,[1] but no distinctive 'anthropology of welfare' has emerged amongst them. This lack is somewhat surprising. Anthropology, despite (or as part of) its colonial heritage, has always had a strong tradition of representing the minority, the underdog, the dependent and disempowered. Durkheim, as Titmuss (1987) points out, long ago argued that individualization and specialization in society make people more socially dependent (Durkheim 1933). Welfare is premised on the assumption that some are more dependent, and needful of help, than others. As Titmuss goes on to say, 'conceptions of "need" and "dependency" have simultaneously been profoundly affected by technological, industrial and social change' (1987: 53). So too have the ways of servicing these culturally defined needs and dependencies, activities which can take place in a number of different spheres: domestic, employment, commercial and state (Jordan 1987: 1). Political and economic forces apart, what 'normalization or optimization' involves (in our definition of welfare above) is also largely socio-culturally defined, as recent debates in journals such as *Critical Social Policy* have testified.

A Durkheimian division into 'simple' and 'complex' societies can be made on the basis of the amorphousness and separation of the spheres in which activities directed towards human welfare can take place, and hence the distribution of welfare within society. 'Simple' societies are marked by all welfare activities taking place as part of the customary, face-to-face relationships of communal living, while 'complex' societies, and welfare delivery, are marked by legally based, impersonal relationships between individuals. However, such a distinction quickly breaks down when subject to scrutiny in any social context, with characteristics of the 'simple' contained in the most 'complex' societies, and the 'complex' increasingly recognized as impinging directly on the 'simple'. The need for welfare is a product of, and provision of welfare a response to, power relationships in society. 'Dependency' occurs regardless of whether the society in question is 'simple' or 'complex'. Policies such as 'community care' within the UK are premised on a view of society that emphasizes its 'simple' characteristics – the face-to-face, family and 'community' relationships in and through which 'care' is primarily to be situated and performed.

A preliminary issue to be grappled with by any effort at developing an anthropology of welfare is the differing 'languages' of welfare used in different parts of the world. In the USA, for example, welfare is defined simply, and quite materialistically, as 'the complex of financial assistance and in-kind goods that sustain those without income or savings' (Glasser 1994: 3). In Britain over the past fifty years, 'welfare', marked by the formation (or, perhaps, reification) of the 'welfare state' with its offer of assistance at the point of need, from cradle to grave, has remained a concern much broader in its scope than American definitions allow.

Questions concerning what welfare provision should entail, and where it should come from, are intensely contested in most industrialized societies. 'Community care' is a largely British attempt from the 1970s to create something of an opposing ideology to prevailing views of what a 'welfare state' is or should be. 'Community care' articulates a romantic, *gemeinschaft* view of 'welfare' and where it will be located. In Britain, 'community' is often pictured in opposition to the state, something which has just disappeared but which, with a little more effort, might be found, or developed, again. It is often used as a gloss for the sometimes chimerical diminution of the powers of the state in favour of local control (McCourt, chapter 3). Thus in the UK in the 1980s the nationally implemented (and hated) poll tax became softened as the (local) 'community charge', 'approved schools' become 'community schools', and the concept of 'community policing' took hold. 'Community care' became in many ways 'a new utopia enchanting society' (Tomlinson 1991: 1), based on 'a cult of localism, [and] rejection of fixed term representative forms of authority' (*ibid.*).

What the anthropology of welfare makes plain is that 'community' as a concept has different meanings both across and within specific cultures. What anthropologists seek to do in exploring these differences is to look beneath the stated (or 'imagined' – Anderson 1991) community to examine the real nature of the 'communities' of which we speak, the localities with their kin, friendship, work and other social networks in which 'welfare' (glossed as 'care') follows its increasingly uncertain trajectory. Often this involves methods such as semantic analysis and long-term participant-observation. Trevillion and Green (chapter 6) point out that in Swedish there is no term for 'community' as such, and in

Portugal, as Aarre's chapter 4 shows, what in Britain might go under the aegis of a policy-driven 'community care' is more appropriately recognized as part of an indigenous 'welfare society'. As Davies suggests in her chapter, 'community care' as a concept has become too politically idealized to be very useful as a heuristic device. For many of its recipients in her case study, community care is seen as just another form of welfare provision. We shall hereafter, for the purposes of this book, treat 'community care' as a locally constructed subset of welfare, not as a qualitatively different phenomenon.

Until recently, there was only a disparate, fragmented literature about the anthropology of welfare, which had not been collated and theorized distinctively. However, the relative paucity of jobs in academia in the 1970s and 1980s meant that many anthropologists in Britain and the US went into 'soft', more applied fields such as social work and community health (D'Andrade *et al.* 1975). In the last ten years or so these scholars have started to publish innovative work in this field, work which has led to interesting new perspectives on issues which have sometimes worn stale in fields such as sociology, psychology or social policy.

Social anthropology, then, promises fresh theoretical and methodological approaches to the subject of welfare. A number of areas of convergence between anthropology and welfare can be discerned. The rest of this chapter will explore the nature of these convergences. There are a number of conceptual areas which we see as key to the active formulation of an anthropology of welfare, namely comparativism, representation, reflexivity, experience, society, culture and application. These, we suggest, are the fundamental concepts and points of convergence which form the dynamic of the anthropology of welfare as reflected in the contributions to this book.

ANTHROPOLOGY AND WELFARE: THE WORLD OUT THERE

Anthropology has traditionally involved the study of 'exotic' peoples in 'other' places, and a key feature of the discipline is that it still is (or should be) cross-cultural and comparative in its scope with regard to the study of welfare (or any other topic). Comparativism is now the fashion in many schools of social policy/welfare (e.g. Ginsburg 1992; Heidenheimer *et al.* 1990; Higgins 1981; Hill 1996). However, much of this work risks an ethnocentric preoccupation with spatial and cultural categories such as 'British', 'Anglo-American', 'Euro-American' or (at its largest extent) the 'western' or 'developed' world. A few authors have begun to cast their net wider than these limiting categories, to incorporate other areas such as 'Europe' or the 'Third World' (e.g. Batley and Stoker 1991; Cannan *et al.* 1992; Dixon and Scheurell 1995; Lorenz 1994; Scharf and Wenger 1995).

It may seem strange, given the roots of anthropology, that the chapters here are all concerned with 'the western world'. This is partly a reflection of where 'welfare anthropologists' have generally practised their craft to date, for a variety of political and economic reasons. This is not to say that 'welfare' is a product of western market capitalism, although it is in western market capitalism, as Durkheim predicts, that institutional arrangements for the provision of welfare are particularly pronounced (and, perhaps, the inequalities which presage the necessity of welfare most marked). However, the chapters in this book also reflect the fact that the anthropology of welfare is in many ways anthropology 'coming home'. In 'kicking around in our own backyard', anthropologists have something of an identity crisis. Social anthropology has to some extent been stigmatized through its past colonial history, its perceived focus on people living faraway, and its reluctance to engage in the activist, political analysis of modern society. As Trevillion and Green argue at the start of their chapter, anthropologists have more to offer welfare theorists than the largely discredited nineteenth-century anthropological theories of cultural evolution and diffusion. They champion the study of meanings, indicating the need to differentiate internally within categories such as 'Europe', 'western' or 'collaboration', and the value of doing so for the development of new and creative institutional cultures.

With their experience of 'exotic' cultures, it might be reasoned that anthropology and anthropologists are best placed to take up areas of concern such as ethnic minority provision. Indeed, such a subject might be seen as the 'specialist' domain of anthropology in the field of welfare studies. However, the papers in this volume also perhaps reflect a reluctance amongst some anthropologists to be limited to the ethnic/ethnological, or to be concerned solely with the concerns of 'other' societies. Instead, anthropologists are actively engaged in research into fields (and groups) based on gender, age or (for example) learning difficulties, in societies closer to 'home'. Just as the categories 'Anglo-American' or 'European' have to be disaggregated and problematized, so have categories such as 'Pakistani', 'women' or 'young people'.

This is not to say that anthropologists are solely concerned with the explication of categories. They are also concerned with how categories are formed, and the power relations which lead to the authority of some over others. The concept of 'empowerment' figures prominently in Lloyd's chapter (chapter 12) on the reasons why older people in retirement housing schemes in the UK have so little voice and influence. His analysis shows the complexity of issues involved, particularly the subtle interplay of forces influencing the exercise of power and authority in such schemes. The felt realities of power and influence are mediated through differing forms of social organization, particularly management policies, and the dynamics of age, class and ability amongst residents. Human issues of frailty and the fear of being consigned to a hospital or nursing home lurk as factors that can stifle residents' voices. Lloyd concludes that managing agencies are crucial in their facilitation and support of appropriate participatory structures.

The elderly are not widely respected or acknowledged in British society (Huby 1992). They are marginalized and, in a sense, are as 'far away' from mainstream experience, both spatially and temporally (cf. Keeling, chapter 11), as the exotic 'others' traditionally studied by anthropologists. The same can be said, in different ways, of the learning disabled, children in children's homes, and the social institutions of the mentally ill, to pick just a few of the topics covered in this volume. In short, the world of anthropology, like the world of welfare, is both elsewhere (out there) and everywhere (at home).

REPRESENTATION AND REFLEXIVITY

Reflections about how groups are represented, and the writer/observer's position in processes of representation, are other contemporary concerns common to both welfare and anthropology. Indeed, it could be said that representing others for cultural, political and ethical purposes is at the heart of each profession's activity. Representations, linguistically and symbolically codified, are seen as creating social reality rather than just reflecting it. This makes the discourse of representation, grounded in political-economic relations of production and consumption, the subject of critical study. The critical analysis of the practice of representation is becoming a major theme in both anthropology (e.g. Clifford 1986; James *et al.* 1996) and welfare studies (e.g. Pithouse 1987; Rojek *et al.* 1988).

Anthropology and welfare practice also converge in the different forms of reflexivity which have become central to the two professions. In social work practice, the need for practitioners who are aware and competent to challenge structural inequalities in society has become an educational requirement in new social work training programmes in the UK (CCETSW 1989). In order to develop an awareness of inequality in practitioners and their educators, these people are expected to reflect politically on the implications of their own structured positions in society. How does the experience of being black or white, male or female, homosexual or heterosexual affect consciousness, values and the micro-dynamics of everyday professional life? Such questions have been opened up for scrutiny only in the last few years. The problematization of the practitioner and the service agency has been a hallmark of recent feminist, anti-racist and socialist critiques of welfare practice (e.g. Jones 1983; Dominelli 1988; Dominelli and McLeod 1989).[2]

While in welfare practice the critical development of structural awareness is designed to sensitize workers to power issues in practice situations, reflexivity in anthropology is focused on the impact of the self in the development of the ethnography. How the implicit self, gendered, sexed and ethnicized, influences the form and content of the ethnography is a clear focus of contemporary concern (e.g. Okely and Calloway 1992). Warren (chapter 10) considers reflexively how her own gendered research role contributed to the final nature of the accounts of social care that she obtained. As Gaynor (1987: 1) writes, we are seeking in these endeavours to link 'biographical and subjective processes to broader structural changes in the society'.

THE EXPERIENCE OF WELFARE

These 'biographical and subjective processes' are synonymous, in much contemporary anthropology, with 'experience', although of course there is a complex interplay between experience and environment. A key point for anthropology is that 'welfare' is not an abstract concept, but translates into, or is transfigured by, the experiences of real actors in concrete situations. These interactions are often powerfully recorded in anthropological writings on the subject, at both individual and institutional levels. Bourdieu's theory of 'habitus' (Bourdieu 1977) is one of the anthropological theories invoked in such accounts to explain the nature of the relationships between the cared for, their carers, and the social, cultural and political-economic milieu in which their interactions take place (e.g. Christensen *et al.*, chapter 2). As their chapter exemplifies, however, such overarching theoretical approaches (the macro-level) are combined with fine-grained description (the micro-level), and the study of process and change predominate. Such combinations are unusual in other social science disciplines.

Anthropology sets great stock by its use of methods for capturing and recording 'experience', in particular participant-observation and other types of small qualitative studies throwing light both upon the perspective of those people studied (variously called 'the actor's perspective' or the 'native's point of view') and upon broader social issues (e.g. Churchill 1994; Spicer *et al.* 1994). Good qualitative research in anthropology is characterized by creativity in its choice and use of techniques and the ways these techniques can be used to access implicit knowledge, or what Geertz (1983) usefully terms 'cultural commonsense'. For example, Edgar (chapter 13) uses humanistic groupwork practices – artwork, imagework, sculpting, dreamwork, gestalt and psychodrama – which are relatively common in some areas of welfare work. He suggests, with examples, ways in which these practices are applicable as innovative methods in social anthropological and other social science research. Such work is exciting because it not only challenges what we regard as the world 'out there', but also involves the researcher or groupworker in the active generation of his/her experiential data.

Warren (chapter 10) reflects on her previous two major studies of frontline carers and older people in the UK. She considers how both anthropological methods and theory have contributed to her qualitative research activity. Like other anthropologists in this book she asserts the anthropological contribution to research methodology as being its ability, through fine-grained ethnography, to articulate the 'taken-for-granted' in human interaction and particularly the difference between what is said and what is done. Moreover Warren asserts that the traditionally perceived 'soft' data that qualitative studies generate can be more reliable and concrete than the manipulated outcomes of quantitative data.

Experience, then, serves to articulate and problematize what may otherwise be simply implied, or ignored. In a number of accounts it is an anthropologist who is on the receiving end of welfare, and writing about it (e.g. Modica 1994;

Brooks 1990). More frequently the analysis is in terms of the experience of others, sometimes those disempowered from talking for themselves. Davies' chapter (chapter 7) looks at how various forms of community care affect the potential for teenagers with learning difficulties to develop supportive personal networks. She uses participant-observation amongst the teenagers and their carers alongside interviews in order to elucidate problems and issues which could not be gleaned from interview or questionnaire data alone.

THE SOCIAL ORGANIZATION OF WELFARE

Anthropology is notable for the felicity with which it can analyse the social structures and organizations involved in the articulation and dispensation of welfare. Welfare is seen as a product of political and economic forces, social structures and cultural norms at the global, national and regional levels. In line with its micro-level and processual interests, anthropology looks particularly at the effects of these forces as they are played out at the local level. However, frequently these levels are not so easily distinguished. Christensen *et al.* (chapter 2) focus on the gendered relationships of dependency, 'the informal caring economy' of a rural farming community in the UK, which paradoxically act to generate independence and against the national policies of community care.

Domestic and state institutions both benefit from the use of qualitative methods in their description and analysis. One important anthropological concept used in the description and analysis of local level informal ties is that of networks (Wenger 1991; Bulmer 1987). Network theory, originally developed by anthropologists such as Barnes (1954) and Bott (1971), and elaborated by Mitchell (1966), Wenger (1991) and Trevillion (1992), has been the basis for the development of a considerable body of work on the interrelationships between people's coping capacities, life event challenges and the nature of actual and potential social networks. Indeed, the heart of the work of the new UK 'profession' of care managers is constructed around the creation and management of personal, voluntary, professional and commercial support systems as set out in the defined 'care plans' for agency users. Network analysis indicates the creativity of people in producing networks even in the most insalubrious settings (such as amongst street gangs (Whyte 1993), and drug addicts (Taylor 1993)). However, as Bulmer cautions, there is a danger in allowing the concept to 'become a blanket term, equivalent to saying that all people have some personal ties and close relationships, but tending to tautology' (1993: 241). Rather than assuming that networks are or will be ubiquitous, we need to look at how they are formed and maintained, with a view to deciding which networks are more effective, and why.

Davies (chapter 7) uses social network analysis as the basis for analysing personal and social development and change brought about by different types of community care. The opportunity for her subjects to work was found to be crucial as a means of promoting the development of optimal social networks for these young people. Parents viewed the 'community' as an ambivalent resource (and one in which their offspring had normally been living from before the advent of 'community care'!), one as likely to endanger as to support their child. Parents saw future social security for their teenage child as residing in the formation of friendships and local social networks of interest and concern.

From the creation of networks, a sense of this elusive thing called 'community' may be born. However, 'community' may not only be a problematic concept for welfare recipients, but also for welfare providers. In considering the reasons for the low uptake of welfare services in rural farming communities, Christensen *et al.* show how the stoicism of such a community in the face of adversity constitutes an aspect of the community's 'habitus' or 'taken-for-granted' way of being. Moreover, they found a sense of self, amongst community members, that was relational and unindividuated. Selfhood was constituted and regenerated through familial and community concepts, historically rooted in land ownership and gendered familial structures and expectations. Such structures of family and community identity were not unproblematic and might lead, for example, to sufferers of mental illness meeting their ambulance transport at a distance from the village and the prying eyes of their neighbours. Christensen and her colleagues argue that welfare professionals need to understand farming communities in culturally specific ways that relate to rural forms of personal and community identity. Sometimes the 'community' is a subterfuge; in McCourt's view (chapter 3), the 'community' in midwifery practice is nothing but the imagined venue for the extension of medical power into the domestic realm.

Anthropologists also study the social organization of the institutions in which welfare is managed (e.g. Aarre, chapter 4, and Baldwin, chapter 8; Foner 1994; Hockey 1990). They look at questions such as how the formal and informal ethos, or indeed the felt 'atmosphere' of an institution, is generated, changed and differentially experienced. Aarre shows the ability of ethnographic analysis based on in-depth participant-observation to 'put the finger' on the reasons for dynamic conflict within a bounded space, in this case the four walls of a very large children's home in Portugal, and the depth of understanding that can emerge from the immersion of the ethnographer within the subtle social interactions of such a place. Staff conflict in the 'home' is effectively analysed as being the result of different conceptions of the child, both in the 'home' and in Portuguese society. Older and original staff view the child as solely an extension of the 'family' leading to the adoption of a familial model of care, one which, ironically, is riddled with favouritism, exclusion and hierarchy. Younger staff, on the other hand, understand children as individuals with basic human rights that are independent of family membership. This engenders a more professional attitude and ideology towards the provision of egalitarian standards of care. Aarre's analysis neatly links the competing ideologies evident in this residential domain to substantive change in Portuguese society as it emerges from the ideological hegemony of the Salazar dictatorship into a liberal social welfare democracy. The contestations beheld within four walls mirror those of the wider society.

Ritual and symbolic practices, such as mealtimes and the use of space in

Aarre's children's home example, are often key variables in the creation of institutions. Hockey (1990) in her ethnographic and comparative study of an old people's home and a hospice shows in detail how markedly different therapeutic environments are ritually and symbolically constructed and maintained. A study of the use of myth, ritual and symbol in a therapeutic community for severely disturbed adolescents in Britain (Edgar 1990) showed that, through the planning of a symbolic care environment, a sense of community identity and cultural originality was created that clearly had significant therapeutic benefits for residents. An awareness of the significance of all parts of the 'treatment world' for residents' self-identity and social ability is an applied manifestation of the value of a holistic perspective, as is also well shown in Baldwin's study of a community mental health centre (chapter 8).

In addition to the institutions per se, anthropologists are well placed to study topics such as the relationship between social services and health services (or social services and local government, as Given touches on in chapter 9), between primary care and secondary health care services or, more generally, between 'the family' (or whatever individual or social appellate is appropriate in a given situation) and 'the professionals/carers'. With the interactions of these people and institutions comes the creation of new social categories – 'care workers' and 'care managers', 'teams' (e.g. in primary health care and social work), 'domestic carers'. Several chapters in this volume directly or indirectly address the question of what experiences and lived realities such labels subsume. They reflect the value of Nader's erstwhile call for anthropologists to 'study up' (1974), to look not only at the recipients of welfare, but at professionals in the welfare world, and the cultures of the organizations they represent.

THE CULTURE OF WELFARE

The 'atmosphere' or 'living ethos' created by the use of ritual, myth and symbols (above) might be synonymous with the 'culture' of the institution studied. However, culture is as much about who does the creating, and their position in the social structure, as it is about the products of the cultural process. As such, culture is perhaps the fundamental concept in distinguishing the unique contribution of anthropology to the study of welfare. It is also one of the most misunderstood concepts outside anthropology (Wright 1994). However, 'culture', properly understood and used, remains fundamental to the anthropological study of welfare policy and practice.

One important aspect of culture, as we have seen above, is its 'taken-for-granted' quality – culture as 'commonsense' (Geertz 1983; cf. Wright 1994). It is this nebulousness which gives it such strength, the filigree 'webs of meaning' spun by different actors in a situation – although Wright cautions against us assuming that 'all people are caught in the same way in one web' (1994: 23). Anthropology can be used to reveal the contested, multiple layers of meaning contained in seemingly straightforward situations.

As Trevillion and Green suggest at the start of their chapter, culture is not a solid 'thing', evolving up a progressive, evolutionary tree, like an organism. Nor is it a thing of 'traits' diffusing from one place to another. However, there are some general cultural principles, ways in which the webs are spun, which can be usefully applied to the study of any situation. Amongst these are exchange and reciprocity, and, as we have seen above, myth, ritual and symbols.

Keeling (chapter 11) looks at the contested nature of the exchange of material possessions within and between generations. In New Zealand the state requires the less than fully able older person requiring residential care to pay for this through the sale of most of their material assets, including the family home. Like their counterparts in many parts of the developed world, New Zealand citizens do not view this request charitably. The emotional and political aspects of this changing situation are well enunciated by Keeling's use of a variety of qualitative research methods.

Given, in his narrative analysis of a 'dump' housing estate in the north east of England in chapter 9, shows in detail the social construction of negative myths about the estate, which have in the long term accounted for its poor reputation and eventual material destruction. Through the medium of an action-research project, Given developed his analysis through a fine-grained consideration of how residents, professionals, officials and councillors talked about the estate and the people. He shows how our stories of 'power and place' inform even our experience of bricks and mortar. At the same time he is critical of social anthropology's historical tendency to mask the political and economic influences on interpersonal narrative and interaction.

Hoecklin's study of a mothers' centre in Germany, in chapter 5, is particularly important in its integration of past and contemporary macro-economic, social and cultural forces, such as the history of class and gender in Germany, contemporary German welfare policy, and normative concepts of the family (particularly the role of the 'mother'), with the micro-analysis of their contested reformulation in an 'alternative' mothers' centre. Her ethnographic work, partly grounded in her own use of the centre, as a mother with a young child, shows how the social anthropological method of participant-observation can illuminate the 'habitus' of historically constructed social values as these are embodied, or played out, in actual group and individual behaviour. Her analysis also shows the generation and creativity of new social and cultural forms, in this case the articulation of specifically German feminist aspirations for new forms of child-care and female/mother support and sociality.

Culture can also be brought into high relief by looking between, as well as within, particular societies. In their chapter on a Swedish HIV hospital social work team, Trevillion and Green (chapter 6) uncover a different philosophical approach towards inter-agency collaboration in Sweden than is found in UK community care practice. In the UK, community care approaches have focused on a consumerist philosophy of task and outcome, but in Sweden, a more open-ended and flexible approach to service provision is to be found, less focused on problem-solving and more concerned with an ethic of social inclusion. Trevillion and Green encountered a Swedish 'imagined community', the 'HIV world', consisting of a tangible social network incorporating agency, worker and client, which was formed and developed through shared philosophical assumptions about personal and social ends. This ability of social anthropology to explicate the partly implicit ethos of a bounded group or culture is well demonstrated in their chapter.

THE APPLIED ANTHROPOLOGY OF WELFARE

The preceding sections have attempted to elucidate key features of the anthropology of welfare by showing the actual or potential points of convergence between anthropology and welfare at theoretical and methodological levels. However, anthropologists do not have to finish there, and a distinguishing feature of this volume is the evident commitment of participating anthropologists to the task not only of articulating but also applying anthropological perspectives to the realities of changing welfare practices and policies. The best work involves the synthesis of the different levels of analysis such as experience, social organization, and culture. Often these perspectives are linked by an understanding of the power relations within which welfare provision takes place.

A good example of such a synthesis is Baldwin's chapter (chapter 8). Her study of a community mental health centre in the USA shows how an institutionally derived, implicit 'folk' ideology runs counter to the therapeutic ideals of the centre itself, so that patients with schizophrenia and those with borderline personality disorder (BPD) are effectively categorized by staff as 'deserving' and 'undeserving' respectively. The different treatment approaches of staff are attributed to the competing 'medical' and 'therapeutic community' models which inform the psychiatric day centre's practice philosophy. Such an analysis links overt and covert ideology with lived experience and creates an anthropological praxis which both explicates and can inform future developments in service provision. Davies' paper is an equally useful example of an anthropologist, by adopting a 'grass roots' perspective, elucidating provision for the learning disabled, with a view to its improvement. From such writings, anthropologists and readers can go on to act as advocates for those underserved by contemporary welfare provision.

Other writers adopt a more openly judgemental or activist stance. Aarre has clear views on the effects of the different models of the child in use in the Portuguese children's home. Keeling has obvious sympathies for the plight of New Zealand elderly forced to choose between 'treasures on earth' and 'treasures in heaven'. Lloyd is actively involved in his research as convenor of the Sussex Gerontology Network's Sheltered Housing Group, and he has co-authored a guide to participation of the elderly in such groups.

For others the activist role is more problematic (cf. Hyatt 1993). Given, in his moving account, is painfully aware that he is writing as part of a local power base, one of 'the new professionals of deprivation'. Even the need to understand the 'dump' housing estate he examined was powered by local politics, specifically the 'not in my backyard' mentality evoked by the estate's destruction and the necessary removal of its inhabitants. However, he uses his personal experience, 'local knowledge', to subvert the myth that the Deans was a model estate in some golden age, a myth which is perpetuated at many levels (not least by the inhabitants themselves). Hoecklin is actively involved in, and presumably helping to shape, the alternative 'mothers' centre' she is studying (in other words she, like the women in her study, is 'equal, but different'). She finds that the centre is not only opposing or subverting dominant views of motherhood but is also, in some cases, playing into them.

Other problematic aspects of the applied anthropology of welfare are touched upon in McCourt's chapter (chapter 3). One is the frequent need for anthropologists to work in multidisciplinary teams in order to be effective. Frequently misunderstood by professionals and the general public, this can be a challenging task. Another is the response to research findings by its sponsors. In the one-to-one midwifery care service her team was asked to evaluate, McCourt reports that health service managers reduced a multifaceted report to a question of economics, the figures of which they then endeavoured to manipulate. Finally there is the potentially therapeutic aspects of the research encounter. In Edgar's chapter (chapter 13), the humanistic groupwork methods he proposes are both research and (in some cases) therapy, and he warns that certain techniques should not be attempted without an experienced and qualified instructor.

CONCLUSION

This volume champions the anthropology of welfare as an emerging subfield in social anthropology. It shows what anthropology can contribute to the study of welfare, the apprehension of welfare institutions, and processes and practices integrating micro- and macro-levels of analysis. It explores the particular theoretical interests which anthropology shares with welfare studies – in comparativism, representation and reflexivity, as well as the experiential methods, social understanding and cultural conceptions which make up the distinctive anthropology of welfare. Finally, it looks at the actual and potential applications of the knowledge that this subfield engenders.

The anthropology of welfare is concerned with the human face of welfare provision, the realities behind the rhetoric, the people behind the policies. It seeks to normalize such accounts in the practice of welfare worldwide.

NOTES

1 See, for example, Chambers (1985), Eddy and Partridge (1987), Messerschmidt (1981), Willigen (1986), Wulff and Fiske (1987).
2 Contributions by anthropologists concerned with race and ethnicity such as Banton

(1988), Cambridge and Feuchtwang (1990), Jenkins (1986), La Fontaine (1986), Wallman (1979) and Watson (1977) have been limited and gone largely unrecognized in welfare studies. Whilst theorists such as Jenkins (1986) and Wallman (1986) have articulated and implemented what Jenkins calls the 'ethnicity paradigm', this approach has barely been considered in welfare practice in the UK.

BIBLIOGRAPHY

Anderson, B. (1991) *Imagined Communities: Reflections on the Origins and Spread of Nationalism* (rev. edn), London: Verso.

Banton, M. (1988) *Racial Consciousness*, London: Longman.

Barnes, J. A. (1954) 'Class and committees in a Norwegian island parish', *Human Relations* 7: 39–58.

Batley, R. and Stoker, G. (1991) *Local Government in Europe*, London: Macmillan.

Bott, E. (1971) *Family and Social Network*, New York: Free Press.

Bourdieu, P. (1977) *Outline of a Theory of Practice*, Cambridge: Cambridge University Press.

Brooks, D. H. M. (1990) 'The route to home ventilation: a patient's perspective', *Care of the Critically Ill* 6, 3: 96–7.

Bulmer, M. (1987) *The Social Basis of Community Care*, London: Allen and Unwin. Extract abridged and reprinted in J. Bornat, C. Pereira, D. Pilgrim and F. Williams (eds) (1993) *Community Care: A Reader*, London: Macmillan.

Cambridge, C. and Feuchtwang, S. (1990) *Anti-Racist Strategies*, Aldershot: Avebury.

Cannan, C., Berry, L. and Lyons, K. (1992) *Social Work in Europe*, London: Macmillan.

CCETSW [Central Council for Education and Training in Social Work] (1989) *Requirements and Regulations for the Diploma in Social Work* (Paper 30), London: CCETSW.

Chambers, E. (1985) *Applied Anthropology: A Practical Guide*, Englewood Cliffs, NJ: Prentice-Hall.

Churchill, N. (1994) 'Welfare-to-work: planners, practitioners, and participants', *Practicing Anthropology* 16, 4: 8–11.

Clifford, J. (1986) *Writing Culture. The Poetics and Politics of Writing Ethnography*, Berkeley: University of California Press.

D'Andrade, R. G., Hammel, E. A., Adkins, D. L. and McDaniel, C. K. (1975) 'Academic opportunity in anthropology 1974–90', *American Anthropologist* 77, 4: 753–73.

Dixon, J. and Scheurell, R. (1995) *Social Welfare with Indigenous People*, London: Routledge.

Dominelli, L. (1988) *Anti-Racist Social Work*, London: Macmillan.

Dominelli, L. and McLeod, E. (1989) *Feminist Social Work*, London: Macmillan.

Durkheim, E. (1933) *The Division of Labour in Society*, trans. G. Simpson, London: Macmillan.

Eddy, E. and Partridge, W. (eds) (1987) *Applied Anthropology in America* (2nd edn), New York: Columbia University Press.

Edgar, I. (1990) 'The social process of adolescence in a therapeutic community', in P. Spencer (ed.) *Anthropology and the Riddle of the Sphinx: Paradoxes of Change in the Life Course*, London: Routledge.

Foner, N. (1994) *The Caregiving Dilemma: Work in an American Nursing Home*, Berkeley: University of California Press.

Gaynor, C. (1987) 'Introduction', in C. Gaynor (ed.) *Social Change and the Life Course*, London: Tavistock.

Geertz, C. (1983) 'Common sense as a cultural system', in C. Geertz *Local Knowledge: Further Essays in Interpretative Anthropology*, New York: Basic Books.

Ginsburg, N. (1992) *Divisions of Welfare: A Critical Introduction to Comparative Social Policy*, London: Sage.

Glasser, I. (1994) 'Anthropological contributions to welfare policy and practice', *Practicing Anthropology* 16, 4: 3–4.

Heidenheimer, A. J., Heclo, H., and Adams, C. T. (1990) *Comparative Public Policy: The Politics of Social Choice in America, Europe, and Japan*, (3rd edn), New York: St Martin's Press.

Higgins, J. M. (1981) *States of Welfare: Comparative Analysis in Social Policy*, Oxford: Basil Blackwell and Martin Robertson.

Hill, M. (1996) *Social Policy: a Comparative Analysis*, London: Prentice-Hall/Harvester Wheatsheaf.

Hockey, J. (1990) *Experiences of Death: An Anthropological Account*, Edinburgh: Edinburgh University Press.

Huby, G. (1992) 'Trapped in the present: the past, present and future of a group of old people in East London', in S. Wallman (ed.) *Contemporary Futures: Perspectives from Social Anthropology*, London: Routledge.

Hyatt, S. (1993) 'Can the anthropology of activism also be an activist anthropology? Thoughts on fieldwork on a council estate', *Anthropology in Action* 16: 19–21.

James, A., Hockey, J., and Dawson, A. (eds) (1996) *After Writing Culture: Epistemology and Praxis in Contemporary Anthropology*, London: Routledge.

Jenkins, R. (1986) 'Social anthropological models of inter-ethnic relations', in J. Rex and D. Mason (eds) *Theories of Race and Ethnic Relations*, Cambridge: Cambridge University Press.

Jones, C. (1983) *State Social Work and the Working Class*, London: Macmillan.

Jordan, B. (1987) *Rethinking Welfare*, Oxford: Blackwell.

La Fontaine, J. (1986) 'Countering racial prejudice: a better starting point', *Anthropology Today* 2, 6.

Lorenz, W. (1994) *Social Work in a Changing Europe*, London: Routledge.

Messerschmidt, D. (1981) *Anthropologists at Home in North America*, Cambridge: Cambridge University Press.

Mitchell, C. (1966) 'Theoretical orientations in African urban studies', in M. Banton (ed.) *The Social Anthropology of Complex Societies*, London: Tavistock.

Modica, L. C. (1994) 'The anthropologist as welfare recipient: views from the inside', *Practicing Anthropology* 16, 4: 5–7.

Nader, L. (1974) 'Up the anthropologist – perspectives gained from studying up', in D. Hymes (ed.) *Reinventing Anthropology*, New York: Vintage Books.

Okely, J. and Callaway, H. (eds) (1992) *Anthropology and Autobiography*, London: Routledge.

Pithouse, A. (1987) *Social Work: The Social Organisation of an Invisible Trade*, Aldershot: Avebury.

Rojek, C., Peacock, G. and Collins, S. (1988) *Social Work and Received Ideas*, London: Routledge.

Scharf, T. and Wenger, C. (1995) *International Perspectives on Community Care for Older People*, Aldershot: Avebury.

Spicer, P., Willenbring, M., Miller, F., and Raymond, E. (1994) 'Ethnographic evaluation of case management for homeless alcoholics', *Practicing Anthropology* 16, 4: 23–6.

Taylor, A. (1993) *Women Drug Users*, Oxford: Clarendon Press.

Titmuss, R. M. (1958) 'The social division of welfare: some reflections on the search for equity' in R. M. Titmuss *Essays on the Welfare State*, London: Allen and Unwin, reprinted in B. Abel-Smith and K. Titmuss (eds) (1987) *The Philosophy of Welfare: Selected Writings of Richard M. Titmuss*, London: Allen and Unwin.

Tomlinson, D. (1991) *Utopia, Community Care and the Retreat from the Asylums*, Milton Keynes: Open University Press.

Trevillion, S. (1992) *Caring in the Community: A Networking Approach to Community Partnership*, London: Longman.

Wallman, S. (1979) *Ethnicity at Work*, London: Macmillan.

—— (1986) 'Ethnicity and the boundary process in context', in J. Rex and D. Mason (eds) *Theories of Race and Ethnic Relations*, Cambridge: Cambridge University Press.

Watson, J. (ed.) (1977) *Between Two Cultures*, Oxford: Blackwell.

Wenger, C. (1991) 'A network typology: from theory to practice', *Journal of Aging Studies* 5, 2.

Whyte, W. F. (1993) *Street Corner Society: the Social Structure of an Italian Slum*, (4th edn), Chicago: Chicago University Press.

Willigen, J. (1986) *Applied Anthropology*, Massachusetts: Bergin and Garvey.

Wright, S. (1994) '"Culture" in anthropology and organizational studies', in S. Wright (ed.) *Anthropology of Organizations*, London: Routledge.

Wulff, R. and Fiske, S. (1987) *Anthropological Praxis*, Boulder: Westview Press.

Chapter 2

'You just get on with it': questioning models of welfare dependency in a rural community

Pia Christensen, Jenny Hockey and Allison James

INTRODUCTION

Drawing on a two-year ethnographic study of the conceptions and practices of dependency, independence and interdependency among farming families, this chapter depicts an anthropology of 'care' in the 'community', through an account of the tensions and paradoxes which surround the provision of welfare in a rural community in the north of England. We focus on one particular area of concern: the limited uptake of services within agricultural communities. For health and welfare professionals this means that problems are often brought to their attention at crisis points or at a late and advanced stage which makes inter-vention more difficult. For the professionals, therefore, the community is regarded as a source of their clients' problems and yet the community also repre-sents the context within which 'care' is contemporarily thought to be best effected. The paradox which this represents can, we argue, be unravelled through adopting an anthropological approach which explores local conceptions of self, family and community and the social practices which sustain them.

The specific agricultural community which we describe is one where local conceptions of the self are, as we shall show, often indistinguishable from those of the family and the community. At a fundamental level, therefore, the profes-sional distinctions usually made between client and carer, between self and family, turn out to be highly inappropriate in this setting. Primarily grounded in the values attributed to the independence and autonomy of the individual in contemporary western society, this model of care is at the heart of traditional biomedical practice and is one which cannot, we suggest, accommodate the all-embracing conceptualization of 'interdependence' which characterizes farming communities. Thus, this chapter lends support to Nettleton (1996) who has argued that, although the new paradigm of health and medicine has apparently shifted its attention to collectivities and groups through notions of 'community care' and 'community medicine', the individual still remains its central focus. When people are simply encouraged to adopt self-care practices in relation to their health at home, little attention is given to the competing social agenda of individuals embedded within the unfolding life of the family and the local community. It may be for this reason, then, that service uptake is low: in the agricultural community which we describe the self is seen as primarily relational (cf. Kakar 1982; Shweder 1991) and the very notion of personal independence is, as we shall show, regarded as a threat to an interdependent 'farming way of life'.

THE RHETORIC AND PRACTICE OF COMMUNITY CARE

An examination of the literature on community care reveals the conceptualizations of social relationships which inform the rhetoric and practice of health and welfare professionals. In this the family is identified as a crucial element in the management of the client's care (Finch and Grove 1983; Twigg 1993: 116) and, as Twigg notes, it can generally be shown that 'care inputs from the informal sector vastly outweigh those from the formal' (1993: 116). In highlighting the importance of family relationships, this literature nonetheless makes a clear distinction between the clients themselves and their families (Barnes 1997). Thus Twigg, in her typology of relationships between public service agencies and carers, cites the 'carers as resources' model as important. This 'places its central focus on the cared-for person . . . the carer only features as part of the background, albeit a vital resource background. He or she is not the main subject of the agency's concern' (1993: 118). Other ways in which agencies might construct their relationship to carers include those such as: the 'semi-professionalization' of informal carers as 'co-workers'; a view of carers as 'victims', 'fellow sufferers', and 'co-clients', whose needs may potentially be prioritized above those of the clients; and the 'superseded carer' who is freed of their burden of caring via the efforts of public service agencies. Yet despite the importance imputed to these 'informal' relationships, each of these models of community distinguishes clients from their carers (usually families) and places emphasis on the potential conflict of interests between them. Through such a view, family relationships are translated into relations of care. This similarly polarizes the roles of family members through the differentiation between 'carer' and 'cared-for'. Most importantly these models thus refuse any engagement with more general questions relating to cultural notions of 'self' and 'family', which, as we show below, turn out to be key elements in understanding the 'habitus' of an agricultural community (Bourdieu 1977).

What we will be exploring in this chapter is the problematic nature of such distinctions in relation to the community within which our study was located. Although local health and welfare professionals clearly voiced the wider rhetoric of community care through such models, and presented it as an important framework for action, their experience of community care in practice was far more problematic. In brief, the complexity of particular local articulations of notions of 'community' and 'family' present professionals with considerable difficulties in defining exactly what and who constitute 'the family' or 'the community'.

TOWARDS AN ANTHROPOLOGY OF WELFARE IN AN AGRICULTURAL COMMUNITY

The challenges to professional practice which are engendered through such localized perceptions of self, family and community came to our attention during twelve months of anthropological fieldwork in an agricultural community in the UK strongly marked by familial connections. The research was carried out through a combination of participant-observation on a number of different farms, and interviews with members of farming families of different generations, teachers working in the local schools, the local vicar and church workers, and health and welfare professionals servicing the community. The latter included a community psychiatric nurse, social and community workers, matrons of residential homes for the elderly, and those running local social services for elderly and/or disabled people such as Meals on Wheels, Darby and Joan clubs and Life Line. While existing studies of relations of dependency have taken as their focus the everyday practical management of disability and acute or chronic illness, anthropological fieldwork sets this within a broader understanding of the social and cultural context. It encompasses, for example, men's working lives and relationships, women's roles on farms and in charitable activities, and the spatial and temporal transitions which go to make up the individual and familial life course. The breadth of an anthropological approach provides a nuanced understanding of 'dependency' and of the responses of 'clients' to the provision of welfare.

The research aimed to explore conceptions of dependency in communities where statutory services are not easily accessible. In particular, it examined the various roles taken on by different family members during sickness, disability and old age. In this respect farming communities turned out to be particularly significant because, as one welfare practitioner described it approvingly, 'nobody has a stronger family influence than the farming community'.

Indeed, over the twelve-month fieldwork period, the importance of the family to the farming community and to the individual became clear. It was made manifest in the mundane and everyday working practices on the farm, as well as at particular times of crisis when the family was more visibly mobilized for support. But gradually, as fieldwork progressed, different aspects of family life were also revealed which suggested that people experienced these strong familial ties to be constraining as much as enabling. As we describe below, 'the family', the supposed bedrock of systems of social and community care and support, was seen as neither necessarily benign nor supportive. Anthropological fieldwork permitted such variations to be noted and explored as a social process. This offered a contrast to more static and idealized visions of what families do, and the concepts of intimacy and privacy through which community life takes place.

A second important feature of the local community was also made apparent through participant-observation fieldwork, a feature which poses a further dilemma for practitioners involved in facilitating community care. Although the local community is in one sense bound together by the strong interconnectedness which exists between extended family members living within the same or neighbouring villages, this does not necessarily engender a wider social sense of community feeling or spirit. As the local vicar remarked, although one might think of 'families forming communities', in practice the idea of the village as a thriving social community 'hasn't [developed] the full potential that it could have'. Between a sense of 'family' and a sense of 'community' there may be, therefore, a wide gulf, even though the local community is constituted, in large part, by extended family and kin relations. During fieldwork it became clear that, at certain times, who exactly constitutes 'the family', in respect of offering help or fulfilling obligations, could both expand and contract. The involvement of 'the family' in the 'community' could also vary in relation to requests for assistance. In this way, then, anthropological fieldwork enabled the complexity of local conceptions of dependence, independence and interdependence to be revealed over time. From a health and welfare professional point of view, therefore, these contradictory practices represent a considerable obstacle to be overcome if the principles of community care and family support are to be fostered in an agricultural community.

'INSIDE' THE AGRICULTURAL FAMILY AND COMMUNITY

As noted above, professional perspectives on family life and models of care often derive from a fixed point of familial crisis when intervention becomes necessary due to the onset of the dependency of one family member upon other kin. However, a broader temporal sweep, which takes into account processes of family life as they unfold across varied sets of circumstances, including those of ill health, yields somewhat different insights.

Central to these is the particular nature of family life within agricultural communities. This is characterized by a strong sense of belonging, whereby individual family members are tied to the land and the farm through the family, extending across the generations. The main responsibility for the farm lies with the family in young or mid-adult life who live in the farmhouse on the land. The older parental generation is often now retired to an adjacent bungalow on the farm or a nearby bungalow or cottage in the village, where other kin relations may also live. Thus, the spatial distribution of land and patterns of residence within the village offer a graphic representation of the interconnectedness of family and kin, and of the hierarchical positions within it pertaining to grandfathers, fathers and sons.

A comparable sense of belonging is also evident in the ways in which family members grow up to embody the interconnectedness of natural, material and social features of their family and work environment. This is revealed in everyday conversations when people characterize themselves and others as belonging to a 'sheep family', or as being an 'arable man' or a 'stock man'. For example, of Grace, a young farmer's wife, her father said: 'she has sheep in her blood, she has that from her mum. They have sheep in her family'. Her brother

Harry's comments on one of his farm workers provide a comparable account of the ways in which 'the farming way of life' is represented as being embodied, or 'in the blood':

> Colin just wasn't a pig man . . . a pig man can see a pig going sick maybe half a day before Colin would see it going sick but the half day could make a difference whether it lives or dies. So, although he is very hard working it just wasn't working out and with the prices being low we decided to get rid of them [the pigs].

In this context, therefore, occupational identities are also seen as family identities which run in the 'veins' across generations. Family relationships are also work relationships mapped onto the land and patterning the local community. Boys, especially, are brought up to see their future in terms of farming. As Harry, a young farmer, explains:

> I was always encouraged to work, so it is partly ingrown. I have just been brought up like that but I do enjoy it. It isn't just a job where you go in nine to five every day and go home and forget about it. It literally can be nearly twenty-four hours a day at certain times of the year.

By using a temporal perspective, therefore, we can see that men's main orientation is the past in the present; that is, the present as experienced through everyday work on the farm, simultaneously connects their personal and familial past with the present in the form of the inheritance of farm and land. Men therefore represent not only their father or their parents in the present, but also the history of the farm and land, and indeed the family's history in the village community. Grace illustrated this in conversation when she explained the important role of her father-in-law for the farm,

> I think it was Ben's granddad that actually bought the farm . . . this is the third generation that has been here and it does help if you have a knowledge of the farm because every field has different bits of land in it, like heavy patches where it might be more clay and then lighter patches. . . . To know the history and the soil type that is one thing that you learn from years of cultivating it. . . . But the boys now they have worked on the farm from a very early age, from twelve, thirteen, fourteen, they weren't going to school very much, they would work on the farm, so by now a lot of granddad's knowledge he will have passed on to the boys and so I would think by now they would know enough about it to carry it and he has passed on all his ideas.

Thus, together men work the land for 'tomorrow'; it is their obligation to hand the land and family name down through the generations. However, they also see their stake in the future as precarious. A piece of farming lore states that 'the first generation makes it, the second generation keeps it and the third generation spends it'. Thus, Dick, citing this piece of wisdom, saw himself as being able to sustain his influence on the farm into the second generation through his son. To this end he would struggle to maintain the values and traditions of the farm. In the third generation, however, this history of hard work on the farm may run the risk of being squandered unless a watchful eye is kept over his grandchildren. Family ties must be tightly drawn. Farming men do not therefore follow a routine, age-based retirement scheme; they simply begin to play a less active role in later life, providing a source of intimate knowledge of the farm and the land and helping out by undertaking less physically demanding farming tasks, such as fetching spare machinery parts. Talking of her elderly, sick father-in-law, Grace illustrates his still significant participation in the farm:

> I mean he was here last night and they [his sons] always discuss what they are going to do the next day and Ben's dad will say, 'Don't you think you should do this?' 'Don't you think you should be getting some muck spreaders rented to spread some muck? Otherwise you are going to have too much work to do maybe in March or' . . . so then Ben will go off and ring the muck spreader man up. It is just another mind to keep things running smoothly. I am sure if he wasn't here they would manage fine but whether things would run just quite as smoothly, I don't know.

The position of women within this community is, however, somewhat different. As young wives who have been brought into the community through marriage, their sense of belonging to the farming family and community is regarded as less dependable, particularly if they are not from farming families themselves. They will not know what the farming way of life entails. For example, as Lucy says, they may lack the knowledge of what is needed to 'back the man up on the farm': that is, the everyday provision of meals, the management of domestic work, shouldering the child care, a willingness to continue childbearing until a son has been provided, and an availability and readiness to help with whatever other tasks on the farm emerge across the working day. Such 'incoming' women represent a danger to the familial and occupational interconnectedness of farming and may even be seen as a potential source of fission through divorce. If this were the case, the farm might have to be split between them. Their particular threat to the continuity of a 'farming way of life' is recognized in the distinction made locally between being a 'farmer's wife' and a 'wife of a farmer'. The first is a woman who lets herself be enrolled on the farm and actively supports and takes a genuine interest in the farm, including keeping an everyday track of the work and progress of the farm. This is seen to be more possible for girls who have been brought up in farming families for they will have an understanding of what is expected of them. The latter woman, by contrast, is seen as more detached and less supportive. She may even oppose her husband's extended family and work patterns, and her practical contribution to the farm may be minimal. Such a woman is more likely not to have been raised in a farming family and is seen as more likely to leave.

Though from a male viewpoint marriage represents an ambiguous necessity for the continuity of the farm and the family, for women themselves it is a point in their life course which they experience as initiating a period of personal vulnerability. As noted elsewhere (Christensen *et al.* 1997) marriage into a traditional farming family usually entails young women leaving their own natal families to join those of their husbands. The new wife joins the established, extended farming family with its own mores and lifestyle. As one of the informants describes it: 'The mother-in-law rules the roost and the young girl had to fit in. It was almost as if she couldn't disturb that pattern because that would then upset things.'

Women, therefore, come to be controlled through their mothers-in-law. Lucy, for example, the 52-year-old wife of a highly successful farmer, speaks of 'drilling in' the demands of a 'farmer's wife' when she first met her new daughter-in-law. Similarly, she also recounts her own first years of marriage as a time of tension. For example, if she complained that her husband did not spend enough time at home or they had other disagreements, Dick would simply leave the house and go to his mother who lived close by. She would then provide Dick with his meals. In this way Lucy's mother-in-law succeeded in keeping 'the family' together. Thus, rather than taking Lucy's part in marital conflicts, she made Lucy realize that if she wanted to keep her husband at home she had to accept his work demands and 'get on with the farming way of life'. Dick's mother's provision of meals can also be seen as a version of another common practice: if a son does not marry, he remains at home and his mother provides many of the 'wifely' services for him instead.

The women's own temporal orientation is therefore towards the future in the present (Christensen *et al.* 1997). Thus the mother-in-law socializes the new wife to perform her necessary part in the continuation of the farm. This includes providing the next generation of farmers. Young women's everyday work therefore revolves around the future, in giving birth, bringing up children and in improving the old farmhouse, often using their own financial capital. Both these activities they see as a literal lifetime investment which will enable the family farm to endure. In the wider community it is women, as is traditional (Finch and Grove 1983; Daley 1988; Nettleton 1996), who take responsibility for the main everyday care of neighbours, elderly or sick family, kin and villagers. In this way women play an important role in creating and maintaining social bonds among locals and across generations and families. In the villages it is mostly women alone who are present during the day. The men work on the farm, in the fields, or in business away from the community, and the children are at school. It is women who ferry children to school and other activities, who shop for friends, neighbours and other family members, who take on small tasks for others, who volunteer their men for an odd job. Though the men contribute financially to community fund-raising activities and other social events, perhaps even helping on a stall, it is women who will organize and conduct most of these services. With the help of some elderly villagers, they run coffee mornings, Meals on Wheels and organize shopping trips, house help or social visits.

CARE IN THE COMMUNITY

In sum, then, both men and women shore up the boundaries of family and community in different ways and with different temporal and spatial orientations. These lead to a complex of different ideas of self, family and community, which we suggest are articulated at times of family crisis such as that induced by the onset of illness. Thus it is this complexity revealed in cultural conceptions and constructs of gender, family and community which we propose is at stake when the practice of care in the community is seen as difficult. Two accounts of rather different illness episodes serve to illustrate these points. They reveal the support which the 'family' can provide an individual in this community, but also the contradictory demands upon individuals which the 'family' makes in relation to 'farming as a way of life'.

Case 1: Neil's meningitis

When Neil Barnes was twenty-one, he collapsed whilst having lunch at his grandparents' house. Their house is built on the farmland where he and his immediate family live. The farm is run by his father, his uncle, his two brothers and himself. The family were all there when he was taken ill. His brother Simon immediately ran out in his socks to fetch their mother, Bridget, from the neighbouring farmhouse. An ambulance was called and Bridget and Simon accompanied Neil in the ambulance with George (his father) and Sandy (his younger brother) following by car. Neil was first taken to the local hospital where the family's GP happened to be on duty. However shortly after his arrival, Neil was transferred to the hospital in the local town, some twenty-two miles from the family home. Later when he was diagnosed as having meningitis he was moved once more to a city hospital about 18 miles from home. During the three weeks he was hospitalized his mother visited him consistently and recalls travelling approximately 1100 miles during this period. However, though the hospital was far away, both family and kin relations, as well as the extensive business networks which link agricultural work and workers, came into play. Whilst in hospital Neil received visits not only from other family members but also from men who had a work connection with his family. When eventually Neil came home his mother was his main nurse and companion. She describes how she made herself available to talk to him, and care for him. Whilst he was ill Bridget gave up the employment which she had, till then, been able to carry out at home. Neil described his gradual return to work on the family farm when he worked a few hours a day before 'getting back into the swing of it' and being able to begin to work full time on the farm some three months later.

For Neil, his extended family played a crucial role during his illness and recovery. The part they played was greatly enhanced by the very nature of 'the farming family'. Tied by both kinship and work relations, the farming family constituted a tightly bound unit. When Neil collapsed not only were his immediate male relatives able to summon his mother very rapidly but they also immediately stopped work on the farm to accompany him to hospital. From the onset of his illness, Neil was surrounded and cared for by his family.

However, the involvement of statutory services in Neil's illness was somewhat problematic. There was no obvious choice of hospital and Neil was therefore sent to first one, then another and finally, when the seriousness of his condition was recognized, he was moved to a specialist ward in a larger city hospital. All these hospitals were at a considerable distance from his home village. Yet the family remained heavily involved in his care through Bridget, his mother, who visited him twice daily. In addition to contact with his father and brothers, his embeddedness in the farming way of life was maintained by their farming associates who stopped by the hospital when passing through. His mother continued an active role in his care when he eventually came home, temporarily relinquishing her own career to look after her son.

Thus, when Neil fell ill the farm work could go on without too much difficulty, precisely because it is work carried out in a familial inscribed community setting. As Neil describes:

> We had nearly finished drilling when I fell ill but anyway one of Dad's friends came and helped out for a day or two . . . and once that was finished they quite easily managed with three of them. They maybe had a bit more to do but they managed quite easily.

For Neil himself, his recovery and return to full health was facilitated by his family and by the flexibility through which they were able to manage and organize their work. As Neil suggests:

> When you start to pick up you want to go and do a bit to see how much you can do before . . . it is no good going from doing nothing to doing a day's work, it like wears you out to start with . . . so I eased myself back into it gently.

This continuum from sickness to well-being contrasts vividly with the urban polarization of illness and health which is marked by receipt of 'sick pay'. In Neil's case, he was able to monitor his own gradual transition from ill health to well-being. He could recommence work early but flexibly with the result that he did not suffer any setbacks by having to return full-time and with a full workload too early.

The second example represents a somewhat different view of the interconnectedness of self, family, work and community and shows how the gendering of illness and care may be a critical factor in such processes.

Case 2: Rosie's leg

One Tuesday morning Rosie, a 27-year-old farmer's wife, stepped on one of her children's toys. By the following day her foot was swollen and too painful to walk on. By Saturday, when her foot was no better, Harry, her husband, called in his mother to look after the children while he took Rosie to hospital for an X-ray. Rosie has three small daughters and as her husband is fully occupied with the work on the farm, Rosie is therefore accustomed to having sole responsibility for child-care. Her marriage to Harry means that she now lives some distance from her own family and cannot readily call on her own mother for assistance. Rosie was surprised when Harry asked his mother for help in this instance. Usually Rosie feels that she does not have first call on her mother-in-law for help, that privilege being reserved for Harry's sister Grace, who lives nearby and has two children of her own. In this emergency, however, her mother-in-law stayed for the weekend as Harry was very busy on the farm and then Rosie's own mother, though herself unwell, travelled north to stay for three days in order to help her daughter.

In Rosie's case family support was more equivocal than that provided for Neil. Though this may be partly explained as a function of the severity of the latter's illness, Rosie's case illustrates the complex set of meanings which 'family' can entail and through which 'care' takes place. Though her mother-in-law was close at hand, recent tensions among the men within her husband's family over farm management and ownership had strained the helping relationship between its female members. In addition, Rosie herself had always been seen as rather an outsider. Although she had occupational training in farming, Rosie did not come from a farming family and thus, as described above, represented a potential source of danger to her new affinal family. In comparison with Neil's illness, this case shows the extended family network poised to contract. The care and support it could offer is acknowledged, albeit in a somewhat circumspect manner, and called upon reluctantly. Rosie herself provided reasons why she would not ask her mother-in-law, Lucy, for help. It was not just that she felt Lucy's daughter Grace, who also has small children, had first call on Lucy's help. 'I don't like to step on her toes,' Rosie says. In addition, Lucy herself did not call on Rosie for help. Rosie recalls the last time Lucy fell ill: 'I didn't know . . . she had real bad flu . . . she didn't ask . . . because I didn't know until Harry said she'd been poorly.'

Rosie's experience of Lucy refusing to ask her for help, or even to let her know when she was ill, hindered the establishment of the kind of reciprocal, interdependent helping relationships through which families constitute themselves in an agricultural community. Thus on another occasion when Rosie and all three of her children had stomach upsets and vomiting, Rosie says, 'I just coped'. After two nights without sleep because she was caring for the children, she became ill herself. She describes what happened in the following way:

> I'd lit the fire and I just lay down in front of it and just . . . I just died . . . and Milly just wrecked the room and just climbed all over me . . . and then Harry came in at tea-time and tried his best to avoid us because he hates being sick . . . he hates being near anyone that's sick.

She went on to spend the night caring for the children again: 'I'd been up three nights on the trot, but when somebody's sick I would never dream of bringing anybody in because they're going to get it, aren't they?'

Consistently, in accounts of her own and her children's illnesses, it is made clear that she does not seek help – 'Well, you just cope, you know . . . ,' Rosie will explain. She does not expect others to care for her or take on her tasks and thus does not see her friends as a source of help. She says 'they've all either got kids . . . of their own, or they're working, to be fair'. Thus, in the case of her leg injury, Rosie made, what was for her, an unusual choice of getting help from her mother-in-law:

> We actually phoned on Saturday morning. Harry phoned his mother to come down to look after these three while he took me to hospital and then Lucy actually stayed most of the weekend and helped me because I couldn't carry Sally.

From this account it is clear not only that she is describing an unusual situation but also that it is Harry who made the initial contact with his mother by his phone call.

It might be argued that Rosie's case is not unusual and that a woman in an urban context might respond similarly, being isolated from family and other sources of support, and with a male partner perhaps being unable to take time off work. However Rosie's refusal to acknowledge her leg injury for four days has to be made sense of in context. She is geographically isolated, which not only makes her inability to walk or drive more serious, but also means that she cannot easily call on a neighbour. In addition, though marriage provides her with close family connections in the community, these are resources which she is reluctant to use. Not only have tensions soured family relations, but the local conceptualizations of family differentiate between consanguineal and affinal kin in such a way that male lines of heredity are privileged. The longest period of help which Rosie received during her leg injury was therefore given by her own mother who travelled some considerable distance even though she herself was unwell.

PROFESSIONAL PERSPECTIVES

In a whole variety of ways – spatially, temporally and socially – this is a community of people who present a stoical self-sufficiency which is, nonetheless, informed by the intense experience of being highly interconnected. It is also a community in which the gendered nature of familial care predominates. Turning now to the perspectives of health and welfare professionals who serve this area, it is clear that they not only recognize some of these features in their experiences of the community but also see them as presenting obstacles to successful professional practice.

In conversations with local school teachers, for example, staff reflected on the different parental expectations of boys' and girls' education. Boys' education, they felt, may receive relatively low priority from the farming point of view, for 'the expectations of all concerned are that son, that family, will come back to that farm and run it for the next generation'. Girls, on the other hand, according to the teachers, are regarded as rather 'second-class citizens in the farming community'. Although they may succeed well academically, and indeed enter further and higher education, it was nonetheless anticipated that they would eventually return to the locality to marry a farmer. This pattern is set, in the teachers' view, early in adolescence: 'Girls go along to the rugby club to meet the boys and wait for them and that's their role in life to pick up and drop off and it all tends to flow in that vein again.'

Thus the teachers are aware of how the important traditions of farming families reproduce themselves in a particular form across the generations and in the locality. In some senses they see this as part of the community's tremendous strength: 'the farming community are very supportive of the family, are very family orientated'. Other professionals observed that, in the village community, 'there's a sort of family feel', so that at times of crisis 'if anybody needed help from farm to farm there was always the help there'. In the case of Neil's collapse and subsequent period of illness, described above, this familial/community support was clearly evident.

However, running somewhat contrary to professionals' emphasis on family/community support and a feeling of togetherness which is engendered through the idea of the family, is a strong perception of the independence and integrity of one family from another. This was variously articulated in professionals' descriptions of clients' attitudes at times of crisis: people are regarded as 'rising to the challenge', 'getting on with it', 'coping very well', 'accepting their lot' and 'hanging on in there'. These stoical attitudes were clearly depicted in Rosie's story and are regarded widely by professionals as the hallmark of agricultural communities. They understand such attitudes to be fostered by farmers' close and daily engagement with the rhythms of the natural world. Reflecting back to farming in the 1930s, through the experiences recounted by old people in the community, the matron of a residential home for elderly people makes this clear:

If the calf didn't live then it was a great disaster financially, but there wasn't any point in grieving . . . you've just got to carry on; the wheel keeps turning and you get on with it really . . . the farming community it was, you know, you got up, you got on with it and you didn't make a fuss.

This attitude, she suggests, fosters a strong sense of familial independence, one family from another. Thus, while farming communities are out of necessity family orientated (since traditionally there was no-one else apart from other family members to rely on), this familial interdependency need not necessarily extend to embrace wider concepts of community.

For example, while professionals praise the support which the family may offer to its individual members, the close-knit nature of village life – a texture partially derived from the metaphoric family which the village represents – can also be seen as working against individuals and individual families. Thus the village 'family' can manifest less supportive aspects of kinship relationships. As one community nurse describes: 'Village communities are very engrossed in each others' lives and although they're busy, they are never busy enough not to notice, flick the net curtain and see what's going on.'

Like the family, the community keeps watch over its members. This may be experienced as the source of a great sense of security and care. When she had flu, Lucy, for example, experienced the friendly support and attention of two of her neighbours. They had each independently noticed that Lucy had not drawn her bedroom curtain as was usual in the morning. One of her friends, Theresa, decided to collect Lucy's dustbin so it would get emptied by the dustmen on their route. Later on she returned the bin to Lucy's back door. Lucy's other friend, Emily, noticed the drawn curtains and called Lucy to ask her whether she was all right and if she needed any help.

By contrast, for someone suffering from mental illness this kind of neigh-bourly surveillance can create serious difficulties in relation to service delivery. The community nurse describes some of these problems: 'They wouldn't know who we were but they would know that farm gets visits from someone regularly . . . strange cars, strange people.' Such surveillance roles are, of course, an integral part of community care but 'looking out for someone' in a caring and concerned fashion could, in the eyes of the community psychiatric nurse, easily become translated into less benign forms of monitoring: 'It's much harder in a small community when you are watched . . . you are watched for better, for worse, but usually for worse.'

Thus, for women with depression, a not uncommon response to the social isolation incurred through being a farmer's wife (Christensen et al. 1997), the community may, from a professional viewpoint, prove to be as disabling as it can be enabling for the women:

It's very much about how you are seen. These women, their self-esteem was really right down in their socks because they knew that the others knew there were problems in the family and that she was not well. It was not talked about but they knew, and she knew they knew.

Alongside the village community, the family too can prove to be a similar constraint. Just as happens within the village, the very interconnectedness and tight interdependencies of family life can, as we have seen, work both for and against individual family members. This partly reflects the enduring form of the farming family which, as a local teacher remarked, can make people just a little bit 'too comfortable' in their families. The family is mostly seen as providing a welcome and supportive framework for its members – for example, at times of temporary sickness or financial difficulties. In particular circumstances, however, from the professionals' point of view, it can not only fail to provide that support but can also actually constitute the problem. We suggest that the family, as a unifying structure, will expose its weakness at those times when the family can no longer literally 'get on with it' and thereby maintain its autonomy as a unit.

For example, in the view of the community psychiatric nurse, it is the family form which exacerbates the onset of depression and other mental illnesses amongst women in farming communities. The traditional and segmented roles of men and women often mean that women spend a great deal of time alone or, when younger, bearing the sole responsibility of caring for young children. But although desperate for company, they rarely make their feelings apparent. In sum, 'they get on with it':

> They were suffering tremendously but in a quiet sort of way, very quiet way and didn't make a big thing about it. But that's sort of northerners, they don't make a big thing about things, you keep it under wraps.

Furthermore, it is precisely the clear gendered divisions of labour which may obscure a wife's illness from her husband's gaze. Only when a crisis occurs – when a wife begins to neglect her household duties or remains in bed for days on end – then a husband's suspicion might be aroused. The community psychiatric nurse explains: 'It dawned on them that they were a bit quiet, but they had never actually looked at their partner.' Only at this often very critical point in the woman's illness would the mental health team be contacted.

GETTING ON WITH IT

It is, we propose, precisely this public revelation of the inability of the family 'to get on with it' which makes care in such communities problematic for professionals and community members alike. In studies of mental illness it has been suggested that the self can be seen as 'an intersubjective public project that can be lost or debased by stigma, rather than by the disease itself' (Herskovits 1995). This means that the experience of 'loss of self relates to the ways that others treat the . . . sufferer' (Sabat and Harré in Herskovits 1995). In the farming community, as we have seen, there is a strong interconnectedness between self and family. In these circumstances the protection of a person's public *persona* becomes all the more important; it is not only the sick person but the whole family that otherwise risks being debased. Thus, for example, our data reveals instances of a woman receiving mental health care who would make a two-hour journey in an unmarked ambulance to the hospital for her daily treatment in order to protect her anonymity and avoid the stigmatization which might follow any public revelation of her emotional state. In other situations, women might walk to a pick-up point outside the village so that the neighbours or even other family members need not get to know about the treatment. For another woman the pressure to maintain the appearance of an unchanged family life entailed rising early to cook and bake for the family before setting off for her hospital appointment. Thus, from these examples, it is clear that the family must visibly be seen to be unchanged as regards the community. Or more precisely, it seems that the changed roles of family members cannot be easily accommodated within traditional farming if such changes entail an inability to be seen to get on with the everydayness of the farming way of life. This can be further illustrated through local peoples' attitudes to two contrasting examples of residential homes for the elderly in the vicinity.

Situated in the heart of one village in the locality, Sunnyside is a small residential home for eighteen old people. Its residents are infirm but not geriatric. Sunnyside aims to have a 'real family' atmosphere and is seen in some ways as a collective granny flat for the village. Kin visit regularly, popping in and out on a daily basis and the home's elderly residents are accorded status within the community. Indeed, the home is in many ways 'the property of the village': as the matron says, 'they always know before we do who's coming in'.

Like Sunnyside, The Elms is located centrally in another village but, by contrast, has over the years increasingly admitted elderly people suffering from dementia. It is ignored by its village community, despite the best efforts of its matron to entice relatives to visit: 'I try getting people here with barbecues, summer lunches, Sunday lunch, anything to get them here, but I'm knocking my head against a brick wall.' In her opinion it is the nature of the elderly people's illness which seems to be the major source of difficulty: 'it's still that "sweep it under the carpet", a failure to acknowledge the changed mental condition of their relative'. However, it is also more than simply a stereotypical response to mental illness that we are encountering here. Sunnyside residents are essentially unchanged; older, more infirm but in essence unchanged. They are carrying along the groove within which they have been embedded throughout life. Residents at The Elms, on the other hand, present visible reminders of what has been lost and altered. It would seem, therefore, that the strength and tradition of the farming family, though providing a degree of flexibility through its very tight interconnections, cannot in the end accommodate radical change. When 'just getting on with it' is no longer enough, then the family itself fragments. One health care professional explains: 'As long as you're well, as long as you can pull together whenever there is pulling and you can be relied on then the family and the community offer tremendous resources.' Should this change, however, isolation will surely follow. Thus for the professionals the paradox they experience is of endeavouring to carry out their professional role within a community where the boundaries between the self, the family and the community are intractable yet ultimately shifting.

CONCLUSION

The stoicism entailed in 'just getting on with it' which was so central in Rosie's account of her illness episodes can be seen as a cultural ethos shared by the farming families in the local community. In Bourdieu's terms it represents a cultural habitus (see Christensen *et al.* 1997). Whether in relation to work or family well-being, 'getting on with it' is an ethos embodied through the life course. Grace, for example, describes this in relation to her early working life on a farm. Prior to her marriage she left her father's farm to work for a while away from home in another part of the country. She recalls:

> At Donald's, Donald put me in charge of a few hundred sheep and he left it to me, it was just up to me and I think I learnt a lot from that, I learnt from being on my own a lot because you learn from your mistakes. I mean Donald was always there if I wanted to ask him something but he was at market a lot of the time. And I just had to get on and do my daily work on my own. . . . Donald was a very robust character, quite rough and down to earth. Just used to get on with the job kind of thing didn't pay much attention to detail. His farm was an absolute dump, just muck everywhere, not neat and tidy like my dad's farm, completely the opposite to my dad's farm. . . . [Dad] used to think it was so rough and while I was there he said that I had got real rough with the way I talked and the way I looked and everything because I worked so hard I never used to get my hair cut or new clothes or anything like that. I really enjoyed it just learning from my own mistakes and working my own way.

Grace demonstrates in her account the interconnectedness which characterizes the habitus of farming life: she learns to stand by herself, to get on with it, at the same time as she becomes tightly bound to Donald's farm, identifying with it and its particular ambience precisely through her presentations of self.

In this sense Grace's account provides further confirmation of the relations between self, family and community which, as we have suggested, lie at the heart of the problems which professionals encounter in the discursive models and practice of community care. This is a locality where the self is not separable from its location in the family or the community, as the rhetoric of community

72513

care and practice would have it. Rather, in this setting, teachers, priests, social workers, health visitors and the matrons of residential homes must take account of the fact that their clients cannot easily be separated out from their families. This constitutes a problem for professionals. They are faced with the challenge of finding different strategies to work around what they see as community and family constraints. What we argue, therefore, is that a model of 'community care' in agricultural communities has to address culturally specific issues relating to personal and communal identities. Following Herskovits (1995), this includes asking fundamental questions about what comprises self and subjectivity in particular local settings.

BIBLIOGRAPHY

Barnes, M. (1977) *Care, Communities and Citizens*, London: Longman.

Bourdieu, P. (1977) *Outline of a Theory of Practice*, Cambridge: Cambridge University Press.

Christensen, P., Hockey, J. and James, A. (1997) '"You have neither neighbours nor privacy": ambiguities in the emotional well being of women in farming families', *The Sociological Review* (forthcoming).

Daley, G. (1988) *Ideologies of Caring*, Basingstoke: Macmillan.

Finch, J. and Grove, D. (1983) *A Labour of Love: Women, Work and Caring*, London: Routledge.

Herskovits, E. (1995) 'Struggling over subjectivity: debates about the "self" and Alzheimer's disease', *Medical Anthropology Quarterly* 9, 2: 146–64.

Kakar, S. (1982) *Shamans, Mystics and Doctors*, London: Unwin.

Nettleton, S. (1996) 'Women and the new paradigm of health and medicine', *Critical Social Policy* 48.

Shweder, R. (1991) *Thinking through Cultures: Expeditions in Cultural Psychology*, Cambridge: Harvard University Press.

Twigg, J. (1993) 'The interweaving of formal and informal care: policy models and problems', in A. Evers and G. H. van der Zanden (eds) *Better Care for Dependent People living at Home*, Bunnik: Netherlands Institute of Gerontology.

Chapter 3

Concepts of community in changing health care: a study of change in midwifery practice

Christine McCourt

INTRODUCTION

This chapter discusses the current policy of community care in the health services in the UK and the ways in which it represents a symbolic or practical return towards 'traditional' forms of health and social care. It explores the concepts of hospital and community drawn on in enacting the policy, using maternity services in the 1990s as a case study. It suggests that changes in this sphere of health care are part of a broader cultural shift in social and health policy, following a period of belief in the progressive nature of large-scale social institutions, towards the models of community and consumerism. This research focuses on the UK in the 1980s and 1990s, but similar movements have been evident in North America, Scandinavia and other European states.

Following the steady incorporation of maternity care into the domain of obstetric medicine during this century, recent reforms have, ostensibly, aimed to reverse this trend. I will draw on data from a large-scale, multidisciplinary study of the implementation of government policy to explore the use of the community concept in the current changes. In-depth interviews with women having babies, observations of professional/client interaction and an ethnographic study of professional responses to the change suggest that there are a number of paradigms and models for public services subsumed within the new community care. The concept of community is drawn on but rarely articulated or explored, particularly from the perspective of the users of such services.

BACKGROUND: HOSPITAL AND COMMUNITY CARE IN THE TWENTIETH CENTURY

From midwifery to obstetrics

The word *midwife* is derived from the old English term meaning *with woman* and the practice of midwifery predates the development of obstetric medicine. The profession of obstetrics, by its nature and with an increasing focus on technological assistance and intervention in childbirth, has largely been hospital based.

Obstetrics developed hand in hand with the hospital as the place for birth. The historical shift away from midwifery practised in the community accelerated from about 1920, with a growing confidence in the capacity of obstetric technology to improve safety in childbirth (Hunt and Symonds 1995). The importance of basic health measures, such as improved sanitation and nutrition, combined with greater awareness of infection control measures in hospitals, were largely overlooked. An overall decline in maternal and infant mortality in the twentieth century was statistically associated with the trend towards hospital care and a causal relationship was assumed (Campbell and Macfarlane 1994; DoH 1980; Allison 1996).

Around the turn of the twentieth century, most births in the UK took place at home. Hospital care was only provided to the affluent and was a sign of that affluence. Paying for the care of a doctor, in a hospital bed, signified greater social status and perhaps promised greater safety and comfort in childbirth, but the rise in hospital birth was accompanied by an alarming rise in maternal deaths (which are thought to have been mainly a result of infection). Ironically, in the early part of the century, despite their poorer general health status, women who were too poor to pay for such services were far less likely to die as a result of childbirth (Tew 1986, 1990). The evidence on safety of birth, which was gathered in the form of perinatal and maternal mortality figures, was largely overlooked in a push towards increasing the availability of maternity hospital beds, trained professionals and antenatal health checks and education to a widening range of women.

In obstetrics and in public opinion, the gradual decline in maternal mortality from the 1930s (after the introduction of sulphonamides and aseptic techniques) and in infant mortality, in line with gradual improvements in social conditions and nutrition, was associated with the establishment of obstetric practice and hospital birth. By the 1970s, policy decreed that all births should take place in hospital and the employment of sometimes life-saving techniques became increasingly routine (Ministry of Health 1970).

Most care at birth was provided by midwives, who, until the Midwives Act of 1902, did not receive formal occupational training but learnt their skills through apprenticeship and experience. After 1902, midwifery training gradually came to be dominated by a nursing model and subordinated to medicine. The now familiar hierarchy of the hospital system – where the different professions constitute a quasi-kinship system of doctor as paternal, nurse as maternal and patient in a childlike role – was embodied in the training of medics, nurses and midwives.

Midwives reacted to these changes in different ways. Some accepted their categorization within nursing and as an adjunct (assistant or handmaid) to obstetrics, while others resisted these changes through interest organizations, such as the Association for the Improvement of Maternity Services (AIMS) and the Association of Radical Midwives, and through re-establishing independent midwifery practices outside the NHS. For many, forms of resistance were more subtle, involving creating niches, or quiet forms of practice within the existing health care system. This practice was assisted by the disciplinary division of roles into care for normal (midwives) and abnormal (obstetricians) pregnancy and birth, but the sphere in which birth was understood or treated as normal was under continual revision in the face of obstetric developments. Additionally, quiet forms of resistance were often carried out as part of a nursing role of hierarchy maintenance within the service structure. Midwives attempted to model their practices around the requirements of protocols, guidelines and routine practices set by others, while, hidden beneath this, maintaining core midwifery principles of working with women and providing watchful support (Kirkham 1990).

Changes in maternity services have also been influenced by the views and wishes of women using them. The availability of pain relief, for example, was one of the main attractions of hospital birth for women, alongside the promise of safer birth. However, since the 1970s, with relative safety in childbirth better established and with increasing withdrawal of alternatives to the dominant consultant-led, general hospital service, the direction of many women's opinions has changed. They have begun to articulate and to challenge the increasing fragmentation, mechanization and depersonalization of care and the lack of choices available to them.

Such views, alongside the critiques provided by social science and midwifery research, fed into the recent policy shift away from the assumption that care in hospital is always best. This rethink was driven partly by increasingly united opposition from women's and midwifery organizations.[1] Women called for the re-establishment of more personalized systems of care. They did not reject technology but called for its more judicious use, allowing them to make choices and remain involved in decisions about their care. Midwives supported this view but also saw the direction of change as one which would allow them to reassert their professional autonomy – a shift away from the restricted, nursing-type role into which they had been steered by hospital practice. By 1993, there was apparent unity on the need for change, encompassing all professional groups (RCOG 1994). Such public unity often masked fundamental differences in perspective. Underlying the professional and consumer-led debates was a struggle for power between different interests (Savage 1986). This was exemplified in the debates over the place of birth, which so profoundly influenced the context and culture in which different balances of power and control were operating.

In the UK, in contrast to other post-industrial states, such as the US and Canada, community midwifery has maintained a solid, if increasingly small, base from which to re-establish its role (Arney 1982). However, community midwives are only involved in birth for a very small number of women, and so are seen to have been de-skilled as an occupational group. Hospital midwives provide the bulk of maternity care, including much of the care for 'normal' births, but the status or meaning of normal birth within consultant units has become increasingly questionable, as fewer and fewer women give birth without intervention or 'active management'.[2] In the division of labour between obstetricians and midwives, normality has traditionally been defined in midwifery in terms of freedom from disease, or being within parameters defined by the concept of naturalness: a physiological labour and birth. Normality was also taken to overlap with and subsume what is common, since pregnancy and childbirth was not traditionally understood to be pathological in most cases. This view was challenged by the placement of maternity services within the acute and secondary (rather than primary) sectors of health care, and an approach to labour care which is akin in many ways to intensive care treatment of those who are defined as sick.

The explicit concern underlying the key trends has been with safety but, as we have seen, developments took place which were in line with group interests such as professional development. While the emerging profession of obstetrics was undoubtedly concerned with safety of childbirth, its capacity to ignore evidence to the contrary suggests that the issues involved were more complex, involving wider cultural developments as well as sectional group interests (Jordan 1993).

In order to illustrate this more general cultural shift in the nature of social institutions, parallel lines can be drawn with the development of other health and social service institutions over the last century in the UK and other industrialized states. The general move towards containment of roles and bodies in what were later characterized as 'total institutions' (Goffman 1968a) has been well described by Foucault (1973, 1979). Although the maternity hospital is unlike a total institution in the sense that women stay for short periods and the boundaries are more permeable, they share many of the characteristics of what are also termed 'people changing organizations' (Alasewski 1986).

The development of community care policy

The conceptualization of the complementary roles of hospital and community as the proper places for, respectively, treatment and care, which is apparent in the recent policy shifts across health and social services, is not described self-consciously as part of that policy. It remains unarticulated in such a way that the shifts towards community care are understood, instead, as produced by technology.

In maternity services, the shift in thinking from the position of 1980 (DoH 1980) with a continuing emphasis on centralized hospital care, to a return towards community-based care (DoH 1993), is seen as made possible through technology ensuring greater safety in childbirth. Effectively, returning certain limited aspects of care to a community setting is regarded as a product of effective technologies and hospital-based treatment, which allow non-medical, community-based care to take its appropriate place.

If we view *hospital* and *community* in this way, as separate domains of activity, characterized by a series of features which are not just about place, but about types of social institution and role, a series of relationships can be discerned in the development of community care policy. The concept of community is not defined in itself, but oppositionally, by what it is not; what it moves away from. Hospital is to community, therefore, as profession is to occupation, treatment to care; male to female. These opposing types are also characterized by different types of activity – the 'doing' active mode of medicine is opposed to the 'waiting and watching' observational mode of midwifery or other forms of social and health care (Jordan 1993). These activities are not only largely embodied by people of different gender, but they are also gender-typed so that, for example, a male carer is understood to be adopting a feminine role. These concepts of community are largely driven by the boundaries of concern and interest used by service-providing institutions and occupations. They also accord with the wider cultural concepts of community, which are associated with notions of belonging, denoted by family, place or other means of connection. Thus the associations of community are generally warm and positive.

The view of most obstetricians remains that, for all but a few carefully selected women, birth should take place in a hospital but most pre- and post-natal care can take place in the community, in local health centres or in the home. This helps to ensure that the more high technology 'acute' care, with birth as 'the main event', remains within the hospital and the sphere of obstetrics, while the longer term, lower intensity care takes place in a separate domain. As Jordan and others have noted, notions of time and duration are culturally situated and may differ widely. Biomedicine tends to impose a functional, institutional construction of time over the physiological and psycho-social sense of time of the childbearing woman (Thomas 1992; Pizzini 1992). Women's concerns and definitions of childbearing are broader, incorporating life history, relationships and changing social roles. Maternity services in the UK are strongly oriented around labour and delivery, which is tightly defined (and temporally limited if seen to be out of time). For example, whereas fifteen years ago women having normal births in the UK were encouraged to remain in hospital for a week following birth, for care and support in recovering from birth and adjusting to motherhood, they are now encouraged to leave hospital twenty-four or even six hours after a short period of recovery, akin to the immediate medical recovery period following an operative birth.

In this new time framework, a 'production line' model still typifies women's experiences of hospital birth but the line now extends to incorporate the community. Pregnancy and birth are treated in the manner of an industrial production process, managed by an obstetric consultant but with parts of the process handled by different people; the pregnant or birthing woman is shifted from place to place and from one professional to another, dictated by shifts and ward-based systems (Davis-Floyd 1994). The reintroduction of community maternity services holds out the possibility of the extension of medical influence or control further into people's lives. Thus, although the associations of the concept of community lead us to view it as generally a good thing – benign, inclusive, and the focus of caring – community health care is understood by professionals and, implicitly, by the wider society, as a product of successful medical development. It is thereby a means of bringing the domain of expertise into those of home, family and locality. The new 'community' created by the health service is envisaged very much with the hospital as its physical and ideological centre.

Changing Childbirth **and the case of one-to-one midwifery**

The report of the House of Commons select committee on health (HoC 1992) gave official recognition to the growing concerns about the maternity services. It was a radical document, which advocated dealing with health in its broader sense, as not just concerned with medicine, which mainly responds to disease or ill-health, but with other influences on health, in particular, the impact of poverty. It advocated wider reforms in social policy as well as far-reaching changes in the character of maternity services to give greater scope for midwives to practice and for women to make choices. The report was not well received by the government of the time, which viewed and promoted both consumerism and community care policy as a means of rolling back the role of the state in people's lives. A classical policy of avoidance by the commissioning of further research was employed. An Expert Maternity Group was convened to undertake further research and to develop a policy consensus. Its remit was narrowed to a focus on childbirth and the provision of maternity services and its membership was largely from within those services, but with a strong midwifery leadership. The resulting policy, enshrined in the document *Changing Childbirth* (DoH 1993), accorded well with the broad policy principles of the time – the promotion of a consumer model for health services, provided within a community base where possible. It set out clear principles – choice, continuity and control for women – and indicators of success for achieving these. The indicators rested strongly on re-establishing the roles of midwives, keeping low-risk care in the community and improving access to information to enhance choice.

This shift in thinking and policy was anticipated by a new model of care – one-to-one midwifery – introduced within one London NHS Trust. This Trust had a strong tradition of obstetric research and a reputation for innovation, for example, in pioneering the use of ultrasound scanning in routine maternity care (Oakley 1993), but this had not previously been midwifery-led. A research-based evaluation was a prerequisite of the development, since it posed a possible radical change, and the service was set up as a pilot scheme, covering two neighbourhoods. This enabled a comparative study to be designed with evaluation of the new scheme alongside the conventional maternity service still operating in neighbouring areas. Conventional care, for women identified as being 'low risk' in the UK is usually known as *shared care*: led by a consultant obstetrician but with care shared between the hospital and the general practitioner (GP). 'High-risk' women usually receive total hospital care. In both settings much of the hands-on care is provided by hospital or community midwives.

In line with the core principles of *Changing Childbirth*, the one-to-one service aimed to be more woman-centred and to achieve this by offering continuity of carer. Continuity of care, provided or co-ordinated by a named midwife, was seen as the key to offering women a coherent service, with choices and a role in decision-making. The development was led by the UK's first Professor of Midwifery, who had been part of the government's Expert Maternity Group. One-to-one midwives worked in a radically different pattern from hospital or community midwives.[3] Each one-to-one midwife carried a personal caseload (forty women per year, with a mix of low and high risk as defined by standard clinical criteria) and worked in partnerships with the support of group practices. Women receiving one-to-one care each had a named midwife who, with a partner, was responsible for her care, which could be led by the midwife, obstetric consultant or GP, depending on medical needs and the woman's choice. Alongside this, care was expected to be more community based, with the one-to-one midwife able to offer maternity care when and where needed.

THE STUDY: AIMS AND METHODS

The research on which this account is based was intended to document the change process, assess its outcomes and survey women's responses to the new form of care. Since studying change was acknowledged to be complex, and the study would involve a wide range of outcomes and issues of concern, this was a multidisciplinary project, incorporating a number of research approaches and methods:

- An ongoing ethnographic study analysing the process of change and its impact on professionals;
- A study of women's experiences and responses to care. This included a large-scale postal survey of women using the service (1400 women), in-depth interviews with a sample of women in the survey, responders (twenty) and non-responders (twenty-five), three small focus groups with local women and a case study of Somali women's experiences;
- A clinical audit of the care provided, clinical standards, intervention and outcomes; and the number of carers seen;
- An economic study of the costs of the scheme and the implications of this for its sustainability.

Studying women's responses to care was a major strand of the research, since the new policy was explicitly oriented towards choice and control for child-bearing women. The survey sample included all women within the relevant areas who had booked for care with this Trust over a one-year period.[4] Questionnaires were posted for self-completion at thirty-five weeks of pregnancy, and at two and thirteen weeks after birth. They included a number of closed questions – for ease of statistical analysis – as well as open questions designed to encourage women to give their views in their own words. Psychological scales and demographic questions were also included to develop a profile of the women in the study and assess whether the form of care might have any impact on their health. Interviews were used to provide a greater depth of response and to avoid framing the issues in the light of the researchers' interests: women were encouraged to tell their stories of pregnancy, birth and the following months and then to comment on what they felt was helpful, or needed improving, in the services offered. These included women who did not respond to the questionnaires, since it was recognized that response patterns may be skewed towards English-speaking middle-class women, who may have different needs and interests from others. We targeted mothers from minority ethnic groups, and those aged under twenty-one, using data recorded in medical notes. An additional six interviews and discussion group were conducted with Somali refugee women, facilitated by a Somali-speaking local community worker.

An original assumption of the research design was that audit of medical records would be used to assess the nature and quality of midwifery practice. It was soon apparent that although such records could reveal important information about easily measured activities or outcomes, such as use of pain relief or method of delivery, the nature of care could not be read literally from such documents. Medical records are texts constructed for a range of purposes and generally respond to the reductive nature of biomedical practice. They tell a particular story which is constructed, partial, and situated within their medical context. Therefore, a further observation study was commenced at the end of the two-year period, to try to gain a fuller understanding of how the midwives practised and the nature of their interactions with pregnant women. We followed a selection of midwives as they conducted the 'history taking' with women booking for maternity care. One-to-one midwives normally visited women for booking in their own homes, while traditional community midwives normally interviewed women at their GP's surgery, and hospital midwives interviewed women in the hospital clinic.

As a multidisciplinary project, the research straddled – awkwardly but productively – the boundaries of different academic traditions. The design of the audit and the structured survey of women's responses drew on positivist assumptions about using research to test and demonstrate direct relationships between interventions and outcomes. An example of this was the concern to test the hypothesis that a new form of care would produce a particular set of outcomes, without particular regard to the contexts in which the care took place, the complexity of organizational change or the agency of those receiving the service. The inclusion of qualitative research reflected sociological awareness of the need to understand the relationship between means and ends, and of the difficulties, practical and theoretical, inherent in any system of measurement. This was a comparative study, not across different cultures, in a traditional anthropological sense, but of a change between systems which are often thought to represent different cultures of care and which, therefore, in the eyes of many of those involved, represent a cultural shift in values, and ways of thinking and acting. In many respects studying change, like cross-cultural research, offers the opportunity to understand core values of a system which might otherwise seem obvious, taken-for-granted or naturally right. Jordan (1993) advocates comparative anthropological research on childbirth because it offers a window into the understanding of systems which are culturally shaped and embedded, internally consistent and therefore appear 'right' and unquestionable. In this case, change efforts had been prompted by awareness of contradictions and conflicts in a system which arose alongside broader social changes, prompted by feminist and postmodern thought.

Situated within the context of policy making and implementation, the project also followed action research principles of relevance and usefulness to research subjects, involving them as partners with the aim of enhancing practice. Although statistically based research requires collection of full data sets before analysis can begin, the research team were mindful of the needs of those providing health services to plan their implementation of the new policy recommendations. Therefore, an interim analysis was conducted and made available half-way through the two-year study, and formal and informal feedback and discussion took place throughout the project.

THE RESEARCH FINDINGS

An overview

The overall findings of the study confirmed those of earlier research on continuity of care and social support in pregnancy and birth (Oakley 1992; Hodnett 1996). In summary, the overall conclusions were that

- women preferred one-to-one care;
- midwives found the role challenging but far more fulfilling than their previous style of work;
- one-to-one care achieved significant reductions in some clinical interventions – in particular, the use of episiotomies and of epidural anaesthesia – without reducing clinical safety;
- the scheme did not increase the cost of the service.

On this basis, it was recommended that the scheme be continued and developed further, under continuing evaluation to study its longer term impact.

The longest section of the research report (McCourt and Page 1996) reflected the complexity and detail of the research conducted. It was about women's responses to care. It provided images, both positive and negative, which invited reflection and debate within the maternity service. The ethnographic study, although incomplete at that stage, raised useful considerations about ways of implementing change and dealing with the problems of resistance and resentment which can arise in a changing organization. Connections were drawn between the complaints of women about the way they were treated in hospital and the feelings of alienation amongst many staff working in the conventional system. The clinical study assured those involved that the new scheme did not compromise safety standards and raised a series of further questions about why change in high intervention rates was so difficult to achieve.[5] The economic study indicated that rather than increasing overall costs, the scheme shifted costs from some aspects of practice to others, in particular reducing in-hospital costs but increasing the costs of midwives working in community settings.

The impact of the change: the meaning of midwifery

The simple model of one-to-one midwifery changed, or at least challenged, a great deal. The midwife's work was to be designed around the women on her caseload rather than around the structures of the institution. As in pregnancy and childbirth, time would not be so easily structured by the routines of shifts and wards, and the spheres of work, home life and leisure would not be so clearly demarcated and bounded (Pizzini 1992; Allison 1996; Leap 1993). The concept of working *with women* meant going back to the origins of midwifery in a more than literal sense. It meant working with women within the context of their families and communities. Most antenatal care was now offered in the woman's own home and women were encouraged to leave hospital as soon as possible after birth, with the midwife providing support at home.[6] Hospital birth remained the norm, but the midwives no longer actively discouraged home birth, and some acted as advocates for women who requested home birth care in the face of medical opposition. Women in early labour were able to remain at home if they wished, with advice and care provided by the midwife.[7] The concept of community operated by the midwives here was, therefore, multi-faceted. It was a concept of place; in particular about the territory which was the woman's – her home and neighbourhood – and the midwife's role out in the community, where they held more autonomy than in hospital. It was also one of structure, in the sense that the services should take their form around the woman in the context of her family and home life, rather than around the hospital as a structure which would mould her experience.

The midwives' view was that most women feel more relaxed and more in control in their own homes. If this is not the case, women can opt for care, provided by the same midwife, at the GP surgery or the hospital clinic. They saw this as empowering women and so the possibility that community-based care, under certain approaches, could imply an extension of medical power within the community and domestic settings was not considered as an issue by the midwifery leaders initiating the project (McKeown 1979). This is also, perhaps, because midwives view their roles, in contrast to those of doctors, as representing care and support, rather than authority.[8]

There is a paradox here for midwives, who also saw the policy shift as a means of reasserting their autonomy and, effectively, their status as a professional rather than occupational group. The one-to-one midwives challenged the new consensus about community care policy because, unlike community midwives, they crossed the boundaries of hospital and community, working with women where needed. They worked around their caseload rather than shifts or routines designed by and for the institution (Frankenberg 1992) and they dropped the symbols of the nursing role – such as uniforms – as they attempted to pull away from the incorporation of midwifery into nursing. In effect, they were not only challenging the boundaries between women and the maternity services – between themselves and the women they care for – but also between themselves and the profession of obstetrics.

Although the assumption that midwives represent care and support, rather than authority, has been substantially challenged by research on midwifery practice (Kirkham 1989; Hunt and Symonds 1995), the leaders of the innovation felt strongly that the caseload model would draw practice away from authoritarian styles to one where a personal relationship with the woman, built up over time, helps to ensure she has a voice and is heard. Although the terminology sounds individualistic, with little hint of family or wider community, it reflected a concern to move away from the assembly-line type systems dominant in hospital nursing and midwifery. In such a system, women (both those using the service and many midwives) described feeling lost, their individuality buried in a system of routinized, often ritual, tasks and with activity divided up into blocks which made sense only in terms of the institutional structuring of relationships and time.

The ambiguities inherent in their changing role were evident in our observations of the midwives' interactions with women at the 'booking' visit. In this inner-city area, midwives often care for women who are reluctant to engage with formal health services for a variety of reasons, as well as women who enthusiastically approach this visit as the first formal recognition of their newly pregnant and therefore changed state. The midwife is required to collect large amounts of information from the woman about her medical history, family and lifestyle, and to provide advice. Information and discussion has been highlighted by pregnant women as an important need; in many ways they are hungry for information; but the midwife has a great deal to do and needs to convey the sort of information which is professionally required of her, mainly health education material and instructions or advice regarding maternity care and the range of screening tests available.

In comparison with previous research on this encounter (Methven 1989), we found midwives, particularly those who have trained recently, far more aware of the need to communicate and to make the woman feel at ease. However, the setting of the visit in hospital in the conventional system constrains communication beyond a straightforward exchange of facts and advice. The interview is conducted around a desk in a treatment room. The midwife is friendly and reassuring but mindful of the need to complete the required parts of the medical notes within the allotted time frame. In many senses, the visit is led, not even by the midwife herself but by the structures within which she operates. When interviewed, hospital midwives were sometimes aware of ways in which they had failed to respond to cues from a woman, explaining this as due to the need to complete the checklist; something requiring a fairly rigid ordering and time schedule. Women's fears or anxieties could disrupt this framework. For example, when a woman began to talk about her previous experiences of pregnancy loss, the midwife stopped her, indicating they would come to this under her obstetric history. This midwife later confided that she was expecting to be told off soon for spending too long on these visits and thereby not doing her fair share of the work (which is measured in number of visits or other activities undertaken). She expressed concern that she had not responded directly to the woman's comments. In another visit, a woman said that she was afraid of a procedure she had experienced during her first labour. This comment was made after the midwife, noticing her own signature in the medical notes but without personal recollection, remarked that she had performed this procedure during the first labour. The midwife, without responding, wrote the woman's comment down and proceeded to her next question.

One-to-one midwives, working in women's homes in most cases, did not suffer such restrictions of time or structure. At first sight, transcripts of their interviews appeared chaotic; unlike medical notes they were full of conversational asides, chatter and memories. Their use of space varied in each visit in ways signalled by the woman and her domestic environment. Family members often continued their daily business, or joined the discussion. Older children were introduced and in some cases midwives were catching up with families where they had assisted with a previous birth. In these cases the child and the details of events were recalled with clarity. The course of the interview was dictated to a greater degree by the woman's interests and questions, with the midwife fitting her objectives into this framework as far as she could. Women seemed more able to admit to difficulties and uncertainties – about the pregnancy or their ability to cope with parenthood, for example – and midwives were more able to respond to them. These midwives also felt obliged to give and collect a great deal of specific information but, due to the continuity of their role, were able to spread the exchange over a longer time period, when need or interest arose. Their main aim was to establish a relationship from which communication and knowledge would flow. However, the potential for contradictions in their role – for example, between using information to 'empower' women or to survey their health and parenting behaviour – remained.

This was illustrated in the process of advising women about antenatal tests. Reflecting the greater awareness of consumer values, information and choice, most of the midwives attempted to offer information and advice about antenatal tests and screening. This is always partial and geared towards explaining tests and procedures rather than exploring the woman's values or the issues which tests may force them to confront. One-to-one midwives provided more information and were more likely than those in the hospital to offer women choice, particularly about tests, such as ultrasound scans, which are not popularly viewed as a form of screening. Yet they still directed women's choices in some ways. For example, after her midwife had described the tests available for Downs syndrome, a woman declined the test. The midwife suggested she think about it and tell her the following week what she wanted, prompting the woman to ask the midwife what she thought she should do. The extension of choice in this case could be viewed as a subtle form of encouraging what is seen by professionals as appropriate use of health care. The midwife later commented on her own ambivalence about her role – she was giving too much information in one go; she preferred to establish a relationship with the woman so that this can follow later and sympathized with the feelings of women who don't really want a lot of the services offered to them. In her view, a lot of it was unnecessary.

Women's responses to maternity care

Our qualitative research on women's responses to care threw detailed light on these issues. Women receiving one-to-one care were happier with the system than those receiving conventional care. Their preferences were reflected in the statistical results of our large-scale survey but explained more fully in their responses to open-ended questions, in-depth interviews and in focus group discussions. Women often felt lost in the hospital system. Although the care provided was ostensibly for and about them, they often felt overlooked and disregarded. These feelings were not necessarily translated into complaints or unhappiness expressed directly about the maternity services. Most women felt grateful for the services provided and the hard work of their carers. Feelings of doubt or failure tended to be internalized and attributed to the self rather than the system – the woman's own failure to cope or the baby's reluctance to feed, for example, rather than lack of, or inappropriate, support.

In contrast to common assumptions about women in different social or cultural groups, the research revealed that women from different backgrounds expressed essentially similar feelings about their experiences of maternity services. The importance of core themes such as dialogue, communication and a sense of confidence or trust were overlaid by particular issues for some women; for example, the sheer difficulty of communicating at all for refugee women who did not speak English and the increased trauma they suffered due to loss of feelings of control over what was happening to them. Maslow's hierarchy of needs (1954) suggests the most basic needs must be attended to before higher level needs can be met, but women suffering other more pressing problems have no less need for social and emotional support. In many ways they receive less.

Women receiving one-to-one care did not experience these problems in the same way, due to the co-ordinating and mediatory role of the midwife. They felt better informed and less exposed in having to deal with such systems. They were also more positive about their birth experiences, due to the presence and support of a known midwife. Interestingly, they sometimes appeared to have accepted their experience, including medical interventions,[9] more easily because they trusted and had confidence in their main carer and felt informed and involved. This can be viewed as a positive outcome for women in coping with the difficult transition of childbirth. It can also be seen as related to the traditionally mediating role of the nurse or midwife in medicine, where she may encourage co-operation and compliance in the woman's contact with the doctor, as well as presenting her interests to him.[10]

Psychological research on childbirth (Green *et al.* 1988; Oakley 1980) suggests that what is important for women's well-being following birth is the degree to which they feel able to influence what is done to them and the degree of control they feel during birth. While the number of interventions women experienced mattered, it was the way in which these were handled which made the most difference. By providing social support to the women, the midwives were increasing the degree of control women felt. This was reflected in women's depictions of the experience of labour. Women in the conventional system were more likely to describe being frightened, feeling out of control, exhausted. In a few cases they described extreme terror, or fear of dying, which was directly connected to the use of medical techniques, including the administration of anaesthesia. The importance of having a person with them, to explain everything, to support their confidence and trust was highlighted repeatedly. Women also described the ways in which midwives 'blocked the door'[11] or bought time for them in some instances, or advised and persuaded them to accept help in others. The mediatory role of the midwife was important to the management of labour and birth and the environment of the delivery suite in the hospital.

Although women's preferences for continuity and personal care were clear in our survey, it was the open-ended data and particularly the personal interviews which revealed the degree of distress experienced by many women in childbirth and in adjusting to life after this. Their accounts indicated that birth in the conventional care system was often experienced in a traumatic way, despite the availability of medical care and pain relief which might be assumed to protect women from unnecessary risk and fear.[12] It appeared that the obstetric approach operating in this context led to heightened feelings of risk, and undermined the confidence of both women and their carers (midwives as well as doctors) in their ability to give birth. Very high rates of medical intervention prevailed, which the one-to-one midwives were able to reduce only within certain limited parameters. As hypothesized, women receiving one-to-one care were more positive about the experience of birth, despite using less pain relief.[13] They felt supported and informed and so appeared to suffer less anxiety. Despite being a group with greater overall socio-economic deprivation than those in the conventional care group, the survey revealed them to be more confident about giving birth and caring for their new babies, even in hospital.

DISCUSSION

The status and role of women as patients or users of maternity care

In maternity services, women are accepted to be healthy and well in most cases. There is nonetheless a tendency in biomedical systems to approach birth, if not pregnancy, as a 'sickness role' (Parsons 1951) in which the patient is separated and removed from her normal responsibilities and rights. The desire amongst many midwives to avoid this role is reflected in their preference for providing care outside the hospital setting and without the use of labelling. For example, in the one-to-one scheme women they cared for were described as just women, not patients. Despite this changing discourse, maternity care is exceptional in the health service, as the only area where care is routinely referred to the secondary health sector.[14] One-to-one midwifery was able to shift this placing of maternity care only to a limited extent.

Pregnancy and birth is an important transition in the life course and social status of a woman, and her family. This transitional state is mirrored by the woman's treatment on entry to hospital, during pregnancy and, particularly, when giving birth. Birth in the modern obstetric hospital is heavily ritualized, as has been described elsewhere (Kitzinger 1993; Davis-Floyd 1994). The rituals of hospital birth during this century, although they follow closely the archetypal features of rites of passage, outlined by Van Gennep (1960), can be closely aligned to the rites of entry into total institutions described by Goffman and others as rites of degradation (Garfinkel 1956). Practices such as shaving, administration of enemas and to a lesser extent, cutting of the perineum (episiotomy – a practice described by Kitzinger as a medical form of female genital mutilation when used routinely) have recently been withdrawn from routine use in the face of research evidence as to their medical ineffectiveness (Carroli *et al.* 1997).[15] Hospital birth, though, still separates the woman from her everyday environment and relationships, and assigns her a special state.

The association between hospital and safety is also pertinent here since people in transitional or liminal states are viewed as both dangerous and vulnerable. In maternity the danger is internalized rather than externalized, seen as threat to the mother and child. The transition of birth is also treated as the point of separation between mother and child, in which the foetus changes its moral and legal state to that of infancy. Such separation of mother and child has particular resonances within a culture which values individualism and independence highly, and this valuation is reflected in the obstetric trend, in recent years in the UK and US towards seeing the identity and moral rights of the mother and baby as separate and possibly opposed.[16]

In order to understand the significance of maternity services as a social institution and the endurance of patterns of care which are not backed by scientific evidence, it is necessary to consider the role of power and gender relationships in the provision of health care and the processes of professionalization which have played a major role in the development, first, of hospital medicine and, more recently, of alternative health care models.

Reflections on community care

What was it about the concept of community care which was so attractive to policy makers, managers, professionals and those using the service, despite their different and sometimes opposing perspectives and interests? Community is a concept which is supposed to bind individuals to social units beyond kinship, the essential material or thread of society and culture. Yet the ways in which it binds are rarely explored and often left undefined. Its amorphism is part of the attraction of the concept, since it allows us to mould its shape to correspond to our own ideas and wants. It is very useful.

The midwives studied in this scheme challenged existing relationships and structures because of the way they crossed the hospital–community boundary in working around the needs of women on their caseload. This pattern of working encouraged them to cross inter-professional boundaries as well as to alter the way in which they conceived of and managed the relationship between domestic and economic domains, between themselves as professional and clients, and between the categories of nurse and doctor within the health service.

Although the midwives transferred much of maternity care to a community setting they changed the physical location of care more than they were able to change the locus of power. Overall power in the service was maintained by obstetric consultants who were firmly located in and dependent on the institutional base of the hospital – the base which has been necessary, in the absence of scientific evidence about the effectiveness of much obstetric technology, to its claims to scientific status.

These were early days in the implementation of this model of practice and time will be needed to judge how far this situation will change. There is evidence from our qualitative work, for example, that over time, the experience of working outside the hospital and closer to the context of women's everyday lives is changing the ways in which midwives approach their work and the power relationships involved in the provision of maternity care. The rate of home births, for example, is gradually rising from a rate of less than 1 per cent before this scheme was introduced, to 3 per cent during our research and now rising further as midwives and women realize that it is possible for them to choose this. The experience of birth at home is very different, since the attendant is a visitor in the woman's environment in the way that the woman is an outsider in the professionals' environment within the hospital. Time will tell whether such changes will be deemed acceptable.

Responses to the research

Writing these conclusions has provided a salutary experience of the policy context in practice, highlighting the degree to which policy makers and practitioners will use, reject or ignore 'evidence' according to how well research results relate to existing beliefs and practices. The drafting of the report on this study, and its timing, was driven mainly by the pressing needs of the local health service. The report had a key local function, as well as being of national policy interest, and the future of the model would – it was said – be influenced by the findings of the study.

Although most of its conclusions were accepted, those on costs contradicted the 'gut feelings' of many professionals, who, although they believed shifting care from hospital to community could save money, felt that this model of care would add overwhelming extra costs to the equation, in a period when each year saw managers grappling with 'cost improvement programmes'.[17] Women were being offered personal care in their own homes, with far greater continuity and more direct professional contact time. This had previously been possible only for women paying for independent midwife care: it was seen as a 'Rolls Royce service' and hence a luxury, despite the evidence of possible long-term health benefits for mothers and babies. Following the circulation of the interim study report, local tensions around the issue of costs increased, manifested in challenges to the integrity and effectiveness of the researchers involved. No specific criticisms were made but the economic analysis in this study looked at the whole system of care, including all health service resources used in the care for these women. However, the study was viewed by decision makers as concerning midwifery alone. Additionally, potential savings from reduced interventions were not considered, since the costs of technology were simply discounted. Researchers and managers differed in their understanding of what was relevant. It was asserted that the scheme was too expensive and so could not be implemented. However, outright rejection of the scheme, although implied, was never seriously posed, since it was also understood to be popular. Although cost was the focus of concern, it also seemed to this researcher that money was a convenient mask behind which to place other feelings of doubt about the changes in structures and relationships the scheme promised to bring about.

The nature of initial local reactions to the final report suggested that while attention is now explicitly given to women's choices, this is understood by managers within a frame of reference which appears to be largely dictated by the concerns of economy. Similarly, for those who are obstetricians, the concern is with maintaining the obstetric role (which incorporates a notion of safety) while achieving economy. To put it crudely, choice is all right as long as people choose the right thing. When a final draft of the research report was circulated, managers requested changes to the economic section: the researchers were informed that unless they stated that the scheme was more expensive they would jeopardize a delicate process of funding negotiation with the local Health Authority. No comments were received on other sections, despite the numbers of issues raised, including some quite serious criticisms. It seemed to the research team that the remainder of the report was accepted easily, even rather uncritically, yet given little attention or weight. To understand these reactions further, it is useful to view this service within the context of philosophical and organizational changes in the health service, changes which are themselves embedded in a wider context of social and cultural change in post-industrial states.

Community care policy as a consensus model and an arena for competing interests

Choice in the NHS and in other public services is now fashionable. With the purchaser/provider split in the health service, patients are now seen in some ways as consumers, but not directly so since services are purchased on behalf of the local community by Health Authorities and in some cases, general practitioners. The NHS is now organized on a market model in which the functions of providing and buying services are split, for the purpose of competition and market discipline, between two facets of the health service. The traditional planning function of the old Health Authorities remains, but conducted in a new manner and in a new relationship with hospitals, now organized as independent NHS Trusts (DoH 1990). The role and representation of *consumers* in this system is formally held by the Health Authorities, but with a duty to consult mediatory organizations such as Community Health councils and specially constituted liaison committees. Choice is seen to be a good thing as long as the choice fits the needs and preferences of the system.

For example, the reforms envisaged and approved by many managers are ones where women receive basically the same type of care but in a different location. Women have more of their routine antenatal visits at the GP surgery and much non-routine care is provided in day-units. This pattern of antenatal care is now preferred by both women and professionals. For birth, most women have care in hospital but early admission to the *delivery suite*[18] is avoided and early discharge from hospital to the visiting care of community midwives is encouraged. Again, women generally prefer this pattern of care but not unquestioningly so, and the complexity of the issues surrounding these choices was highlighted in our study. Little allowance is made in this system for women's needs for considerable care and support during and following labour and birth. Reductions in hospital lengths of stay were wanted by women, who wished to avoid institutional treatment and to adjust to parenthood in a relaxed, comfortable environment, but they have been driven largely by economic considerations, masked by the rhetoric of choice. In a similar fashion, the closure of psychiatric institutions, and the shift towards community mental health care, was driven by an uncomfortable and largely unacknowledged coalition of otherwise opposing philosophies (McCourt-Perring 1993). Part of the attractiveness of the concept of care in the community lies in its potential to draw together competing political and ideological perspectives and groups.

Despite the stated concern of current policy with the principles of choice and control for women, in this local context, of an obstetrically led and oriented maternity unit, the issue of power remained largely unarticulated in the research design and analysis. This perhaps reflected a new optimism about reform, encouraged by the apparent consensus of views about the role of midwifery and the value of community-based care. It was also influenced, however, by the ways in which the dominant biomedical model defines and limits the research paradigm. Traditionally, health services research has adopted a positivistic framework and has been led by clinicians. The role of social scientists has been marginal, and midwifery research is a developing but still relatively low-status field. In this environment, research designs are expected to provide clear and replicable evidence of direct connections between input – new treatment – and outcomes – improvement or not. The processes by which change occurs or the context in which change is introduced are seen as less worthy of investigation, even though, in much research of this type, the change is essentially an organizational one, involving people, rather than a controllable intervention. This research environment makes it more difficult to deconstruct what is going on and what underlies the findings. It was clear to the research team that the context and processes of change were significant for the outcomes and effects, hence the inclusion of an ethnographic study, but nonetheless, issues such as power and gender relationships have only been touched upon.

The research does, however, throw light on some of the undercurrents I have noted. One is the attempt, by midwives, as part of the *Changing Childbirth* agenda, to re-establish the autonomy which had been the norm before the rise of hospital-based obstetrics for all women.[19] Effectively, the current changes represent a means of identifying themselves as a professional group, with their own identity and areas of practice and expertise. However, the way in which this has taken place is very different from the processes which characterized the established professions such as medicine and law. It could perhaps be described as a more feminized model of professionalism, focused on co-operation and mutuality with the client and discomfort with the individual exercise of power. The midwives are conscious of the dilemmas they face in trying to offer choice to women while holding their own, learned, ideas about what is good for them, or of encouraging women to depend on them while also purporting to offer them empowerment.

Practice in the community was important to the midwives' achievement of autonomy since, in a hospital setting, even in more midwifery-led units, they are part of an obstetric team. In more obstetrically led units, the hospital midwives are treated as playing a nursing role and as an occupational rather than a professional group. They work around rotas and shifts, procedures and guidelines, with little opportunity to exercise judgement. To empower women who are using the services while working in this manner represents a double challenge. Conversely, the traditional community midwives had no clear role or authority within the hospital setting yet their work was still compartmentalized along lines set by the hospital system.

The one-to-one midwives were able to overstep this boundary, and work to their own, woman-centred routines, but they still worked as part of the same obstetric team and the same hospital system. The power struggle in which they were effectively engaged required change within that system. At the same time, they faced the paradox of trying to establish a professional role within the maternity care system, while also wishing to establish a different type of role and relationship with the women they provide care for, which entailed a shift in philosophy away from the professionalism of medicine (Freidson 1970).

CONCLUDING REMARKS

The implementation of *Changing Childbirth* through the one-to-one scheme illustrates well the differences in understanding as to what is meant by community care. These follow from a tendency, at the level of government policy, to gloss over complicated issues. Looking back at the formation of this policy, for example, there has been little comment on the shift from the arguments of the Winterton committee, which looked at women's health in its broader context and meaning (HoC 1992), to a document which focuses primarily on childbirth (DoH 1993), viewing the transition in the lives of women within a narrower and more short-term frame of reference.

Midwives' understanding of the principles of *Changing Childbirth* are concerned both with greater choice and control for women and for themselves as a group. The one-to-one midwives, those who stepped forward to try out the most radical model of practice linked to *Changing Childbirth* felt strongly that working with women in their own environment would be empowering for both groups. The obstetric response to this model appeared ambivalent – on the one hand it posed a threat of taking influence over practice away from them, while on the other, it promised to separate the domains of care so that the clinical domain remained the core of obstetrics, with key activities remaining within the hospital, while the domain of care and support could be appropriately shifted to the periphery: to community and midwifery care.[20] Similar arguments can be applied to the acquiescence of many psychiatrists to the closure of the old asylums: much psychiatric work was transferred in this process to the preferred setting of the district general hospital, with nurses providing ancillary medical care in community-based clinics.

I have also suggested that it is possible to view the re-establishment of community care, which is assumed by many professionals to be a product of technological and medical advancement, as a means of extending the powers of biomedicine, and of the state, further into domestic and community settings. While this was certainly not the aim or approach of the one-to-one midwives in this study, the aims and intentions of practitioners are not uniform and are not equivalent to the aims or effects of public policy.

The policy of community care in the UK is now widespread, and despite negative recent public reactions, is widely accepted by professionals. I have suggested that this consensus is one which masks quite deep-seated differences of understanding and philosophy. It is also one in which the concept of community employed in policy remains vague and largely unstated. In policy terms, it is increasingly allied with the trend towards consumerism as a model for public services, grounded on our popular economic understanding of the market-place. The complexities and the difficulties of viewing service users as consumers are glossed over in policy but they emerge as conflicts in local practice. The case of maternity services is one in which the service users can most easily view themselves as consumers, even though in practice the choices they make are constrained by lack of knowledge and lack of access, as individuals, to decision-making processes. The findings of this study suggest that the issues of choice and control are far from clear-cut, even with the introduction of the new caseload model, with its emphasis on the relationship between midwife and woman and her family. The response to those findings, so far, indicate further, that the concept of choice remains limited to those choices which are acceptable to an existing set of interests. The conclusions of research, like the views of women, are likely to be ignored if the issues they raise are uncomfortable ones.

NOTES

1 Maternity service user groups have been vocal and well organized. There has been a tendency among some professionals to dismiss their views on the basis that they are mainly middle class and therefore unable to represent what most women want. Such arguments have also been levelled against other service user groups but were not backed up by our research (see also Green *et al.* 1988).

2 Active management is where technological or pharmacological intervention is employed to ensure labour conforms to statistically defined norms, primarily regarding time (see also Pizzini 1992).

3 Who, as I have noted, still work in the UK. However, in urban areas in particular, where the larger teaching hospitals are concentrated, their roles had become increasingly restricted, and largely confined to antenatal and post-natal checks, rather than birth care.

4 Women who booked for care after twenty-eight weeks of pregnancy, or who moved into or out of the local area or gave birth before twenty-eight weeks of pregnancy, were excluded.

5 Although it may seem reasonable to conclude that such lack of change reflects basic medical need, the rates of operative and assisted births vary widely in different health settings without bearing any relationship to outcomes for mothers and babies. Rates vary widely in different UK hospitals as well as between different countries which have well-funded and developed health care systems (Jordan 1993; Audit Commission 1997).

6 I have argued that shorter hospital stay after birth was an existing trend, but in this model it was accompanied by a higher degree of social support at home than is usual in health services where strong community midwifery has not been maintained.

7   Pankhurst has noted, in a study of a similar scheme, that women were distressed by the experience of presenting themselves to the hospital as a 'false alarm' or not in established labour. The feeling that they had failed to judge the appropriate point of entry to hospital for the event of birth undermined their confidence (Pankhurst 1997).

8   This is, inevitably, a stereotyped view, since individual doctors may in practice be equally or more caring and supportive than individual midwives. The midwives were generalizing to a type which represented the majority of those with whom they worked. The stereotype also involved gendered assumptions about caring roles in which female doctors are classified as part of a male group rather than identified in common with midwives who fulfil a female-type role.

9   Although these midwives were able to reduce significantly some important interventions, such as use of episiotomies, the overall rate of medical intervention in birth remained high for the UK.

10 I use the word advisedly here as representing a gender role rather than individual obstetricians who may, of course, be female. Similarly, although there are a few male midwives, they are seen as exceptional in terms of the gender role of midwifery.

11 Women's own comments and observations of professionals on the delivery suite revealed that midwives use a range of behavioural ploys to avoid medical contact with women at certain points. As suggested above, these can be a subtle means of maintaining, or appearing to maintain, existing hierarchies and protocols, in order to exercise independent clinical judgements and facilitate women's choices.

12 For a related discussion, see Gottleib (1995) and responses to this.

13 Women were able to choose methods of pain relief but women receiving one-to-one care were significantly less likely to use epidural anaesthesia and more likely to use no pain relief.

14 The primary sector of health care is run by general practitioners and associated paraprofessionals who are normally based in community health facilities such as clinics or surgeries. Primary health care providers act as gatekeepers to secondary services, which are hospital based and usually managed by medical specialists.

15 Some routine use of episiotomy remains, since different institutions vary greatly in their use of this practice. Midwives in the one-to-one scheme were able to reduce the rate of episiotomy from 30 per cent to 19 per cent of all births, without increasing the rate of tears experienced by women. There has been little exploration in the research on episiotomy of whether or how far it has a ritual role. By ritual I do not imply an empty or meaningless act, as is common in popular English usage, but an activity loaded with symbolic meaning (Jordan 1992).

16 Clear examples of this philosophy are provided by the foetal rights movement in the US, the model of the foetus as a parasite recently developed by a professor of obstetrics at this NHS Trust (N. Fisk, interviewed for BBC television) and the spate of court-ordered caesarean sections in the UK during the 1990s.

17 Cost improvement is a euphemistic term for the annual 3 per cent saving required of health service managers, which they are expected to make through increased efficiency, thus avoiding 'cuts' to the service. In practice, such savings are usually made through reduction of staff grades or numbers, and are overwhelmingly applied to the less powerful professional groups.

18 The change in language used here – from *labour ward* to *delivery suite* – reflects the changing discourse of maternity care, which emphasizes the passivity of women and their dependence on technological assistance.

19 For an interesting discussion of the situation of the loss of African-American midwifery traditions in the US, where midwifery was effectively outlawed in the historical period I have covered, see Fraser (1995).

20 Again, my argument here is about groups. A minority of obstetricians were more

actively supportive of these changes and advocated changes in the training and socialization of medical students through placement with midwives in the community.

BIBLIOGRAPHY

Alasewski, A. (1986) *Institutional Care and the Mentally Handicapped*, London: Croom Helm.

Allison, J. (1996) *Delivered at Home*, London: RCM Press.

Arney, W. (1982) *Power and the Profession of Obstetrics*, Chicago: University of Chicago Press.

Audit Commission (1997) *First Class Delivery: Improving Maternity Services in England and Wales*, London: HMSO.

Campbell, R. and Macfarlane, A. (1994) *Where to Be Born*, Oxford: National Perinatal Epidemiology Unit.

Carolli, G., Belizan, J. and Stamp, G. (1997) 'Episiotomy policies in vaginal births', in M. K. Enkin, M. Renfrew and J. Neilson (1995) *Cochrane Collaboration Pregnancy and Childbirth Database*, Oxford: Update Software.

Davis-Floyd, R. (1994) 'The ritual of hospital birth in America', in J. Spradley and D. McCurdey (eds) *Conformity and Conflict. Readings in Cultural Anthropology*, New York: HarperCollins.

DoH [Department of Health] (1980) *Second Report from the Social Services Committee, Perinatal and Neonatal Mortality (the Short Report)*, London: HMSO.

—— (1990) *National Health Service and Community Care Act*, London: HMSO.

—— (1993) *Changing Childbirth, Report of the Expert Maternity Group*, London: HMSO.

Foucault, M. (1973) *The Birth of the Clinic: an Archeology of Medical Perception*, London: Tavistock.

—— (1979) *Discipline and Punish: the Birth of the Prison*, Harmondsworth: Penguin.

Frankenberg, R. (1992) '"Your time or mine": temporal contradictions of biomedical practice', in R. Frankenberg (ed.) *Time, Health and Medicine*, London: Sage.

Fraser, G. (1995) 'Modern bodies, modern minds: midwifery and reproductive change in an African American community', in F. Ginsburg and R. Rapp (eds) *Conceiving the New World Order: The Global Politics of Reproduction*, Berkeley: University of California Press, 42–58.

Freidson, E. (1970) *Profession of Medicine: a Study of the Sociology of Applied Knowledge*, New York: Harper and Row.

Garfinkel, H. (1956) 'Conditions of successful degradation ceremonies', *American Journal of Sociology* 61: 420–4.

Gennep, A. van (1960) *The Rites of Passage*, London: Routledge and Kegan Paul.

Goffman, E. (1968a) *Asylums. Essays on the Social Situation of Mental Patients and Other Inmates*, Harmondsworth: Penguin.

—— (1968b) *Stigma. Notes on the Management of a Spoiled Identity*, Harmondsworth: Penguin.

Gottleib, A. (1995) 'The anthropologist as mother', *Anthropology Today*, June.

Green, J., Coupland, V. A. and Kitzinger, J. (1988) *Great Expectations. A Prospective Study of Women's Expectations and Experiences of Childbirth*, Cambridge: University of Cambridge Childcare and Development Group.

HoC [House of Commons] (1992) *Second Report on the Maternity Services*, (The Winterton Report), London: HMSO.

Hodnett, E. (1996) 'Support from caregivers during childbirth and continuity of caregivers during pregnancy and childbirth', in Enkin *et al. Cochrane Collaboration Pregnancy and Childbirth Database*.

Hunt, S. and Symonds, M. (1995) *The Social Meaning of Midwifery*, London: Macmillan.

Jordan, B. (1993) *Birth in Four Cultures. A Crosscultural Investigation of Childbirth in Yucatan, Holland, Sweden and the United States*, Illinois: Waveland Press.

Kirkham, M. (1989) 'Midwives and information giving in labour', in S. Robinson and A. M. Thomson, *Midwives, Research and Childbirth*, vol. 1, London: Chapman and Hall.

Kitzinger, S. (1989) 'Childbirth and society' in I. E. Chalmers and M. Keirse (eds) *Effective Care in Pregnancy and Childbirth*, Oxford: Oxford University Press.

—— (1993) *Ourselves as Mothers*, London: Bantam.

Leap, N. (1993) *The Midwife's Tale: An Oral History from Handy Women to Professional Midwife*, London: Scarlett Press.

Maslow, A. H. (1954) *Motivation and Personality*, New York: Harper and Row.

McCourt, C. and Page, L. (1996) *Report on the Evaluation of One-to-One Midwifery*, London: Centre for Midwifery Practice, Thames Valley University.

McCourt-Perring, C. (1993) *The Experience of Psychiatric Hospital Closure: An Anthropological Study*, Aldershot: Avebury.

McKeown, T. (1979) *The Role of Medicine: Dream, Mirage or Nemesis?*, Oxford: Blackwell.

Methven, E. (1989) 'Recording an obstetric history or relating to pregnant women? A study of the antenatal booking interview', in S. Robson and A. M. Thomson (eds) *Midwives, Research and Childbirth*, vol. 1, London: Chapman and Hall.

Ministry of Health (1970) *Domiciliary Midwifery and Maternity Bed Needs: The Report of the Standing Maternity and Midwifery Advisory Committee*, (the Peel Report), London: HMSO.

Oakley, A. (1980) *Women Confined. Towards a Sociology of Childbirth*, Oxford: Martin Robertson.

—— (1992) *Social Support and Motherhood*, Oxford: Blackwell.

—— (1993) 'Obstetric ultrasound as a case study in learning from history', in A. Oakley, *Essays on Women, Medicine and Health*, Edinburgh: Edinburgh University Press.

Pankhurst, F. (1997) *Caseload Midwifery: an Evaluation of a Pilot Scheme*, Brighton: University of Brighton, Centre for Nursing and Midwifery Research.

Parsons, T. (1951) *The Social System*, New York: Free Press.

Pizzini, F. (1992) 'Women's time, institutional time', in R. Frankenberg (ed.) *Time, Health and Medicine*, London: Sage.

Royal College of Gynaecologists (1994) *The Future of the Maternity Services*, London: RCOG.

Savage, W. (1986) *A Savage Inquiry: Who Controls Childbirth?*, London: Virago.

Tew, M. (1986) 'The practices of birth attendants and the safety of birth', *Midwifery* 2, 1: 3–10.

—— (1990) *Safer Childbirth? A Critical History of Maternity Care*, London: Chapman and Hall.

Thomas, H. (1992) 'Time and the cervix', in R. Frankenberg (ed.) *Time, Health and Medicine*, London: Sage.

Chapter 4

The child welfare debate in Portugal: a case study of a children's home

Karen Aarre

INTRODUCTION

The idea of a state-run welfare system is still new in Portugal, but legislation is changing fast. The concept of state responsibility for citizens and citizen rights has only developed since the end of the Salazar regime (1974). Portugal has been described as a 'welfare society' (Santos 1993) rather than a 'welfare state'. Briefly, this refers to a welfare system which is heavily reliant on the family and private institutions and organizations. The Portuguese 'welfare society' did not develop in response to a planned policy such as a notion of 'community care', but is rather an informal system which has continued to work alongside and in conjunction with the welfare policies of the democratic state. The question which will be addressed towards the end of this article is whether or not the Portuguese 'welfare society' is a form of modern sociability, altruism, reciprocity and face-to-face solidarity, or is in fact a premodern sociability, characteristic of a badly functioning 'welfare state' creating differentiation, hierarchy and exclusion. I will argue that the Portuguese welfare system is one going through profound changes bringing about conflicts between the old and the new generations of welfare practitioners.

Drawing on material gathered during fieldwork as a volunteer in a Portuguese children's home for three months in 1995, I hope to illustrate the conceptual changes taking place in relation to the welfare system at large, and will address the attitudes towards child welfare and the idea of responsibility and rights: who is ultimately responsible for the child – the parents, the family or the state?

The focus of my study is the conflicts between the members of staff in the children's home where I worked over what the home provides, or should provide, for the children who live there. The conflict is primarily between the founders of the home and the new members of staff. The home was founded in 1948 when there was no state welfare provision for homeless or abused children, and when poor and marginalized people had to rely on charity. The founders still emphasize that they are a charitable institution (although the home now receives state funding) and believe that the home should be seen as an extended family. This idea leads them to treat the children as extensions of themselves. The new members of staff are younger and professionally trained, and believe the home should be a professional institution which looks after the children for the state, the emphasis being on the rights of the child. The model to which the staff subscribe affects the way they treat the children, how they view the Portuguese welfare system and their ideas of 'family', 'responsibility', 'charity', 'rights', 'duties' and 'the individual'.

METHODS

More in-depth anthropological studies of the Portuguese welfare system are needed. Several Portuguese sociologists and social policy analysts are looking into the changes and status of the welfare state at a macro-level, but few are working on the micro-level. In the field of child-care the result is that, while statistics on the number of children in care, the proportion of institutions receiving state funding, etc. are readily available, there is a lack of in-depth studies showing how people are affected by welfare policy and how they interpret and manipulate it. More in-depth, anthropologically informed studies of the Portuguese welfare system are needed. Participant observation provides the qualitative data needed to understand and interpret the already existing quantitative data.

In my fieldwork I found that participant observation gave me insights into the children's home I would not have obtained through a study of social policy or statistical data alone. I did, however, find such quantitative data interesting to analyse in relation to my in-depth case study. The quantitative data portrays changes in welfare policy as a uniform development, whereas anthropological research shows how these changes are interpreted and debated by the people who are affected by them. I lived in a children's home in one of Portugal's largest cities for about three months in 1995 and shared a bedroom with a member of staff. During the day I helped out with the care of the children between the ages of nought and twelve in a variety of ways, from organizing activities to helping out with their personal hygiene. I had all my meals with the staff and had opportunities to speak to them and observe their work at various times throughout the day. For ethical reasons I will use fictional names for people and places, and will refer to the home as 'the Lar' which means 'hearth', 'fireside' or 'home' in Portuguese. A residential institution is often referred to as a 'Lar'.

THE LAR

The Lar was set up in 1948 by a Baptist minister, Papa Ferreira, and his wife Mama. They had five children of their own, and started taking street children into their home. The word spread, and soon more and more children started to turn up at the Ferreiras' doorstep. Papa and Mama's policy was never to turn a child away, and soon their house became so crowded with children that they had to buy another house, with money collected through the local church and gifts from Baptist churches in Canada. Mama Carla, an unskilled woman, was employed on a voluntary basis in 1949 to help out. The Lar continued to expand and they had to move a second time to its present site. Most of the money for the buildings and for the running of the Lar came from Baptist churches in Portugal, Canada, Britain and Germany. Since 1992 the Lar has received money from the state to pay for the upkeep of eighty of the around 110 children who live there. Receiving state funding has meant that the Lar now has to take the children which the social services send them, if they have space. Apart from that, the Lar still operates as an independent, private institution. It has to comply with government regulations and must allow inspections by the social services, but the regulations are general and inspections rare, so it has a great deal of independence. In short, the Lar has grown organically since its beginning. It was never planned and set out as a large institution, but instead grew in relation to needs.

The staff

Mama died four years ago, but Papa, who is ninety-two years old, is still working. His two middle-aged daughters, Paula and Sonia, and Mama Carla act as the directors of the Lar together with Carlos, a man in his early thirties who was brought up there. Papa is still the principal director. The other employees are a mix of volunteers who have worked there for a long time, people who grew up in the Lar, and professionally trained staff. Apart from the directors, the staff to whom I will refer are Tania, a nursery school teacher in her twenties; Catherine, an English woman in her forties who originally came to the Lar as a volunteer sixteen years ago, after she had finished Bible school in England; and Brian and Ann, an English couple in their late sixties, who came out to the Lar to set up a pottery after Brian retired as a Baptist minister in England three years ago. When I inquired about how many people worked in the Lar, no-one was able to tell me, not even those responsible for the accounts and the payments of salaries. Tania explained to me that this was because they remembered who worked there as persons rather than as numbers. I had difficulty identifying who was employed and who was not, because a lot of people brought up in the Lar now work there full- or part-time, and there are a lot of volunteers who come and go intermittently. It was also difficult to find out who was responsible for which tasks as many of the staff are involved in several areas.

The children

There were about 110 children in the Lar when I was there. The staff were not able to tell me the exact number because some children had just arrived, whereas others had just left, quite apart from the problem of defining who were 'children' among the oldest ones. The ratio of girls to boys is roughly 45:65. There are 'children' of all ages, ranging from nought to thirty. As already mentioned, some of the children never leave, but stay on to work for the Lar once they are adults (I counted at least thirteen who were over eighteen years old who lived and worked in the Lar). However, most of the children leave around the age of seventeen to twenty. Most of the children come before they are nine years old. The Lar is reluctant to accept older children, because they tend to have more difficulty in adjusting. This is in conflict with their otherwise 'take all' philosophy.

The children come from a variety of backgrounds, and are sent to the Lar for a variety of reasons. Some stay there for years, others for a few months. For some the Lar is their home, whereas for others it is a temporary address while problems are being sorted out with their real families. In order to get some overview of the backgrounds of the children, I decided to make a study of their files. This turned out to be less than helpful as the files were disorganized, vital papers were missing from several of them, and most of the official papers were written in such general terms that it was difficult to understand the children's backgrounds from them. No records were kept on the children after they had entered the Lar. This corresponded with the staff's apparent lack of interest in the individual child, demonstrated by their reluctance to employ a social worker or a psychologist. Children and staff spent no time talking about the children's problems. Either the staff did not find talking to the individual child about his or her problems important or useful, hoping that the children would solve their personal traumas through religious teaching as well as through just living in the Lar, or they felt that they could only provide a minimum for a maximum number of children. There was a growing awareness among staff about the importance of getting individual counselling for the children, but it was not entirely believed in, proved by their reluctance to employ professionals to provide this service. A point I will get back to is that this might be a reflection of the Ferreira family's idea of the Lar being an extended family, and within this family discourse there is no place for professional help. None of the staff understood my reasons for wanting to know about the backgrounds of the children; for them it was of little importance. Another possible reason for the lack of faith in counselling among the older staff could have been the idea that religion already provides the necessary support for the children. This was not something I was told, however.

Whereas the children's files (where these existed) could tell me very little about the children's backgrounds, staff were better sources of information. In a sample of children I picked, certain factors were common: alcoholism, drugs, incest, violence in the family, prostitute parent, parent in jail, death of one or two parents, or abandonment by one parent. In most cases, the children were in the Lar for a variety of reasons, for example the father had abandoned the mother, who could not afford to keep the child alone.

The family model versus the institutional model

Underlying the relationships between the staff in the Lar I found that there were many conflicts which emanated from a deep-rooted disagreement about what the Lar was and what it should be. Although this conflict was not spelled out to me, nor necessarily understood or disentangled by the staff, I have interpreted it as being between two opposing models, which I shall call 'the family model' and 'the institutional model'.[1] I believe that the conflict in the Lar represents a similar debate in Portuguese society at large, concerning how to conceptualize 'the child'. This will become clearer in the final section.

'The family model' views the child as principally an 'offspring of parent' (Munday 1979). Where the parents fail the child, no-one has responsibility for the child; hence those who do choose to support such a child do so out of charity and generosity, and this support must be viewed as a gift to the child. Those who subscribe to this model are the Ferreira family and Mama Carla, as well as some of the children who have been brought up in the Lar and now work there. They see the Lar as replacing the biological family of the children, and providing a harmonious, extended social 'family' for them.

'The institutional model' focuses on the child as 'non-adult', that is as an individual per se, and not in reference to the family bond. The child who is failed by the parents is seen as a vulnerable victim for whom all members of society are responsible. The focus is on universal 'rights' and responsibilities. The new members of staff act on this model, and view the Lar as a place for the children to stay while problems are being sorted out in their families. It should deal with the problems of each child. The new members of staff view the Lar as a chaotic and unprofessionally run 'institution'.

At a more concrete level, the conflict was about whether the Lar needed to change or not, emanating to a large extent from the new staff's frustration with the continued authority of the Ferreira family and Mama Carla. The conflict was also related to power and pride: the Ferreira family and Mama Carla, who had set up the Lar originally, and who have always run it, were proud of their work and did not want newcomers criticizing or changing anything. In the following, I will give a few examples of issues creating conflict between the two models in the Lar.

Space

A study of the spatial layout of the Lar gives a good indication of the conflicting models held by the staff about what the Lar is: a family, or an institution. The most striking feature of the Lar is the difference between the staff's and the children's living spaces. The adults' living spaces are clean, decorated and given a personal touch through photos and decorative objects. The children's living spaces have no decorations, and are simple, functional and usually dirty. The children have no private spaces where they can keep their belongings and be alone. They sleep in over-crowded rooms in bunk beds with up to twenty-two children per room. The children's living quarters are divided into a boys' side and a girls' side and this segregation is very strict. This is contrary to the way boys and girls are treated in normal families. Cutileiro (1971) writes that in some poor families, brothers and sisters may share a bed until the boys are about twelve years old.

The adults, on the other hand, all have private rooms, and the Ferreira family even have their own flat. The semi-private space of the adults which the children can see, namely the adults' dining room and the administrative parts, are all dominated by objects belonging to the Ferreira family. This division between private and public space is paralleled by a distinction between 'family' and 'institution'. The Ferreiras recreate the 'family' in their own living quarters, whereas the children's living quarters resemble an 'institution'.

The children have to eat out of metal bowls and drink out of metal cups, and are not accompanied by adults during their meals. The boys and girls have separate dining rooms. The Lar does not attempt to recreate the 'family meal' in the children's dining rooms as it does in the adults' dining room, where the table is laid with china and Papa gathers his family around him at table and treats all others as if they were guests in his home.

Property

The children's lack of respect for property in the Lar was an issue of controversy among the staff. The children break their toys almost immediately after receiving them, and many of the children steal what they can get their hands on. The Ferreira family and Mama Carla interpreted this as bad behaviour and believed the only way to deal with this was not to decorate the children's living spaces, and not to have communal toys. The new members of staff interpreted the children's behaviour as natural in a place where there were so few adults and so little supervision – the behaviour was therefore seen as a rational way of coping with the 'survival of the fittest' ethos among the children. The new members of staff thought that by decorating the living spaces and creating a sitting room and a toy room for the children, they would come to respect communal property. What was particularly interesting about this conflict was that those who liked to think of the Lar as a family were also the ones who wanted to keep the Lar a materially sterile place, whereas those who supported the institution model, wanted to see the Lar changed into an attractively decorated place 'like home'.

Politics

In a political argument in the adults' dining room one evening during the election campaign, the older members of staff argued fiercely against state-provided welfare. Their main argument against it was that 'people just want more and more for nothing instead of recognizing all the things they have already been given by the Social Democrats'.

The Lar was set up during the Salazar regime as a charitable institution which received no state funding and no guidelines from the state. It was set up according to Christian ideas of charity. The centre-right Social Democratic

Party headed by Cavaco Silva, had been in government for twelve years by the time I did my fieldwork. It encouraged the continued running and building of charitable institutions by offering grants. The so-called 'IPSSs', literally private social solidarity institutions, receive funding from the government and are supposed to comply with government regulations. Since regulations are few and often ill-defined, the IPSSs exercise a lot of freedom. The Lar became an IPSS five years ago when it decided to accept funding for eighty children. Funding was given for the number of children the social services recommended that the Lar house but, as noted, regulations are vague and inspections rare, so the Lar continues to house thirty more children than recommended. Since there are fewer children's homes than needed, the social services have not criticized the Lar for exceeding the recommended limit. On the contrary, they continually refer more children there. There are also a lot of children's homes which do not receive state funding because they prefer to avoid any kind of state interference. These children's homes (and usually also the IPSSs which need to top up the government contributions) raise funds by selling handicrafts produced by the children in the homes, by selling newsletters, and through various other fund-raising activities such as flea-markets, collections in churches, and associate membership schemes. The Social Democrats (and now the Socialists) have allowed the IPSSs and the private institutions a lot of freedom because they have not been able (or willing?) to significantly expand the welfare system. (One reason for this may be the commitment on the part of Portugal to pursue fiscal austerity in line with criteria for monetary union within the European Union.) State-provided welfare and universal rights to welfare threaten charitable institutions and the way they are run today, and hence the Ferreira family and Mama Carla felt threatened by the rhetoric employed by the Socialist Party during the election campaign, which demonstrated a commitment to state-provided welfare.

Mama Carla and the girls' side

Mama Carla was until five years ago the person responsible for the care of all the girls in the Lar. Tania, who came to the Lar five years ago, believed that Mama Carla had too many responsibilities and was not able to look after the girls properly. She therefore started to get involved with the care of the girls, which created a conflict between the two women.

Tania started a project to rid the children of lice, but Mama Carla was not co-operative and not happy about the 'intrusion', so Tania had to give up. She has continued to give the little children showers when she can, and also makes sure they clean their teeth. Mama Carla does not like anyone to get involved in what she considers her domain, so the teeth-brushing case is illustrative. As Mama Carla is the one who organizes the meals and distributes the evening snack, she is the one who decides when and if the children will be able to brush their teeth in the evening. She cannot openly prevent Tania from doing this, as she recognizes that brushing teeth is a good thing, but she can assert her continual authority by manipulating the snack time and preventing the children from cleaning their teeth if the snack is late.

This conflict between Tania and Mama Carla is also apparent in the medical care of the children, where Tania has taken responsibility for making sure the children get their vaccinations. Mama Carla asserts her authority by 'forgetting' to hand her the vaccination cards. She has worked in the Lar for forty-eight years and considers it her home and the girls her own children. The interference of a new young woman therefore feels like an intrusion into her private space. Tania, on the other hand, entered the Lar five years ago as a trained nursery school teacher and sees the Lar as an institution. For her the important thing is for the children to be clean and healthy regardless of who does it, as long as it gets done properly.

Another source of tension between Tania and Mama Carla is the latter's favouritism. She has some girls whom she treats as her own children and blatantly favours. One of these at the moment is four-year-old Iris, who came to the Lar as a baby. She is the youngest of a family group of five children who were sent to the Lar because their father had died and their mother could not afford to keep them. I believe the mother still has custody over the four older children, as I know that she took one of the other daughters home for two months the previous year. Iris was covered in very bad eczema caused by negligence when she entered as a baby, when Mama Carla became her legal guardian. Since then Mama Carla has not allowed Iris to see her mother, although her brothers and sisters frequently do so. Iris sleeps in Mama Carla's room, gets special clothes, eats in the adults' dining room, gets up later than all the other children and has baths in Mama Carla's bathroom, has no lice and is always protected by Mama Carla, or by Mama Carla's other favourite, Susanna, who is eighteen years old. When Iris is allowed to join in activities with the other children, Susanna is sent to look after her. Iris seldom comes to the playroom for nursery school because she is allowed to sleep late. This favouritism makes Tania very angry, but the Ferreira family accepts it. They cannot criticize Mama Carla for creating a family for herself when the Ferreira family themselves are an exclusive family unit within the Lar.

The directors rent a house in the Algarve every summer, where they spend their holidays. Mama Carla went there for two weeks while I was in the Lar in July, and she invited Iris, Susanna and Teresa (another favourite) to go with her. Mama Carla has also been known to reject children whom she once favoured. One of these was Liliana. She was a favourite until she went home to her family for almost a year. When she came back, after her father had been murdered, Mama Carla rejected her. She also did the same to Sofia (now twelve) who came to the home as a baby, but who went back to her mother for six months a year ago. When she came back, Mama Carla had found a new favourite to replace her. It is clear that she felt rejected by the children she had treated as her own, because they went back to their biological parents. Her family life is her job, and therefore she has not developed an attitude of professional objectivity or distance. Tania, on the other hand, used to tell me that the children were better off in their natural families, and that the Lar should work towards reintegrating them into their families where possible.

From child to adult

The fact that the Ferreira family and Mama Carla treat the Lar as a family is reflected in the fact that the children are not obliged to leave at any specific age. As long as the children behave well they can stay. Filipa was eighteen years old when I was there, and she had had a baby three months before my arrival. She is one of the most outgoing and toughest looking girls, yet when I asked her when she would leave the Lar she told me that she would stay until her baby was seven or eight years old. I asked her why she would not leave now that she had got her own child, and she replied that she did not dare to be on her own, and that the world 'out there' was so dangerous that she would not know how to cope. Two 21-year-old twins, who left the Lar to do military service, returned later to work there. They were surprised by my questioning them as to why they had come back, and responded that 'this is our home – we have no other'.

The English woman, Catherine, frequently expressed anger about the fact that the children are not encouraged to leave at eighteen. They are scared to leave the Lar because it does not prepare them for adult and family life, she claims. Hence a lot of the children stay on and start working in the Lar, although a lot of them are unhappy and frustrated there. Seen in the context of Portuguese families, this is quite a normal order of things. Children will stay at home until they have saved enough money to get married and buy a house, and those who never marry may stay at home all their lives (cf. Cutileiro 1971; Pina-Cabral 1986). This begs the question of the definition of childhood: when does a child become an adult? There are two different definitions of childhood in Portugal: in the context of the Portuguese family the child becomes an adult when he or she marries, but according to Portuguese law, a person becomes independent and ceases to be a minor at the age of eighteen. The older members of staff adopt the first definition which explains why it is difficult to say how many 'children' there are.

Sex

Sex seemed to be a great taboo in the Lar. The children were not given any sex education. Filipa was the first girl to become pregnant. She came back to the Lar after a holiday in Lisbon, and announced that she had become pregnant by mistake but did not want to marry the father of the child. She was angry with the directors for not teaching her about the facts of life, but their reply was that 'we didn't tell you about sex, but also we didn't tell you to go out and have sex, so the responsibility lies with you'. The directors were very angry with her and there was a debate about whether to kick her out or let her stay. The reasons for expelling her would be to teach her responsibility – that she was now a mother and must look after her child herself. But Mama Carla decided to let her stay. I asked Catherine and Tania about whether this incident was used as an example to teach the other children in the home, but they both replied that, as usual, it was not talked about. I was interested to hear from the older children that they all thought Filipa had been stupid to get herself pregnant. Tania told me that the girls are not even taught what menstruation is, and that what they know they have learned from each other.

The issue of sex education demonstrates the conflict over the aims of the Lar between the Ferreira family and Mama Carla, and the new staff. The new staff felt strongly that the Lar should educate the children to become responsible in relation to sex. The Ferreiras and Mama Carla took the view that teaching the children about sex would corrupt their minds, and that within the concept of 'the family' it would not be appropriate to discuss such matters.

Public/private

On Sundays the children had to dress up to go to church. This is part of the public/private divide which is so apparent in the Lar. Every time we took the children out they would dress up in nicer clothes than they would wear in the Lar. This was to show the outside world that the children were well cared for by the staff. This is parallel to what Cutileiro writes of the parent-child relationship in the Alentejo (Cutileiro 1971). If a child is scruffily dressed it reflects on the mother and signifies that she does not take proper care of her children. The tours around the Lar given to visitors, such as that given to me by Papa on my first day, were focused on the parts which were new and well-equipped. The areas which the Ferreira family normally show visitors are the workshops, the playroom and the study rooms. The new staff expressed anger about the fact that the Ferreira family had originally been opposed to these building projects/renovations, but after the new staff had completed them anyway, the Ferreira family claimed the credit. Brian told me that he considered the workshops to be semi-autonomous, run separately but used by the children of the Lar.

Whereas the new staff were indifferent to the volunteers who came during the summer, the Ferreira family, and especially Papa, treated them as guests in his house. They were served desserts every day and the food was generally better. I always had to kiss Papa when I entered the dining hall, and only the Ferreira family and Mama Carla had their own places at the table. The meals were considered a family occasion and Papa would not eat until his daughters had arrived. Tania told me that she could not stand the atmosphere of the dining room, and the fact that she never wanted to turn up to meals upset the Ferreiras greatly.

I also was treated as a guest throughout my stay. No-one had thought about what my role would be when I arrived; I was just expected to get on with it, and to 'learn on the job'. The fact that the volunteers are treated in this way is linked to the Ferreiras' attitude towards charity. Just as the Lar should not have a say in what aid it receives but should accept everything with gratitude, so the volunteers are treated as gifts on the one hand, and guests on the other. The fact that I was not given a specific job from the start also reflects the 'family' way of organizing the work within the Lar. No-one has defined jobs, and people are referred to by their names rather than by their positions. Even the spaces within the Lar are not divided up into professional categories such as 'the administrative area' versus the living quarters. Although the spaces are divided up and the staff perform different tasks, there is a definite hierarchy. The Ferreira family does not recognize this but rather treats the Lar as a bounded whole, a family.

Although the Ferreira family and Mama Carla talk about the Lar as an extended family, the children themselves do not consider the staff and the other children as family. They were very concerned to tell me about their biological families, about when they were at home last, and who their siblings are within the Lar. Although many of the children live in the Lar for several years and develop the feeling that it is their home, all the children I spoke to were very aware of the fact that they were not living with their families. Symbolically, however, there are many ways in which the Lar does function as an extended family. But although it is organized in ways which are similar to those of a family, the fact remains that there are certain fundamental differences which allow the new staff to reject the 'family' concept and to complain about the Lar as a badly run institution.

THE CHILD WELFARE DEBATE IN PORTUGAL

The conflict between the 'family model' and the 'institutional model' in the Lar illustrates the conflicts in the public and the private arena as to how the child should be considered in contemporary Portugal. I propose that individuals' concepts of 'childhood' and 'the child' differ, and that this is illustrated in the discrepancy between public policy and practice. Policy makers have adopted the United Nations' language in relation to children: children are seen as *individuals* with rights to protection by the state where the family fails to provide adequate health care or moral education for the children. The focus is therefore on the physical and psychological aspects of the child. The rights to a mentally and physically 'safe' environment are the foci of these child-centred regulations.[2]

On the practical level, however, these intellectual ideas are not necessarily followed by action. An example of this is the conflict between the social services and children's homes. The social services in Portugal complain that children's homes are badly run: there is sexual abuse in several of them, and many of the homes do not provide adequate care for each individual child. The new staff in the children's homes, on the other hand, complain that the social services never check up on the children who have been referred to them, and never do their job properly in trying to solve the problems in the families. So on both sides, the people responsible for the care of the children are neither prepared or numerous enough to handle the number of cases. As a result they each blame the other for the failure to follow the new expectations and pressures by the state. The fact that the staff of the children's homes and the social services are both blaming each other is also an illustration that there is a growing and changing awareness of the needs of children, but that neither side has fully recognized its *own* responsibilities accordingly. The idea of childhood itself is being questioned and manipulated on all sides, as is the issue of responsibility.

I suggest that conceptual differences concerning the child in Portugal run parallel to a series of changes at the political level which can be simplified as follows:

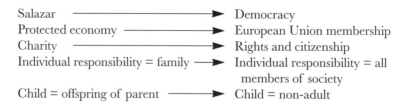

Pre-democratic Portugal **Democratic Portugal**

Salazar ————————▶ Democracy
Protected economy ————▶ European Union membership
Charity ————————▶ Rights and citizenship
Individual responsibility = family ——▶ Individual responsibility = all
                                        members of society

Child = offspring of parent ————▶ Child = non-adult

The change from the Salazar regime to democracy has challenged existing concepts of 'the individual', 'the state', 'responsibility', 'charity', 'the gift' and 'the child'. Although the change from dictatorial rule to democratic rule happened quickly, the formulation of democratic laws and regulations did not change people's values overnight. I believe that the political jargon of democracy in Portugal has preceded culturally held values, and that values are being transformed, reformulated and debated accordingly at the moment.

With the development of democratic ideals come concepts of citizenship and rights, and the equality of every individual. Once people believe that every individual has rights, particularly in relation to social welfare, every individual becomes responsible for the well-being of all others (cf. Scheper-Hughes 1987: 24). When there was no developed system of welfare in Portugal, people had to rely on the charity of others and, more often, on the charity of family rather than strangers. The family and the household was the basic unit of social solidarity and any help to others beyond this sphere was considered an act of charity. The solidarity within the family created a sense of shared substance, the idea that the family was a self-contained unit. Within this unit, roles were defined by gender and age. Social policy directed at the family has dramatically challenged these basic structures and concepts of hierarchy, rights, duties and responsibility as well as gendered and age identity. If all citizens have the right to social welfare, then each member of society is entitled to receive from others when in need. From being responsible for family members, people are now obliged to look after everyone in society. The formulation of citizens' rights dissolves the exclusive sphere of the family and includes all members of society in an 'extended family'.

During the 1980s the concept of the 'welfare society' or *Estado-Providência* was formulated to account for social practices and relations which provided a degree of social protection and welfare, but which were not provided by the state as in other European countries which had well developed 'welfare states'. In 1993, Santos described Portuguese 'welfare society' as the networks of reciprocal help which exist between people, based on the links of parenthood or neighbourliness. These small social groups exchange goods and services based on a principle of reciprocity similar to the relations of the gift studied by Mauss (Santos 1993: 46). This 'welfare society' is not an easy 'object' to study because of its many factors and informality, asserts Santos, but it is definitely a system of welfare rather than the residues of premodern sociability (Santos 1995). Instead of defining the 'welfare society', Santos opposes the characteristics of the system with those of the Portuguese 'welfare state'. He argues that whereas the 'welfare state' is absent, distant and insufficient, the 'welfare society' is informal, it is an integral part of people's relations, it is multi-dimensional and autonomous, and the logic of inter-personal action is spontaneous. Santos argues that the 'welfare society' in its old form is going through a crisis and that new forms are emerging which are more formal, more functionally differentiated and with more links to the 'welfare state' and the market. An example of this new form of 'welfare society' is the flourishing of the private institutions of social solidarity: IPSSs such as the Lar.

Whereas Santos presents a rather benign picture of the Portuguese 'welfare society', Nunes (1995) is critical of it. He asserts that whereas the 'welfare society' used to be seen by the left and the right as a premodern protection system which was destined to disappear with urbanization, modernization and the expansion of regulation by the market and by the state, now the 'welfare society' is given the new label of being a postmodern phenomenon, a response to social solidarity problems in the disorganized capitalist era and the transfer to civil society of protective functions earlier held by the state. The recent excitement about this 'welfare society' or 'community care' as it is known in Britain and in the United States, is linked with a tendency to ignore problems which studies of its virtues and limits have revealed in countries such as Portugal, argues Nunes. In Portugal, where the state has been insufficient in providing complete welfare, a large part of the functions which respond to risk and care situations are covered by solidarity networks of family and friends. Nunes argues that the 'welfare state' cannot be substituted by the 'welfare society' or vice versa, simply because they respond to different problems and needs. Relying on a 'welfare society' leads to differentiation, hierarchy and exclusion because it does not allow for solidarity between strangers. It works within the given frameworks of the family and social organization and therefore reproduces the sexual division of labour, family organization and the power structures within the family. Nunes is therefore sceptical of 'care in the community' as a response to the crisis in the welfare states of other countries. In Portugal it is not a new system of welfare, rather it is a left-over of a system developed when there were no state means of social protection. The current governments, instead of getting rid of the already developed system of a 'welfare society', co-operate with the existing structures by giving financial support to those who wish and qualify for it. This can be viewed as a cheap way of providing state welfare, or it can be seen as a conscious policy of protecting and encouraging the 'welfare society'.

Dolor Comas d'Argemir (1994) raises the issue of how to conceptualize support and care within a modern state, because although these have a material aspect they are also linked to emotion. Care is linked to love, and it is therefore difficult to locate this in the division of labour. The issue is interesting here because it raises the question of whether or not care can be public or if the two are mutually exclusive. Is care linked to love, and if so, can there be public care? How is this made possible? First, one has to ask, like Richard Titmuss (1970), 'who is my stranger?' Following Soledad Garcia, who one's stranger is in the new complex world is linked to who is included and who is excluded from citizenship:

> 'Citizens' – said Aristotle – 'are all who share in the civic life of ruling and being ruled in turn.' Since the old Greek republican experience of city democracy, the effects of two Revolutions and a declaration of human rights by the United Nations have modified considerably our conception of what a modern citizen should be. Today we think of citizenship in relation to 'national identity', 'sovereignty', 'community', 'participation', 'entitlements', and to some extent 'equality'. The common denominator of these issues is that they all refer to the experiences of 'exclusion' and 'inclusion'.
>
> (Soledad Garcia 1994: 255)

Taking into account that children cannot participate in political decision making, and are dependent on adults to provide care and make decisions for them, to what extent is the child a citizen? As long as children remain partly excluded from full citizenship, do they remain strangers? According to Titmuss, in a modern welfare system, they do not. Dependency is in fact one of the basic principles of the welfare system, upon which the system relies (Titmuss 1976: 53). The welfare systems 'reflect contemporary opinion that man is not wholly responsible for his dependency, and they all accept obligations for meeting certain dependent needs of the individual and the family'.[3]

Children under the Salazar regime had to rely on charity where the family failed them. Their identity was linked to their family; without their family children had no rights and others had no moral or legal obligation to look after them. This tight link between the family and the child is particularly well illustrated in Cutileiro's work, where the issue of honour and shame is discussed. How children act and present themselves reflects on the family – if a girl is promiscuous, her parent's honour is damaged in the eyes of others. If a child is scruffily dressed, this signifies that her mother does not take proper care of her family. The children are clearly seen as extensions of the parents, and likewise brothers and sisters, and husband and wife, are extensions of each other. Together the members of the family represent a unit with different facets which are all part of the same 'organism'. Munday's (1979) conceptual category of child as offspring of parent is indicative of the traditional Portuguese view of the child. With the development of children's rights, however, the child is seen as an individual separate from the family, and the emphasis is placed on the child as non-adult, that is, as a vulnerable *individual*. But internalizing these ideas happens gradually. This is the crux of the conflicts in the Lar: namely the differences between traditional and new ideas of 'the child'. What is debated is what separates 'the child' from 'the adult'. How should 'the child' be conceptualized – as offspring of parent, or as non-adult? Who should be responsible for the child – the parents, the family or the state? What has not been included in this discussion is the extent to which children themselves define childhood (cf. James and Prout 1990, Kessen and Siegel 1983).

CONCLUSION

Since the democratic revolution in 1974 the Portuguese welfare system has been going through profound changes. From relying on charity, Portugal, to some extent, has developed a state welfare system. This change has brought about conflicts between the old and new generations of welfare practitioners. Whereas the old generation regarded helping the underprivileged as an act of charity and generosity, the new generation typically believes in the rights of all citizens to social protection. From there being no notion of responsibility for those beyond one's immediate environment, younger professionals believe in the responsibility of all for their fellow citizens. This debate is clearly illustrated in my case study. The founding family built up the home along the lines of an extended family. Employees of the new generation prefer to view it as a professional institution. The core of this debate lies in the opposing concepts of childhood to which the two sides subscribe: those believing in the family model see the child as the offspring of its parents whose rights should be defined, granted and protected by its family; those supporting the institutional model view the child as an individual whose rights should be defined, granted and protected by the state.

The child welfare debate in Portugal shows that the welfare system is in a hybrid phase between a 'welfare society' and 'welfare state'. Though the state has adopted much of the legislation and rhetoric of a classical 'welfare state', it continues to rely heavily on charitable institutions to deliver social protection, thereby causing this internal conflict.

NOTES

1   I have also found a strikingly similar debate among staff in the Catholic children's

home where I am currently undertaking fieldwork. This home was also founded in the 1940s and grew organically in relation to need. This home has currently about the same number of children as the Lar.

2   Stephens (1995: 14) asserts that 'modern children are supposed to be segregated from the harsh realities of the adult world and to inhabit a safe, protected world of play, fantasy and innocence'.

3   Although all social welfare systems recognize and deal with dependent needs of citizens, and there are different kinds of welfare systems and thinking (cf. Esping-Andersen 1990), ultimately social welfare is a value concept (cf. Forder 1984).

BIBLIOGRAPHY

Comas d'Argemir, D. (1994) 'Gender relations and social change in Europe: on support and care' in V. Goddard, J. Llobera and C. Shore (eds) *The Anthropology of Europe*, Oxford: Berg.

Cutileiro, J. (1971) *A Portuguese Rural Society*, Oxford: Clarendon.

Esping-Anderson, G. (1990) *Three Worlds of Welfare Capitalism*, Cambridge: Polity.

Forder, A. (1984) 'Explanations of poverty', in T. Caslin, R. A. D. Forder, G. Ponton and S. Walkate (eds) *Theories of Welfare*, London: Routledge and Kegan Paul.

Garcia, S. (1994) 'The Spanish experience and its implications for a citizen's Europe', in V. Goddard, J. Llobera and C. Shore (eds) *The Anthropology of Europe*, Oxford: Berg.

James, A. and Prout, A. (eds) (1990) *Constructing and Reconstructing Childhood: Contemporary Issues in the Sociological Study of Childhood*, London: Falmer.

Kessen, F. S. and Siegel, A. W. (eds) (1983) *The Child and Other Cultural Inventions*, New York: Praeger.

Munday, E. (1979) 'When is a child a "child"? Alternative systems of classification', *Journal of the Anthropological Society of Oxford* 10, 3, 161–72.

Nunes, J. A. (1995) 'Com mal ou com bem, aos te atém: as solidariedades primárias a os limites da sociedade-providência', *Revista Crítica de Ciências Sociais* 42, 5–25.

Pina-Cabral, J. (1986) *Sons of Adam, Daughters of Eve. The Peasant Worldview of the Alto Minho*, Oxford: Clarendon.

Santos, B. de S. (1993) 'O Estado, as relações salariais e o bem-estar social na semiperiferia: o caso português', in B. de S. Santos (ed.) *Portugal: um retrato singular*, Porto: Afrontamento.

—— (1995) 'Sociedade-providência ou autoritarismo social?', *Revista Crítica de Ciências Sociais* 42: 1–7.

Scheper-Hughes, N. (ed.) (1987) *Child Survival*, Dordrecht: D. Reidel.

Stephens, S. (ed.) (1995) *Children and the Politics of Culture*, Princeton: Princeton University Press.

Titmuss, R. M. (1970) *The Gift Relationship: From Human Blood to Social Policy*, London: George Allen and Unwin.

—— (1976 [1958]) *Essays on 'the Welfare State'*, London: George Allen and Unwin.

Chapter 5

'Equal, but different'?

Welfare, gender ideology and a 'mothers' centre' in southern Germany

Lisa Hoecklin

INTRODUCTION

This chapter introduces an anthropological and gendered perspective to 'welfare' and 'community care' in Germany. I consider three levels: 1) the 'welfare state' (*Wohlfahrtsstaat*) as an ideology and a system of stratification which carries particular cultural assumptions about women's and men's identities, duties, needs and rights; 2) some of the structural consequences of those gendered assumptions; and 3) the construction of 'private initiatives' as 'communities' to negotiate and contest those consequences.

'Welfare systems' are not discrete *moral* institutions separate from and correcting for inequalities arising from a particular *rational* economic system. Like educational systems and other institutional structures, 'economic systems' and 'welfare systems' are constructed with assumptions about people's roles and relations in society. They are connected to and directly affected by other social institutions, discourses and ideas. Embedded in the structure of welfare systems, like economic systems, are assumptions about the identities, duties and needs of women and men. West Germany's welfare system is noted as a complex scheme which effectively maintains status differentials based on class and occupation.[1] In recent years some sociologists, political economists and feminist scholars have offered important insights into how gender has been neglected in mainstream welfare-state theories and have shown some of the effects of different welfare systems for women and men (Sainsbury 1994; Lewis 1993). In this chapter I will explore some of the assumptions about gender and the family embedded in West German social policy and their concrete consequences for different groups of women. I show how the division of labour between women and men in a very specific model of 'family', reflected and produced through social policy and other institutions, is connected to ideas of what needs are legitimate, who should satisfy them and where this should occur. In West Germany, religious organizations, 'private' families, and 'private' initiatives are given the roles of 'carers' and 'communities'. 'The market' and to some extent 'the state' are (and historically have been) largely regarded as opposed to 'the social', resulting in a comparatively underdeveloped service sector to meet 'social' needs (except health care).

Social policy rewards those who fit the model of 'the family' with which it is constructed, penalizes those (particularly women) who do not, and thereby attempts to standardize and justify 'normal' gender behaviour.[2]

From my fieldwork in Bavaria, I offer ethnographic insight into some of the different understandings of gendered needs and rights, and into the construction of 'communities' to respond to those needs. In West Germany in the 1980s, there was a wave of 'new social movements': environmental and peace groups, self-help projects and 'private initiatives' addressing a number of issues. There are an estimated 2,700 private initiatives in West Germany organized by and for women to meet needs relating to family life and parenting. About 410 deal specifically with the needs of women in their first years as mothers (Runge 1992). Much of the literature on such private initiatives and self-help groups discusses the importance of a *Vernetzung* (network) –

> to weave a community of individuals with similar interests to move a part of their individual every day life out of the confined space of the nuclear family into other relationships. . . . The collective self-determination of the arrangements of their living conditions is the unifying factor in these groups.
>
> (Runge and Vilmar 1988: 20f. in Runge 1992; Reyer and Müller 1992)

Below, I describe how a group of women have created a private initiative, the *Eltern/Kind* centre in Lambach to legitimate and negotiate their needs as mothers.[3]

The four women who founded the centre explained to me that it was initially conceived of as a way for women to escape the isolation brought on by the role of motherhood; a place for mothers to meet outside of private homes and to establish social contact.

The reaction to their initial attempts to establish a mothers' centre to meet the needs of mothers evoked dominant normative expectations for women in this role, and led to denial of physical space and funding. Subsequent appeals in terms of 'good Lambach families' and on behalf of children, were much more successful. This 'constructed community' meets various contested needs for different members – contact outside private households, building skills to help members re-enter the workforce, and structural support (such as initiatives for hourly child-care and lunchtime child supervision in schools). These needs are only slowly becoming legitimated in social policy. Though some of the norms and gender discourses of the centre I describe are noticeably different from what is generally observable elsewhere in the field, and different from the assumptions and norms constructed in social policy, the group continues to reconstruct the dominant ideas of gender difference. I trace historically some of the strands of these social ideas of gender difference embedded in the fabric of current social policy, as well as in the reactions for and against it.

Comparative social policy research often focuses on answering the question of whether individuals are 'commodified' or 'decommodified' in and by different systems. 'Gendering' this research tends to mean detailing the specific material outcomes of policies for different groups of women. The anthropological approach offers an additional perspective to this important 'gendering' work, by exploring the gendered ways in which ideas of 'welfare' and 'community' are constructed, understood, manipulated and contested in institutional structures originating in specific political, socio-economic and historical contexts. Furthermore, anthropological methods can highlight some of the culturally specific ways in which women experience these ideas at a personal level, and the political processes and terms in which they are able to contest or impose their own meanings. It also tries to show how these ideas are connected to other social 'truths' to show the 'logic' of a particular 'welfare system'.

METHODS

I have been conducting fieldwork in Lambach since August 1994, with the exception of a six-month stay in Oxford in 1996. I chose Lambach because it was also a location in Germany where my husband, who is German, found suitable employment. The move coincided with the birth of our first child, and our second daughter was born in Lambach in 1996. My research interests in gendered assumptions in social policy, their structural consequences, and the growth of 'mother centres', grew partially out of my situation as a new mother and many of the difficulties I encountered in that role. The non-existence of any formal child-care options and the initial difficulty of meeting people and becoming part of any social network within which to conduct research, made the *Eltern/Kind* centre the only immediately accessible group of informants. Rather than an obstacle to it, my baby became part of the research and facilitated my rapid inclusion into this 'community'. My informants include over twenty members of the centre, numerous neighbours, employees of local employment and welfare services, politicians from various parties, members of the local tennis club, as well as my husband's work colleagues and relatives. I have attended seminars, lectures and discussion groups on a range of issues (from the criminal justice system to implications of the European Monetary System to various *Frauentag* (Women's Day) events), and participated in many local ceremonies and festivals. As the issues I was interested in changed over time, I did not use a standardized interview schedule, but have explored ideas of gender, child-care, socialization, national identity, European integration and social policy.

'WELFARE' AS IDEOLOGY AND AS A SYSTEM OF STRATIFICATION

The notion of a welfare system as a discrete moral institution, as a liberal panacea for the negative social consequences of capitalism, is more an ideology than reality. Many industrialized countries have constructed social welfare systems based on the core idea of social citizenship, usually taken to mean universally guaranteed social rights. Direct comparisons of 'welfare systems' assume that the ideas and categories usually regarded within 'welfare' – equality, full employment, family, needs and rights – are unproblematic and comparable in different national contexts. However, assumptions about gender, models of family, and ideas of citizenship organize and inform each nation's notions of 'social rights', as do socio-economic exigencies. The grandfather of welfare in continental Europe, Otto von Bismarck, introduced mandatory social insurance in Germany in the 1880s for particular people (those with labour market status), not primarily with the idea of equality and protection of all citizens, but essentially to appease socialist opposition after his anti-socialist laws of 1878 proved ineffective (Carr 1991: 136). This is one of many examples of welfare as *Realpolitik*, not the promise of 'equality', within a specific political, socio-economic and cultural context.

A 'welfare system' can be analysed as a system of social reproduction, representing, expressing and reproducing certain kinds of social persons with particular relations. Like the individual physical body, social (institutional) bodies are used to represent social values. Welfare systems are constructed with particular assumptions about people's appropriate roles and relations in society, and are manipulated according to (or at least accompanying a discourse of) changing economic requirements. Forms of difference and especially power differences, precisely because of their embeddedness in everyday structures and discourse appear 'natural', inevitable, and even 'god-given'. Power differences between men and women, or between different racial, ethnic or socio-economic classes, are made to appear 'natural' by virtue of the fact that they seem to unfold out of our personal daily experiences (Yanagisako and Delaney 1995). They are reproduced not because individuals are passive recipients of the definitions created by others, but because people perceive, construct meaning and strategize within their social context. As Henrietta Moore so aptly put it in relation to gender differences:

> It is not that the material world, as a form of cultural discourse, reflects the natural division of the world into women and men, but rather that cultural discourses, including the organisation of the material world, actually produce gender difference in and through their workings.
>
> (Moore 1994: 85)

I describe below some of the gendered assumptions embedded in Germany's social policy system and in the structure of the labour market, and go on to show some of the material consequences of these assumptions for different groups of women. I then give an account of how a group of women in Lambach organized themselves into a community of mothers to renegotiate some of these material conditions.

GENDERED ASPECTS OF WEST GERMANY'S SOCIAL POLICY

Recent comparative research on welfare systems offers a broad typology of the stratification different welfare 'regimes' (re)produce (Esping-Anderson 1990, 1994). Along with France, Austria and Italy, Germany is classified as a *conservative regime* characterized by status differentiation and social rights connected to status and class.[4] The other two regime-types in this typology are *liberal regimes* (examples are the United States, Canada and Australia) in which means-tested benefits dominate, and *social democratic regimes* (primarily Scandinavian) which provide many universal benefits as social rights based on citizenship and financed by taxes.

The strength and combination of two critical aspects of the German social welfare system differentiate it from most other welfare systems. First, social rights in Germany are more closely linked to employment and contribution records than in any other system, so that what you get out of it largely depends on what you paid in over a 45-year period of continuous employment. The social welfare system is also differentiated among occupational groups. It is the prototype of a system connecting social provision and security with social status. It is 'a system powerfully dedicated to income maintenance for those who have "earned" it' (Esping-Anderson 1990: 224; Schiewe 1994). Policy is based on maintaining existing status – especially for the haves. 'Capital and labor, civil servants, white or blue collar workers as well as men and women are perceived as having distinct status and complex schemes have been developed which provide for these different statuses to be treated differently' (Ostner 1994: 135). Social rights are differentiated by one's social status and thereby the system both justifies and reproduces the status differentials on which it is based.

A second important organizing aspect of assumptions about the gendered order and family/state relations is that Germany's system is based on the principle of subsidiarity: treating women and social services (except health care) as belonging to the domain of the family. There are two sides to this. First, social security focuses on male heads of household and grants derived benefits to wives and widows. Second, the system requires that those closest to the need in question, the family or the community, in most cases have to be the first providers of help. Only when this capacity is exhausted and/or in need of support will the state intervene. I have been told that the first question you are asked when you apply for welfare is, 'Don't you have any family?' Any intervention on the part of those less close to the person with the problem has to be justified.

Some of the origins of the Catholic principle of subsidiarity in German social policy have been traced to the Weimar Republic, during which the powerful Catholic Centre Party stressed Catholic social ideas and focused on relations between institutions and on related individuals in their family roles, rather than on separate individuals (Kaufman 1989 in Ostner 1994). Later, Adenauer's reconstruction government, especially the first Minister of the Family – the militant Catholic Franz-Josef Würmeling – treated the family, with its differential roles and statuses as the foundation and model for the wider society (Moeller 1989). The *Hausfrauenehe* (housewife family model) with women as dependents became the Cinderella of German social policy (Moeller 1989). Instead of class, the family became the object of social policy in postwar West Germany. It was regarded as an intimate, inviolable sphere which promised protection, security, and organized self-help and survival in the face of the collapse of other sources of constituted authority. Single and working women, children and non-marital relationships were ignored (Borneman 1992). Families without a male earner were (and still are) commonly referred to as 'incomplete' or 'half' families (Janicke 1994). This was at a time when nearly one-third of the slightly more than fifteen million households in West Germany were headed by divorced women or widows. Defined as temporary aberrations created by World War II, the problems of groups which did not fit policy makers' conceptualization of 'the normal family' were addressed only by short-term solutions (Borneman 1992).

Women and men are assumed to have different 'natural' roles in society which combine in the *Hausfrauenehe* to ensure the social and economic reproduction of the family and society. Rather than abolish such 'natural' dependencies, family policy should support women to live out their female potential, that is, to live a different but comparable life with different obligations and occupations (Ostner 1994: 132).

SOME CONSEQUENCES OF THE ASSUMPTIONS IN SOCIAL POLICY

Assumptions in West Germany about a 'natural' gendered division of labour within a private, self-maintaining family unit have led to policies which define the identities, duties, social rights and spatial location of women first in terms of their roles as wives and mothers. Policies discourage labour participation of married women and mothers. High social transfers (for example, generous local and state payments for the birth and maintenance of each child) encourage women with children to stay at home; there is high taxation on a second family income; and little to no public provision of social services (especially child and elderly care), which are seen as 'private' family responsibilities . Relative to other European countries, Germany offers the most generous benefits for women to remain at home after childbirth (Commission of the European Communities 1994), the highest taxation on a second income, and the lowest percentage of children three years of age and younger in formal day care in the European Community or North America (3 per cent, compared with 50 per cent in Sweden and Denmark, 40 per cent in the US, 30 per cent in France and 5 per cent in Italy) (Zimmerman in Esping-Anderson 1994; Kahn and Kamerman 1985).

Comparatively few options for child-care

Social policy assumptions in West Germany, locating child-care within the domain of the family and specifically as the duty of the biological mother, translate into almost no public options for care outside the family for children under three years of age. While structural conditions between East and West Germany are slowly converging since reunification in 1990, there are still some significant differences for women left over from the previous system. State-run child-care for children under three covered 2.7 per cent of all children in West Germany in 1995, compared with 68.9 per cent of all children in East Germany (Bundesfamilienministerium in Focus 1996). The fact that 40.6 per cent of married women with children under three in Germany were in formal employment in 1992, and 55.5 per cent of single women with children, testifies to the reliance on other 'private' child-care solutions. In 1994 there were 3,500 places in Bavaria for under threes in a state with a population of 11.8 million and these places exist almost exclusively in the largest cities (Statistische Jahrbuch Deutschland 1994). For children three to six years of age, 77.3 per cent were in kindergarten in the West and 97.3 per cent in the East. Kindergartens start accepting children when they are three years old, however there is a shortage of kindergarten places numbering in the hundreds of thousands. In many areas a child will not get a place until he or she is four or five. In 1995, 63.2 per cent of school-aged children in East Germany were in an organized after-school programme, while only 5 per cent of West German children were in such care (Bundesfamilienministerium in Focus 1996).

The child-care programmes that do exist in West Germany, like all social services, are either public or voluntary (primarily religious). According to one OECD report on child-care, there are no proprietary, for-profit child-care facilities in Germany (Kahn and Kamerman 1985). According to policy makers (Bayerisches Staatsministerium für Arbeit und Sozialordnung, Familie, Frauen und Gesundheit 1994), surveys of many West German parents (Reyer and Müller 1992; Pfau-Effinger 1993), and to my informants, there is a mistrust of for-profit organizations providing 'care' functions. This aversion to satisfaction of 'private' needs by for-profit professionals is often clear in arguments against various demands for state provision of child-care. For example, arguing against making child-minding a certified and government regulated profession, the CDU German Minister for the Family said that this would give 'caring' the character of being transportable from family to family (Focus 1996: 85). Parents' aversion to such care may be changing, though. I recently read a report about a 'children's hotel' opening in another city in Bavaria that will offer hourly or overnight care for children over five years of age. Two female teachers came up with the idea and will run the 'hotel' themselves.

Other structural factors mitigate against formal employment of women with children. There are few multi-generational households – 83 per cent of all households in Germany have three or fewer members, 66 per cent have two or fewer (Statistische Jahrbuch Deutschland 1994). Small family size, the lack of regulation of private child-minders, and the social norm that the biological mother cares for a child at home until the age of three add to the difficulties.

Structure of the educational system and labour market

The assumptions embedded in the complex status- and gender-specific system of social policies are also visible in the structure of the educational system and labour market. A critical aspect of social control in reinforcing the gendered division of labour in the family, and between the family and the state is school hours. Opening hours for kindergartens vary, but are typically only from 8 am to 11:30 am, while schools tend to be in session from 7:30 to 12:30. Lunch is served in very few schools in Germany. For young children, someone must be available to pick the child up from kindergarten and make them lunch. This simple fact has enormous consequences for controlling women's activities. The German emphasis on consuming lunches prepared by the mother in the privacy of the family is connected to a preference for all 'private' needs to be met within 'private households'. According to my informants, the duty of a mother is always to be there for the child and to meet all of his/her needs (*da sein und alles tun*).

The social ideas of subsidiarity and cultural assumptions about gender and the family have also led to a particularly structured labour market. The male wage in Germany has developed as a family wage with the expectation that it supports a non-employed spouse and children. There are very high fixed costs to employers for each incremental employee, and little job mobility both because of this investment and because social contributions are based on a 45-year continuous working career. Both sides, therefore, try to minimize employment uncertainty. This is one reason for the inability of the low-wage service sector to develop, which has typically been one important way female labour has expanded in other de-industrializing countries (Sgritta 1989; Commission of the European Communities 1994). Also, measures to protect the family's privacy and non-work time create limited opening hours for shops, offices and schools, that both operate as social controls on women and prohibit a flexible, low-wage service sector to employ them. Furthermore, in that private family needs are supposed to be met privately within the family or the community, and because of tight fiscal measures, employment in social services, another immensely important female job sector, is also stagnant (Esping-Anderson 1994).

Female labour participation – low and part-time

In social policy and the labour market, women are treated as part-time and occasional workers. The rate of female workforce participation in 1992 was 40 per cent for all women over fifteen years of age in Germany – 39.2 per cent in West Germany and 43.6 per cent in East Germany (Statistische Jahrbuch Deutschland 1994: 117). Of this total, 37 per cent of women employed in West

Germany are part-time workers compared with 0.037 per cent of men in West Germany and 15 per cent of women employed in East Germany (Statistische Jahrbuch Deutschland 1994: 117). This percentage of women in part-time employment is one of the highest in the European Union behind the Scandinavian countries and Great Britain, which have much higher overall rates of female labour participation. There are few skilled part-time jobs available. In cross-national comparisons, women in Germany are exceptionally concentrated at the lower end of personal and 'junk' services relative to other industrial countries (Esping-Anderson 1990). Single and divorced mothers are more likely to be formally employed than married women with children, especially when the children are over fifteen years of age. While 40 per cent of married women with children under three years of age are in employment, 42 per cent of divorced women and 55 per cent of single women with children in this age group work outside the home. Employment for mothers of older children increases only slightly for married women, while it reaches 74 per cent and 78 per cent for single and divorced mothers of children between fifteen and eighteen years of age respectively (Statistisches Jahrbuch Deutschland 1994: 118).

Birgit Pfau-Effinger (1993) reports that in a representative survey of West German families, very few women accept the idea of both parents working full-time if dependent children are still at home (Bertram 1991; Weidacher and Bertram 1991, both quoted in Pfau-Effinger 1993). In a recent Allensbach polling survey, a sample of West German women aged twenty-one to sixty-five were asked: 'Without regard to your current living situation, in which role would you feel most satisfied as a woman?' While 35 per cent responded '*Hausfrau* and mother', 48 per cent thought they would feel most satisfied as 'mother, who on the side is occasionally or part-time employed'. '*Hausfrau* and mother' was chosen most frequently by women over sixty and women with the lowest form of secondary education. Women under thirty with higher levels of secondary education were much more likely to add part-time or occasional work to their preferred role. About 6 per cent of all women responded that they would feel most satisfied as a mother employed full-time, and 8 per cent as a full-time employed woman with no children (Allensbach 1991).

In the community of Lambach and its neighbouring villages, only 17.6 per cent of women over fifteen years of age are 'officially' employed, i.e. earning over 610 DM per month in so-called *sozialversicherungspflichtigbeschäftigte Arbeitnehmer* (in which workers are required to pay social insurance contributions) (Bayerisches Landesamt für Statistik und Datenverarbeitung 1994). In my circle of informants, I have only met or heard of two married women with children who admit to working outside the home except those who are paid for their time at the mother centre I describe below.

Women in 'hidden' and unsecured employment

The official employment rates do not present the whole picture. There is a whole category of hidden workers in the so-called '610-Mark jobs' – fewer than fifteen hours per week and earning less than 610 DM a month – who are not required to pay taxes, unemployment insurance, social security or any other social taxes. Proponents of '610-Mark jobs' argue that these are part-time, often seasonal, jobs that provide flexibility to employers and employees in an otherwise rigid and expensive labour market. Opponents argue that these jobs are generally low-paid, low-skilled jobs taken up by those most in need of social protection: women. The head of the local *Arbeitsamt* (employment office) explained that these jobs are filled primarily by women, either those without an education or married women with school-aged children who do these jobs to earn what he called 'a little pocket money'. Estimates place the number of workers employed in unsecured employment (no social payments and therefore no entitlements) at about 4.5 million, with 70.5 per cent of these being women. From 1987 to 1992, the number of these 610 DM jobs rose by an estimated 36 per cent (DGB-Bundesvorstand 1997). Many of the current social policy and labour market reforms being debated in Bonn centre around the perceived need to make the labour force more flexible and less expensive in order to remain globally competitive. This trend points toward even more 610 DM unsecured jobs. Kirsten Schiewe reports that this highly gendered construction of unsecured employment has been challenged as indirect discrimination against women under EC law on equal treatment in social security and that a few cases are pending before the European Court of Justice (Schiewe 1994: 135).

Financial and social consequences for women not conforming to the *Hausfrauenehe*

Because most women work discontinuously, often part-time and for low wages, and only for a total of about twenty years, their pensions (because they are based on earnings and continuous contribution periods) are small: for white collar workers in West Germany, 48 per cent of a man's wage and for blue collar workers, 39.3 per cent (Schiewe 1994). About 62 per cent of women pensioners received less than 500 DM per month compared to only 10 per cent of male pensioners. Benefits are closely linked to family status and in most cases, widows' pensions derived from the male income (60 per cent) are higher than those based on the number of years women spent employed. Pension differences along gender lines are greater than along occupational lines. Women's low insurance pensions are a notorious feature of the German pension system (Schiewe 1994: 145). As a consequence, mainly women in low-wage or unsecured jobs, single mothers, widows of husbands in low-paid jobs and divorced women from short marriages risk being dependent on welfare benefits (Scheiwe 1994); i.e., those not conforming to the *Hausfrauenehe*. The social status of *Sozialhilfeempfänger* (welfare recipient) is by all accounts *ganz Unten* – the very bottom of the social scale.

How do different women understand and construct their identities within these material conditions? An interesting case is the remarkable growth of 'mothers' centres' in West Germany since the 1980s. Part of what is often called the 'new social movements' of the 1980s, a wave of 'self-help groups' and 'private initiatives' have been constructed by groups of individuals with the common goal of 'self-determination of their everyday living conditions' (Runge and Vilmar 1988: 20f. in Runge 1992).

In my fieldwork with the mothers' centre in Lambach, I have been exploring the struggle over one group's claims to their needs and rights as mothers, the terms under which their claims are legitimated, the alternative norms of the centre, and how the group contests some of the normative consequences of women's identities constructed in social policy and other institutions. It is understood as a 'community' based on the social role of mother.

CREATING A MOTHERS' CENTRE IN LAMBACH

Lambach is a city with a population of about 30,000 located in Bavaria. The state of Bavaria is the largest in land mass and second most populous of sixteen German *Länder* (states). In this part of Bavaria the physical environment presents a picture of orderliness, cleanliness and beauty. The idea of establishing a mothers' centre in Lambach grew out of a research project conducted by a psychologist, Frau Carmen Singer, who moved to the area from Berlin. Divorced with two young children, she arranged funding from a not-for-profit foundation to study the situation and needs of families with children in the region. In her year-long study, she interviewed politicians, kindergarten teachers, social service officers, paediatricians and mothers to find out what kinds of social support existed for families with young children in Lambach, and what were the perceived needs.

Carmen explained to me that the gap between what local politicians and clergy thought was needed for young families, and what mothers with young children expressed a need for, was great. While most 'officials' (all men) thought there were already enough services on offer for families, in her conversations with mothers, many diverse needs were expressed. She explained some of them:

> When children don't come into kindergarten until they are four or five, that means that women have to stay home with them and this is difficult when they are alone, with no grandparents. But it was more complex than just that problem. In one area it seemed that more kindergarten places were needed, in another that there was a need for somewhere for school-aged children to go after school, in another the women felt completely isolated because at the moment they have children they said, they fell completely out of social life. They wanted to be able to meet and exchange ideas and experiences with other women.

The need for contact was especially urgent among single parents, all mothers of course, who often had no way of becoming integrated into their community, and among people who moved to Lambach from elsewhere in Germany and not only were without relatives, but had difficulty making contact with 'normal' local families.

The main themes in Singer's study were:

- oppressive isolation of many young mothers;
- increasing numbers of single mothers in very difficult living situations (financial and social);
- foreign children and their families disadvantaged and ostracized;
- increasing poverty, especially in families with many children;
- overall pessimism that anything would be done to create child-care options or allow a meeting place for mothers and children.

In the course of her work, Singer met other women whom she said she motivated to do something about the situation. There were initial disagreements among some women about whether addressing the needs of mothers was the responsibility of the state or of private initiatives. Those that were adamant that they should only put pressure on the state to construct a mother-care facility did not become involved.

About ten women actively participated in establishing the centre. I asked each member of the initial group separately to describe the responses they encountered most often in their efforts to find physical space for the centre and at subsequent phases of its development. They all responded with a similar list of responses they heard from local politicians, church leaders and various others with whom they discussed the project:

- 'There are norms for families here that a man and woman maintain.' (*Hier gibt es Normen der Familien, an die Mann und Frau sich halten.*)
- 'Who makes offers, awakens needs.' (*Wer Angebote macht, weckt Bedürfnisse.*)
- 'It is best for children under three years old to be cared for in the family.' (*Kinder unter drei Jahren sind am besten in der Familie aufgehoben.*)
- 'Private initiatives don't work. We just don't do that sort of thing here.' (*Initiativen funktionieren nicht. Sowas tut man hier nicht.*)
- 'There is no need for such an initiative. This is an idea for larger cities, it would not take hold here.' (*Es gibt keinen Bedarf für solche Initiative. Das ist eine städische Idee, die hier nicht Fuss fassen wird.*)

One member of the group told me that when she described the centre as a *Treffpunkt* (meeting place) for mothers to members of the city council, the typical response was 'why do you need that? When my wife meets other women she just goes to their home for coffee'. It was perceived as a *Kaffeeklatch* (a group of women gossiping over coffee). The attitude was 'why can't you just meet your friends elsewhere, *privately*?' One 32-year-old woman explained, 'these men thought that we should all just do our job and stay at home with our small children, crouched within our own four walls, and be happy that we were provided for financially by our men'. Two women who were single mothers 'not in particularly good financial circumstances and without a husband to support us', reported that the city council's attitude, that they were a group of wealthy women wanting to 'dump' their children, was especially infuriating. In a review of the written statements of purpose used to access funding over the first two years of the centre's existence, the messages no longer stressed the idea of a meeting place for mothers, but became increasingly focused on providing space for children and 'good Lambach families', as a place for learning parenting skills, and to further the community life of families.

Current location, membership, leadership structure and services of the centre

It took many meetings and a well-executed media campaign for the group to succeed in gaining access to physical space for a mothers' centre. They negotiated a five-year, rent-free contract with the Lambach city council for a 100m² room in the ground floor of an old block of low-income flats on the other side of the train tracks from the city centre. The deal was conditional on *Eltern/Kind* renovating the space at their own costs.

The space was completely unusable in its original condition. It took the group one year of enlisting help from other private initiatives and local clubs who, once persuaded that this was a useful project for 'good Lambach families', agreed to send members to work on weekends and evenings to renovate the rooms completely. Currently, the space is divided into two equal size rooms connected by a small kitchen in one throughway, and a small hallway with a bathroom in the other. One room has two small tables with children's chairs which are used for arts and crafts activities or for snack time. There is a corner with a sofa, adult-size chairs and a coffee table, which is used for *Eltern Runde* (round-table discussions) on Tuesday and Thursday mornings. Any parent can bring a topic for discussion. There is also a desk with a filing cupboard in the hallway across from the bathroom where a *Dienstmutter* (a mother who is 'on duty' that day) takes money for open sessions where anyone can come and pay 2.50 DM per hour (about £1).

The organizational structure of the centre consists of a three-person *Vorstand* (executive committee) and a four-person subcommittee which shares the workload. In the past year, it has become evident that with the national and state budget cuts, the Bavarian funding for mothers' centres will disappear by 1999. In response, *Eltern/Kind* went through a six-month process of trying to develop a consensus among all members for the direction the centre should take. The *Vorstand* group explained the financial situation in detail to all members who chose to attend three separate meetings, asking for input, ideas and comments.

Since then, the twenty-five members who decided to take a more active role have formed themselves into six additional subcommittees to look at alternative funding sources.

Total membership of the centre is 150, with approximately one-third single and divorced parents (this is an estimate, as there are no written classifications into single, married or divorced members). Other than differences in marital status and class, the membership is quite homogeneous. All regular members are white, twenty-five to thirty-eight years of age, with one to three children, and German citizens (except two Americans and one English woman). There was one Turkish woman who lived in the rent-subsidized block of flats where *Eltern/Kind* is located, and who attended the centre regularly when I first joined in 1994. However, the building was vacated in 1995 to prepare for renovations, and she did not come back. All of my informants from the centre have been either members of the Green political party or the Social Democratic party.

Over the past seven years, the group has succeeded in introducing some activities that they initially thought would be impossible due to resistance by the city council. Two qualified child-care specialists (*Erzieherinnen*) are on duty during opening hours. They offer hourly child-care two mornings and one afternoon per week for children over two years of age. To date, the child-care has not been intended to enable mothers to take a part-time job, but simply to run errands on their own or to have a break from their children. The group is currently attempting to expand its child-care facilities to enable certain women to go into part-time employment. Plans include arranging lunch-time child-care at local primary schools and creating a child-care facility operating from 8 am to 3 pm with ten places for children aged two and over. Both these projects are described as primarily enabling single mothers to earn an income and thereby not to be forced to deal with the humiliation at different welfare agencies. The leaders of the group are already planning how they will sell the idea of care for children under three to local officials who have to give approval. There is, however, already some opposition within the group to offering more than occasional hourly care for children under three, as it goes against norms that children this young should be cared for at home by the mother.

Eltern/Kind also offers its members financial compensation for some work in the centre. Every morning and afternoon session there are two mothers who are on duty to open the centre, assist the child-care specialists, set up for snack time, take money, and clean at the end of a session. Currently, they receive 10 DM an hour (£4), but it has ranged over the years from 6 to 12 DM depending on the annual funding. Forty mothers (no fathers) participate in this work.

For the university-educated, middle-class, non-Lambach women who founded the mothers' centre and who are still active in the executive committee, it is partly a socially acceptable professional project, a domain where they can exercise their professional skills while constantly being with their children and earning a small income during their period of active mothering. Without their skills, knowledge, combined networks, and 'outsider status', establishing the centre would most likely not have been possible. In addition, two of the founding members were single parents who reported having had great difficulty becoming integrated into any social network. For them and other women not in a 'normal' family situation *Eltern/Kind* was and is a way of constructing a 'community' for themselves. Other individuals involved in the centre have other interests. For some mothers, it is a place to receive advice on accessing social benefits and returning to employment, or where they can earn a small honorarium for their duties at the centre and socialize with other mothers.

ALTERNATIVE NORMS OF THE CENTRE

There are a number of ways in which the centre has developed some alternative norms for mothers, and, more generally, alternatives to normative concepts of hierarchy, order and specialism. This is evident in what members say the centre is, and to a large extent the group's behavioural norms are confirmed in my observations.

Informal, non-hierarchical and flexible

The centre is informal and non-hierarchical. People immediately use the informal *Du* instead of the usually obligatory and formal *Sie*. There is a policy that anyone can contribute their particular skills and ideas, or develop them according to their interests. Recently, a group of mothers met to discuss how the new fundraising groups should present themselves to the other members and request volunteers to assist. All six women present stressed that this had to be done in a non-hierarchical manner, with everyone feeling on the same level and operating as teams. One 36-year-old mother of two commented that people are more creative and things work better when everyone is on the same level. The leaders of the groups, another 28-year-old woman said, should be referred to as *Ansprechspartnerinnen* (contact persons), not as leaders. The group worked by consensus to decide which issues to address during the meeting and how they should be presented.

This is contrary to the highly specific training required for almost every job in Germany, which generally makes one an 'authority' in that particular task. For example, in the extensive apprenticeship system in Germany, over 400 specific courses are offered teaching how to sell clothes, bake bread, work a cash register, wait tables and so on. One can move from the status of *Lehrling* (learner) to that of *Meister* (master) in any particular trade. Furthermore, the flexibility of the centre, such as reacting to members' needs by creating a mix of offerings (childcare, play groups, courses and advice) reportedly created discomfort, distrust and misunderstandings for local officials. Several members of *Eltern/Kind* have explained to me that they have a hard time describing the centre to people without others becoming confused. One 30-year-old told me that she is often asked, 'well is it a kindergarten or not?' There are generally clear rules for specifically labelled things.

A community of families

Another conception of the initiators of the centre is that it should be an accessible source of information and advice for 'alternative families', i.e. single and divorced parents and their children. In addition to providing information and advice, they offer to accompany a single parent to the various agencies and offices to help them apply for assistance. Not only are government agencies notoriously segmented and hierarchical, according to a wide range of informants, but they also have a widespread reputation for being intolerant of 'abnormal' families. Obtaining information and assistance is therefore usually a difficult and intimidating process. This is widely reported in the press and confirmed by my own contact with various social agencies. This centre is intended to create a 'community of families' where even these 'abnormal' families can gain contact and assistance. Several single and divorced women I have spoken with describe how difficult, if not impossible, it is for them to make contact with 'normal families'. Through the centre, though, I have observed that single, divorced and 'normal' families undertake a number of activities together outside the centre. Summer picnics, Christmas parties, celebrations of local holidays, and children's birthday parties are organized at various members' homes with a mix of people from different social classes and from different family situations. The emphasis, they say, should be on creating a 'family friendly community' in what is generally perceived to be a 'child unfriendly' society.

CONSTRUCTING IDENTITIES AS MOTHERS

Members of the mothers' centre seem to be primarily involved in negotiating the immediate structural consequences of norms for mothers (isolation, physical confinement to private homes, the unacceptability of having personal needs or employment while children are young, and poverty for many mothers not in 'normal' families). None of the members seem concerned with a radical political resistance to ideas of the gender division of labour or to norms for children's upbringing. Generally, the role of mother is recognized as a serious, difficult, and important if frustrating job/profession (*Beruf*), to be taken with pride. There are frequent discussions at *Eltern/Kind* of the idea of *nur Hausfrau* (only a housewife) that they say they hear from childless career couples and young professionals. In response, the group builds its counter-discourse of mothers as capable and hard-working professionals. This *nur Hausfrau* idea, several women have explained to me, is part of a shift in societal values to increasing individualism, materialism and consumerism. 'Where does the Hausfrau and mother fit within this *Leistungsgesellschaft* (achievement-oriented society)?' one 34-year-old mother of two asked me.

In response, women in the centre construct an identity and 'community' against the negatively perceived values of individualism and consumerism. This includes a romanticizing of the association of motherhood and nature. An illustrative example is another key goal of the centre: being and teaching children to be *umweltbewusst* (environmentally conscious or aware). One group of five women I discussed this with described this idea as having two aspects: 1) teaching/inspiring a respect for and harmonization with nature, and 2) practising an environmentally conscious way of living. There are regular activities where children (usually aged between one and four years) 'experience' nature. For example, one morning one of the teachers brought in a large pumpkin. The children were each encouraged first to touch it all over with their hands, to smell it, and to tap on the outside to see what it sounded like. Then, the teacher cut it open and had the children look inside and describe what they saw, to take the seeds out with their hands, to rub them, taste them and smell them. When they had 'experienced' the pumpkin, they baked the seeds and ate them. Similar activities are developed every day, for example planting and picking herbs in the garden, or in games where the children imitate the sound of rain and thunder by pounding on the floor. The other aspect of this environmental awareness is apparent in many aspects of the centre. For example, everything that can be is recycled, and many of the members ride their bicycles or take buses to the centre regularly instead of driving. While some do not own cars because they cannot afford them, many do not use their cars when they can use other forms of transportation for 'environmental' reasons. One 29-year-old woman, who cycles to the centre pulling her two sons (aged two and four) behind her in an attached wagon, told me that she rarely uses her car because of the damage it does to the environment, and because she feels much freer on a bike than in a car. The 42-year-old psychologist who initiated the idea for the centre explained that in her view, 'learning the cycles and rhythms of nature is so vital because we (humans) are part of it. With the culture of consumption and individualism,' she added, 'people have lost their connection with nature. This disconnectedness from nature leads to illness and disease.'

I recently saw a documentary about a newly built 'environmental kindergarten' called 'Noah's Ark' in Bavaria, built for sixty-nine children at the cost of 2.5 million DM. This project is to serve as a model and pilot programme for 'environmental education'. In an interview with the mayor of the town, he said that the importance of this project is to teach the children an understanding of the environment, which is necessary to work against increasing materialism and mechanization in our industrial age. Dismayed, he said, 'we are living in an age where children can name more makes of cars than they can animals'. Many aspects of the kindergarten and the examples of games and projects shown, were very similar to what I have observed at the *Eltern/Kind* centre.

The opposition of 'the family' and mothers' role within it to materialism, industrialization and individualism has a long history in Germany. Louis Dumont (1994) argues that the 'idiosyncratic' formula of German ideology, 'community holism plus self-cultivating individualism' (*Bildung*), is widely encountered in German authors from the eighteenth century (Dumont 1994: 42). Far from being incompatible, Dumont says, the ideology actually works in the way that the individual develops through his/her service in and for the whole. Through industrialization, many German writers of the nineteenth and twentieth centuries characterized Germany as a *Kultur* (cultural) nation against 'that thing of the west' which was characterized as *Zivilisation* (civilization). 'Civilization' was material progress, common to all and international, while Germany was the repository of spiritual values, of *Kultur*, which was peculiar to her (Mann in Dumont 1994: 57).

I take up the more recent versions of this discourse in the next sections. The points I would like to leave the ethnographic material with, however, are two important ideas being reconstructed in the *Eltern/Kind* centre: 1) of this level of 'community', and of motherhood, as closer to nature and as healthier than higher levels of society, which are negatively regarded; and 2) the idea that the job of 'mother' is regarded as a different, but equal profession which deserves social recognition. These are ideas that are embedded in broader German social policy, other institutional structures and material conditions in Germany.

HISTORICAL AND CURRENT IDEAS OF GENDER DIFFERENCE

The construction of gender difference in terms of different, but equal duties and spheres for men and women, and of the symbolic opposition of women in the roles of wives and mothers to industrialization, materialism and individualism has been a continual historical process. These social ideas can be traced through nineteenth-century industrialization, early twentieth-century German feminism, the gendered division of labour and gender symbolism under National Socialism, postwar reconstruction of 'traditional morality' in West Germany, and the current discourse about the perceived economic crisis.

The work of industrialization in Germany, as elsewhere, was structured within a social context of a simultaneously developing 'feminization' of the household and increasingly segregated and detailed gender roles (Quataert 1986). Through their roles as bearers of children and guardians of the household, women as wives and mothers became a symbol of the 'traditional' order during a period of social change and mass migration (Dasey 1989). The values women symbolized within the sentimentalized family were increasingly set against the symbols of industrialization. William Paterson (1989) reports that environmental groups have existed in Germany since the late nineteenth century and that their appeal was usually based on the expression of explicitly anti-industrial values. Tönnies' late nineteenth-century articulation of the dichotomy between the 'natural' *Gemeinschaft* of the family, opposed to and threatened by the artificial *Gesellschaft*, represents the intellectual context in which industrialization in Germany proceeded. Fritz Stern, in *The Politics of Cultural Despair*, argues that there was a mood of pessimism accompanying industrialization in Germany; a search for a truly German character and resentment of everything western. The family in Germany symbolized how they were different from the west, and they wanted to be different (Stern 1974).

In Weimar Germany, the maintenance of gender difference and the theme of 'Mütterlichkeit' (motherliness) were advocated by both bourgeois and radical feminists, though there were other deep divisions between the two movements. For bourgeois feminists, 'motherliness' designated difference between women and men, and should characterize the grounds on which women should participate in public life: 'not as equals to men, but as strong individuals with distinctive qualities capable of humanising the increasingly mechanical and bureaucratic world' (Chamberlayne 1991: 208). 'Radical' feminists often used 'motherliness' in a biological sense to argue women's suitability for certain types of work. Though bitter political enemies, these groups' common ground was a shared commitment to women's roles in the family and to ideals of female duty, service and self-sacrifice. Deference to the larger community and the ideology of separate spheres for women and men were basic assumptions behind their demands (Bridenthal *et al.* 1984).

National Socialist policies focused on restoring 'traditional morality' by redefining appropriate social norms. The Weimar image of the 'new women' – who voted, used contraception, obtained legal abortions, and earned wages – was a symbol, employed by the National Socialists along with race, for the cause of all of the misery and hardship of the ensuing economic disaster. While promising to restore women to the realm where they could regain the dignity and security eroded by modern life, they linked women's safety and defence to the family and their roles of *Hausfrau* and mother within it (Koonz 1986). Nazi women of the period wrote that men and women were of equal value to society and insisted that a division between masculine and feminine activities be maintained. Images of family life linked feminine roles to a healthy, 'natural' order (Koonz 1987).

After World War II, women's status was again placed on the political agenda in the name of restoring 'traditional morality'. Healthy families were to serve as a bulwark against Communism. Policy makers in West Germany concluded that all women worked, though for the Minister of the Family, only women in Communist countries worked outside the home (Borneman 1992). Mothers were supposed to preserve and transmit to children the values that would abate the worst excesses of unbridled competition and would prevent West Germany from becoming a materialistic nation (Moeller 1989).

In explaining how West German feminism differs from 'western' feminism, Ilona Ostner reports that the former never wholeheartedly embraced *Emanzipationslogik*, egalitarian policies which promote full-time paid work for women. Feminist debates have pointed toward policies based on difference, rather than equality, advocating policies which consider unpaid care and other domestic activities as socially vital, and as a peculiar sort of work that should be publicly rewarded and compensated (Ostner 1993). She describes West German women's preference for a patchwork or zigzag life trajectory – 'they want to commute between the domestic and market worlds'. The theme of 'different but equal' can be found across the political spectrum. Chamberlayne (1991) analyses the 'Mothers' Manifesto' issued by a section of women in the Green Party in 1987. This constituency within the Greens has argued against equating emancipation for women with participation in the public domain on equal terms with men. Disenchanted with the values of competitive, individualistic, industrialized society, they advocate that mothers' qualities of sharing, intimacy and uniting body and soul, which has been all but destroyed by 'reason', must be returned to the centre of society for the sake of humanity (Stopczyck 1989: 112 in Chamberlayne 1991: 201).

In the 1990s, the issue of changing demographics (the lowest birth rate in the world and a rapidly ageing population structure) often appears in the popular press in terms of a financial and moral crisis. Who will pay social security for the millions of individualistic people who are choosing not to have children? This question is sometimes posed in terms of images of the hard-working, stable, sacrificing, 'traditional' family versus the materialistic, hedonistic and individualistic double-income couple who are only taking from society and giving nothing back (Gardiner 1993: 116; Gerbert 1993: 93; Krumrey 1995: 68–74). The difference between the two opposed images is a symbolic association of the *Hausfrauenehe* as natural, moral and positive versus two employed individuals living together without children as individualistic, selfish and threatening to the public good. The labour of the woman is the obvious difference between the two pictures. This is also vivid in the popular dichotomy *Kind oder Konsum* (child or consumption).

There is a sentimentalizing of the *Hausfrauenehe* family as the social institution creating moral and economic order and stability. The decline of this traditional value is creating 'an ego-society', 'a moral vacuum', 'a value crisis' and 'the dissolution of society' (Gerbert 1993: 203–8). Most recently, one prominent CSU (Bavarian affiliate of the Christian Democrat Union) politician published his reading of one of the major causes of the economic crisis of the *Sozialstaat*: 'the destabilisation of the family and changing values have a tremendous impact on the rising social costs . . . and on the problems of the labour market.' 'A major cause is the divorce rate,' he says, 'above all women with children who are dependent on social welfare. . . . Private problems become a task of the state' (Focus 1997).

Certainly, there are alternative discourses and responses by different groups. The point is, though, that the *Hausfrauenehe* family model, and women's duties as wives and mothers within it, have been and continue to be symbolically associated with the moral survival and well-being of society as a whole in dominant social discourse. At times of perceived social or economic crises, this rhetoric has tended to accompany and justify policy changes.

CONCLUSIONS

The 'welfare system' is connected to other institutions, ideas and discourses. It represents, justifies and reproduces broader social ideas about social persons and appropriate social relations. The identities it gives and the structural conditions it creates materially and socially penalize those not conforming to the model of the family with which policy is conceived, and their appropriate gendered roles and duties within it. 'Women' in the roles of wives and mothers within a particularly defined *Hausfrauenehe* have been assigned the duties of social reproduction and defence. They have been symbolically associated with nature, which is central to notions of individual and collective health. 'Sickness' contracted in the larger *Gesellschaft* is treated with nature. This dichotomy between the 'natural' community of the family (*Gemeinschaft*), characterized by love and morality, versus 'fictive', threatening social ties of *Gesellschaft* is very much a part of the folklore of German self-consciousness (Dahrendorf 1967). Dominant discourses of the family in West Germany have repeatedly reconstructed morality and personhood in these terms. The *Hausfrauenehe* family as the natural *Gemeinschaft* is conceived of as a place for social recovery and order, it is where one experiences being a person and being humane (*Mensch sein*) (Bundesministerium für Familie und Senioren 1994).

Twentieth-century Germany has been (re)presented internally as a battleground between 'modernity' and 'tradition' (Habermas 1984). Over time, tradition (represented by one model of 'the family' and by women as wives and mothers) has been conceived of as a unit of defence against the hostile and destructive threats of industrialization; of 'alien races' and the 'new women' of the 1920s; the communist East; and most recently against materialism, 'hedonistic individualism', 'pure capitalism' and 'the shareholder value concept' (*Der Spiegel* 1997). It is women as *Hausfrauen* and mothers who are 'humanizers' against the 'mechanization of modernity'.

'Private initiatives', such as the constructed private 'communities' of mothers' centres, can be better understood within this context. For my informants in Lambach, ideas of the separateness and opposition of private domains of family and community from public domains of state and market combine with a pessimism about changing anything 'above' from 'below'. The interaction between the two is largely regarded as undesirable. Rather than relying on partial funding from local government (commonly referred to as *Stadtväter und -mütter* – city fathers and mothers), the group is actively seeking other sources of finance to 'become independent of government control'. Women as mothers are the clients and providers of the care in their separately constructed community. While attempting to legitimate some of the needs of mothers, and to change some of the consequences of normative expectations for mothers, they also reconstruct a discourse of motherhood as 'different, but equal'. The group is trying to create some options for child-care, for example, but this is intended for single mothers so they do not have to interact with welfare agencies. The child-care is not intended for middle-class women within 'normal' families. Furthermore, the role of mother is connected to 'nature' and the environment and as defence against individualism, consumerism, illness and disease.

The gender ideology of 'different, but equal' has been manipulated and negotiated by different groups at different times for various purposes. Materially, however, it is social reproduction of gender difference, as well as class and status difference, which characterizes the German 'welfare system'. In the current economic circumstances (including the highest rate of unemployment since 1938 and the changing demographics), there are calls from all political parties for major structural reform. It will be interesting to follow the development of the gendered discourse accompanying reforms and their material outcomes for different groups, as well as the role of mothers' centres such as the one described here in these changes.

NOTES

1   Where I write 'West Germany' and 'East Germany', I am referring to the former West and East German states. I am simply omitting 'the former' for ease and clarity.
2   After World War II, East German policy makers started with different assumptions about 'normal' gender behaviour, which resulted in different consequences for women's life courses.
3   The names of individuals, the city name of Lambach and the mother centre's name of *Eltern/Kind* are pseudonyms.
4   Since reunification, West German social policies have been extended to the new Länder (former East Germany).

BIBLIOGRAPHY

Allensbach (1991) *Familie Umfrage* [Family Survey], Bonn: Allensbach.
Bayerisches Staatsministerium für Arbeit und Sozialordnung, Familie, Frauen und Gesundheit (1994) *Familienpolitik in Bayern: Berich der Bayerischen Staatsregierung* (Family Social Policy in Bavaria: Bavarian State Government), München: Bayerisches Landesamt für Arbeit und Sozialordnung, Familie, Frauen und Gesundheit.
Bayerisches Landesamt für Statistik und Datenverarbeitung (1994) *Gemeinde Daten* [Community Data], München: Bayerisches Landesamt für Statistik und Datenverarbeitung.
Borneman, J. (1992) *Belonging in the Two Berlins: Kin, State, Nation*, Cambridge: Cambridge University Press.
Bridenthal, R., Grossman, A. and Kaplan, M. (eds) (1984) *When Biology Became Destiny: Women in Weimar and Nazi Germany*, New York: Monthly Review Press.
Bundesministerium für Familie und Senioren (1994) 'Materialien zur Familienpolitik der Bundesregierung' [Family social policy resources of the federal government], Bonn: Bundesministerium für Familie und Senioren.
Carr, W. (1991) *A History of Germany 1815–1990* (4th edn), London: Arnold/Hodder Headline Group.
Chamberlayne, P. (1991) 'The "mothers' manifesto" and the concept of Mütterlichkeit', in E. Kolinsky (ed.) *The Federal Republic of Germany: The End of an Era*, Oxford: Berg Publishers Limited.
Commission of the European Communities (1994) *Social Protection in Europe 1993, Directorate-General Employment, Industrial Relations and Social Affairs*, Luxembourg: Office for Official Publications of the European Communities.
Dahrendorf, R. (1967) *Society and Democracy in Germany*, Garden City, New York: Doubleday.
Dasey, R. (1981) 'Women's work and the family: women garment workers in Berlin and

Hamburg before the First World War', in R. Evans and W. R. Lee (eds) *The German Family: Essays on the Social History of the Family in Nineteenth and Twentieth Century Germany*, London: Croom Helm.

Der Spiegel (1997) 'Das neue deutsche "Wirtschaftswunder" . . . Arbeitslose' [The new German economic miracle: unemployment], *Der Spiegel* 12.

DGB-Bundesvorstand (1997) 'Nicht auf unserem Rücken: geringfügige Beschäftigungsverhältnisse Trend zu sozial ungeschützter Arbeit auf dem Rücken der Frauen' [Not on our backs: the trend toward low-wage, unsecured employment on the backs of women], January Issue, Düsseldorf: DGB-Bundesvorstand, Abteilung Frauenpolitik.

Dumont, L. (1994) *German Ideology: From France to Germany and Back*, London: University of Chicago Press.

Esping-Anderson, G. (1990) *The Three Worlds of Welfare Capitalism*, Cambridge: Polity Press.

—— (1994) 'The continental European welfare states: labor reduction and the emerging crisis of social insurance', unpublished paper presented at July 1994 International Sociological Association meetings, Bielefeld, Germany.

Focus (1996) 'Ein täglicher Balanceakt: Der gesetzlich verankerte Rechtsanspruch auf einen Kindergartenplatz hilft Eltern nur wenig – Deutschland bleibe eine Betreuungswüste' [A daily balancing act: the legal right to a kindergarten place is little help to parents – Germany remains a child-care desert], *Focus* 38.

—— (1997) 'Standpunkt: Keiner traut sich an die Tabus heran' [Viewpoint: no one dares to talk about the taboos], *Focus* 12.

Gardiner, A. (1993) 'Die Sehnsucht nach Familie' [The longing for family], *Brigitte* 18.

Gerbert, F. (1993) 'Familie: Abschied von einem Traum' [Family: farewell from a dream], *Focus* 7.

Habermas, J. (ed.) (1984) *Observations on the Spiritual Situation of the Age: Contemporary German Perspectives*, translated by Andrew Buchwalter, Cambridge, MA: MIT Press.

Janicke, C. (1994) 'Situation Alleinerziehender im Bodenseekreis: Voraussetzungen, die Familienzentren brauchen, um ihnen Unterstützung anzubieten' [The situation of single parents in the Bodensee region: the need for family centres to offer them support], Diplom-Arbeit für die Staatliche Abschlußprüfung im Fachbereich Sozialwesen, Katholischen Fachhochschule, Köln.

Kahn, A. and Kamerman, S. (eds) (1985) *Child-care Programs in Nine Countries; A Report Prepared for the OECD Working Party on the Role of Women in the Economy*, Washington, DC: US Department of Health, Education and Welfare.

Koonz, C. (1986) *Mothers in the Fatherland: Women, the Family and Nazi Politics*, London: Jonathan Cape.

—— (1987) 'Nazi women before 1933: rebels against emancipation', *Social Science Quarterly* 23.

Krumrey, H. (1995) 'Gesellschaftskrieg: Singles contra Familien' [Societal war: singles against families], *Focus* 33: 68–74.

Lewis, J. (ed.) (1993) *Women and Social Policies in Europe: Work, Family and the State*, Aldershot: Edward Elgar.

Moeller, R. G. (1989) 'Reconstructing the family in reconstruction Germany: women and social policy in the Federal Republic, 1949–1955', *Feminist Studies* 15, 1.

Moore, H. (1994) *A Passion for Difference*, Cambridge: Polity Press.

Ostner, I. (1993) 'Slow motion: women, work and the family in Germany', in J. Lewis (ed.) *Women and Social Policies in Europe: Work, Family and the State*, Aldershot: Edward Elgar.

—— (1994) 'Independence and dependency: options and constraints for women over the life course', *Women's Studies International Forum* 17, 2/3.

Paterson, W. (1989) 'Environmental politics', in G. Smith, W. Paterson and P. Merkl (eds) *Developments in West German Politics*, London: Macmillan Education.

Pfau-Effinger, B. (1993) 'Modernisation, culture and part-time employment', *Work, Employment and Society* 7, 3: 383–410.

Quataert, J. (1986) 'Teamwork in Saxon homeweaving families in the nineteenth century: a preliminary investigation into the issue of gender work roles', in R. B. Joeres and M. J. Maynes (eds) *German Women in the Eighteenth and Nineteenth Centuries: A Social and Literary History*, Bloomington: Indiana University Press.

Reyer, J. and Müller, U. (1992) *Eltern-Kind-Gruppen: Eine neue familiale Lebensform?* [Parent-child groups: a new family living form?], Freiburg im Breisgau: Lamertus Verlag.

Runge, B. (1992) 'Frauen-Selbsthilfe und Frauen-Projekte' [Women's self-help and women's projects], in C. Faber und T. Meyer (eds) *Unterm neuen Kleid der Freiheit das Korsett der Einheit: Auswirkungen der deutschen Vereinigung für Frauen in Ost und West* [Under the New Dress of Freedom the Corset of Unity: Effects of German Reunification for Women in the East and West], Berlin: Sigma Rainer Bohn Verlag.

Sainsbury, D. (ed.) (1994) *Gendering Welfare States*, London: Sage.

Schiewe, K. (1994) 'German pension insurance, gendered times and stratification', in D. Sainsbury (ed.) *Gendering Welfare States*.

Sgritta, G. (1989) 'Towards a new paradigm: family in the welfare state crisis', in K. Boh, M. Bak, C. Clason, M. Pankratova, J. Qvortrup, G. Sgritta and K. Waerness (eds) *Changing Patterns of European Family Life: A Comparative Analysis of 14 European Countries*, New York: Routledge.

Statistische Jahrbuch Deutschland [Statistical Yearbook of Germany] (1994).

Stern, F. (1974) *The Politics of Cultural Despair: A Study in the Rise of the Germanic Ideology*, Berkeley: University of California Press.

Yanagisako, S. and Delaney, C. (1995) 'Naturalizing power', in S. Yanagisako and C. Delaney (eds) *Naturalizing Power: Essays in Feminist Cultural Analysis*, London: Routledge.

Chapter 6

The co-operation concept in a team of Swedish social workers

Applying grid and group to studies of community care

Steve Trevillion and David Green

INTRODUCTION

The influential Griffiths report defined community care in terms of enabling people 'to live normal lives in community settings' (Griffiths 1988: 3.1, 5). For those involved, like ourselves, in what has become the massive industry of community care policy and practice, it is easy to lose sight of the simple but deeply radical shift involved in supporting individuals in the community rather than seeking to remove them from it. Any system which aims to 'design and arrange the provision of care and support in line with people's needs' (Griffiths 1988: 3.4, 5) is going to be very different from one which simply seeks to slot 'problem individuals' into a range of preordained services frequently provided only within highly stigmatized institutional contexts.

While more has been written about community care than any other twentieth-century welfare policy initiative, some of its most basic features are still under-researched. In particular, although almost every kind of financial, organizational and even interpersonal feature of community care has been the subject of government sponsored research, there has been little attempt to find out what it means to those actively involved, and to society as a whole. Ten years after the publication of the Griffiths report in the UK, this chapter is an attempt to develop an anthropology of community care and thereby, reinsert the question of meaning at the centre of the community care debate.

Our subject is 'collaboration', or the process of working together with others to assess need and deliver services. We see this as important because community care is utterly dependent upon the development of new collaborative cultures in place of the old institutional ones and it is here, also, in the exploration of cultural creativity, that we think anthropology has much to offer.

To date, the problem is not that anthropology has had no influence on research into collaboration, but rather, that an unacknowledged nineteenth-century anthropology has continued to distort our perceptions of the subject. We begin, then, with a critique of the nineteenth-century assumptions underlying current approaches to collaboration and move on to develop a new framework for thinking about the meaning of community care in general and 'collaboration' in particular. This consists largely of a reinterpretation of Mary Douglas' work on 'grid and group' applied to the analysis of the shift from institutional to community care. We use this framework to illuminate an ethnographic account of the process of 'co-operation' as it was described to us by a group of Swedish *kurators* and members of their 'co-operative network' in the course of a short-term but intensive period of fieldwork in Stockholm in 1996.

COMMUNITY CARE: NINETEENTH-CENTURY MODELS AND TWENTIETH-CENTURY PRACTICES

For anyone aware of the history of anthropology, one of the most striking features of the current debate about community care is its implicit endorsement of discredited nineteenth-century ideas about the development and spread of cultural practices. Much of the debate about community care appears to revolve around a set of paradigms virtually indistinguishable from those associated with nineteenth-century 'evolutionism' and 'diffusionism'. These need to be challenged before we can begin to mark out a terrain in which anthropology can help us to understand this important development in twentieth-century social welfare policy and practice.

'Evolutionism' has been described as the desire 'to arrange the peoples and social institutions of the world in an evolutionary series, from a theoretical primordial man to the civilised human being of mid-nineteenth century Europe' (Leinhardt 1966: 8). 'Diffusionism' has generally been associated with the ideas of Clark Wissler and the *Kulturkreis* school who held that cultural artefacts of all kinds have diffused outwards from a relatively small number of innovative 'culture centres'. Although long abandoned by anthropologists these simplistic cultural models continue to exercise a strong influence on the way in which community care is represented.

Who would now defend Morgan's division of history into three stages: *savagery*, *barbarism* and *civilization*? Many years ago such ideas were condemned as 'unhistorical' and 'unscientific' (Leinhardt 1966: 12). And yet, community care is usually described simply as a reaction to and against the inefficiency and barbarism of the 'great confinement' (Foucault 1973: 38–64) of marginalized populations in 'total institutions' (Goffman 1968: 13–22), a feature of prewar social policy across Europe. For example, in a recent book on care management, the authors, while trying to locate community care within an historical context, end by declaring that it is a 'happy combination of sound economics . . . and common humanity' (Orme and Glastonbury 1993: 10).

In the UK and within the context of this kind of discourse, successful community care initiatives are frequently represented as tokens of or signposts to an idealized communitarian future (Benn 1982). In contrast, the divisive features of institutionalization are seen as distasteful relics of the past – either morally flawed (Wagner 1988) or 'unfit' to survive because they are found wanting by the Audit Commission on one or more forms of quality measurement (Audit

Commission 1992).The Audit Commission makes direct use of the concept of 'fitness' in its work and regularly declares institutions or policies 'unfit' in relation to the tests of 'efficiency' and 'effectiveness'. In recent years it has applied this approach directly to the evaluation of inter-agency arrangements particularly those intended to generate co-ordination between health and social care organizations (Audit Commission 1992: 10–12). Studies of collaboration have in this way become dominated by a neo-Darwinian paradigm.

Diffusionism, too, is alive and well in social policy, particularly in the relatively new field of comparative social policy where, all too often, ideas and policies are seen as spreading across continents or around the globe mainly as a result of their inherent superiority. This is reminiscent of the way that the *Kulturkreis* theorists saw superior cultures exporting their ideas to inferior ones.

There is a tendency to see the spread of community care practices as merely the inevitable result of the adoption of morally superior and more professionally advanced theories and concepts generated by a small number of innovative welfare cultures, most frequently Anglo-American ones. This ignores the fact that where diffusion does take place, it is often dysfunctional, testifying to the power of ideology rather than to the superiority of ideas. For example, within the UK, many of the problems of community care in the period since the passing of the NHS and Community Care Act in 1990 can be traced back to the slavish adoption of American case management models developed to solve different problems in a different context (see Griffiths 1988), while more relevant European models and experiences were largely ignored.

What these tendencies have in common is a belief in a relationship between community care and progress which is not only highly questionable in its own right but also tends to prevent us from asking many of the most interesting questions about community care. In particular, by convincing us that the spread of ideas about community care is historically inevitable, they prevent us from inquiring into the way in which community care emerges in the context of individuals and groups trying to make sense of their relationship to one another in a rapidly changing, local, national and global environment, in which 'traditional' solutions to welfare problems no longer seem to work or to be desirable. This is the context in which we should be thinking about the vexed question of collaboration.

The ways in which the collaborative ideals of the NHS and Community Care Act have failed to materialize have by now been exhaustively documented (e.g. Hudson 1992). In part, the failure to find a solution to this long-standing problem may be connected with the way in which studies of collaboration have been dominated by a specific 'narrative' of progress (Trevillion 1996a: 96). In some cases, efforts have even been made to arrange 'types' of collaboration or inter-agency partnership into an explicit evolutionary series. So it is alleged that communication is the earliest stage of a process which leads inexorably through co-operation to co-ordination and finally, at the apex of the evolutionary pyramid, to total merger (Payne 1986).

But what we now know is that there is an enormous gap between this kind of 'talk' and the ways in which individuals and groups actually go about the process of building community care networks and making sense of what they are doing. If we are interested in exploring these processes, we would do better to think in terms of cultural creativity rather than narrow cultural determinism and to make use of a very different kind of anthropology to understand both the nature of community care and the processes associated with collaboration.

THE COLLAPSE OF THE INSTITUTIONAL GRID

Welfare systems are undergoing massive levels of change and nineteenth-century anthropology cannot help us to see what is going on. Drawing on the work of Douglas and Turner on ritual boundaries, spaces and categories, and Goffman and Foucault on total institutions and disciplinary regimes, we can identify a whole range of issues which have little or nothing to do with either evolution or diffusion. One of the most obvious of these is the shift from a mode of social and cultural practice generating segregated, marginalized, medicalized and controlled living spaces (such as asylums and hospitals) to one associated with the progressive removal of the physical and symbolic boundaries separating these spaces from other, more 'normal' ones (Wagner 1988). In short, an anthropological perspective suggests that community care is, in part, concerned with what could be called 'the normalization of space'.

The same point could be made in relation to time and power relations. For example, in community care individuals will be able to choose when they have breakfast or even whether they have breakfast at all. They will have control over their own daily routines in ways which are impossible in an institutional environment (Seed and Kaye 1994). This restructuring of space and time is therefore directly related to the empowerment of individuals and families, and the dismantling of institutional systems of power and control (Collins 1989).

Community care can consequently be defined in anthropological terms as *a process of restructuring time, space and power relations*. But unless we want to repeat the evolutionist error of assuming that change is unilinear it is important that we view this process of restructuring in a more complex and open-ended way than we might otherwise do. Mary Douglas' work on 'grid and group' (Douglas 1973: 77–92) makes it possible for us to begin to do this. The concept of 'grid and group' was inspired by Bernstein's concept of restricted and elaborated codes, but in Douglas' hands it became a powerful tool for thinking about types of control systems linking cosmological characteristics with degrees of conformity.

At its most basic, grid and group analysis involves four quadrants generated by two pairs of oppositions. One axis consists of the opposition between a completely shared public system of classification and a completely private system of classification. The other axis consists of an opposition between a situation where the group has total power over the individual and one where this group pressure is completely absent and the individual is able to exert pressure on others him/herself (Douglas 1973: 84).

By adapting this matrix to our own purposes, we can create a model which both describes the process of cultural change associated with community care and which allows us to map different kinds of community care systems in a comparative manner (Fig. 1).

The bottom right quadrant is largely irrelevant to our present discussion and is applicable only to those societies where there is no legitimate authority and no commitment to welfare but only a militarily strong and self-seeking tyrant or dominant elite: Mobuto's Zaïre springs to mind. The bottom left-hand quadrant describes an extreme form of market dominated welfare in which everything is for sale but there is no shared system of values.

We are principally concerned with the two upper quadrants. Community care implies some common values, although, in some cases, the level of shared classification may be very minimal. Community care lies above the horizontal line but always closer to it than institutional care. If institutional care is associated with a welfare culture characterized by strong grid and strong group structures, both rejecting and oppressing those who do not match up to the demands of conventional behaviour, then community care is associated with a movement away from this towards a welfare culture in which there is a high level of social change, and in which norms and values are constantly renegotiated.

Thinking in these terms enables us to see more clearly why the process of delivering community care has proved to be so troublesome. Much can be explained in terms of the difficulty of imposing any values, including those of community care, in the context of a relatively weak grid. Moreover, it is easy to see how attempts to do so tend to swing the cultural system back towards strong grid and the kind of institutional controls which are antithetical to community care. Community care therefore relies upon the maintenance of a classificatory grid strong enough to make new policies and practices widely acceptable, but not so strong as to undermine the flexibility of systems and the empowerment of individuals which are critical to its identity.

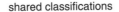

shared classifications

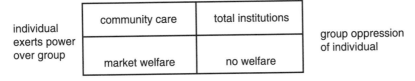

	community care	total institutions
individual exerts power over group			group oppression of individual
	market welfare	no welfare

privatized meanings

Figure 1 A grid and group analysis of welfare systems

For any society, this is a risky enterprise. A complete fragmentation and privatization of meanings can only be averted if new kinds of cultural strategies are developed to reinvent some kind of consensus about meanings, goals, etc. In the new cultural conditions associated with community care, a public classificatory system can no longer simply be imposed on groups and individuals.

This is the context in which we need to understand the current preoccupation with the problem of 'collaboration'. 'Collaboration', or the process of working across organizational, professional or role boundaries, emerges in anthropological terms as a reconfiguration and reinvention of the classificatory grid associated with a shift in power from the large-scale corporate group to smaller and less formal groups and networks. This puts us in the position of being able to explore both the process by which rigid classificatory boundaries are dissolved and the responses to it by which new forms of 'connectedness' (Bott 1971) are generated between individuals and groups previously separated from one another by the strength of the institutional grid.

Another way of putting this is that, as we move from the top of the institutional quadrant to the bottom of the community care quadrant, we also move from social situations dominated by highly organized and enduring social groups, which impose patterns of social interaction on their members, to ones characterized by relatively open-ended, fluid social networks whose existence is constantly being negotiated and renegotiated. From this perspective, *collaboration is nothing less than the process by which social reality is negotiated in and through community care networks of various kinds.*

A range of possible collaborative configurations are conceivable, from those involving a minimal commitment; to shared norms and values and minimal interference in individual or agency autonomy; to those involving much higher levels of sharing and mutual responsibility. However, as it is impossible to conceive of the development of new classifications without subverting old ones, collaboration can also be seen, in anthropological terms, as a *transgressive* cultural practice, apparently undermining accepted boundaries and identities in its search for new ways of thinking about and practising welfare.

Interestingly, community care in general, and collaboration in particular, has emerged as a laboratory of cultural innovation in which attempts to dissolve and rebuild the world of welfare are constantly going on. In this context, it is time we began to ask how these 'experiments' are being conducted in different countries and to identify where on the continuum of cultural configurations they lie. This is not so much an orthodox comparative project as a way of exploring collaborative cultures which may be very different to one's own, and the process begins to fill in the top left-hand quadrant with good quality ethnographic data. This is likely to raise some interesting issues and questions. For example, some forms of collaboration will be close to the boundary of the vertical axis indicating major differences in levels of power and control, while others will be close to the horizontal axis indicating a highly privatized and individualized set of arrangements.

But it is difficult to see how a highly privatized and individualistic world view is compatible with the kind of social relationships that make collaboration possible. Collaborative cultures lying in the bottom left-hand corner of the community care quadrant might therefore be taken as the outer limit of collaboration. Likewise, collaborative cultures lying near the top right corner of the quadrant might be seen as containing so many quasi-institutional control features that they also constitute the limit of collaboration. In contrast, one might expect the most 'successful' examples of collaboration to be found near the centre of the quadrant, where there is a commitment to building a shared world view combined with opportunities for participative interaction.

One useful way of analysing some of these differences is in terms of the extent to which 'connectedness' or high levels of mutual interaction exist and are associated with an 'imagined community' of 'carers' (Anderson 1983). In such a situation, the networks to which the individual belongs represent to that person a meaningful collective entity regardless of the lack of formal group or organizational boundaries.

Collaboration cultures where there is little evidence of an 'imagined community' are likely to lie in the bottom left-hand corner of the community care quadrant. But in the centre and towards the right of the quadrant, one would expect any tendency towards diversification and fragmentation to be counteracted by a commitment to an 'imagined community' within which to negotiate shared meanings that bind individuals and groups to one another on a voluntary basis. If we are interested in applying anthopology to the development of social policy, it seems clear that any examples of collaboration which can be located in the centre/right of the community care quadrant are likely to be of considerable interest.

BACKGROUND

For many years we had been working on various aspects of the question of collaboration, often through detailed discussions with individual practitioners. Bur we had become critical of many aspects of contemporary British approaches to collaboration and wanted to see if alternative approaches were being developed elsewhere.

Why Sweden? The choice of Stockholm was partly opportunistic. We would have been prepared to work with professionals from any of the European Union countries. But the literature on Sweden made us aware that some of the issues associated with the transition from a state welfare culture to more complex and negotiated patterns of welfare would be very likely to be present. One significant factor was the way the Swedish literature demonstrated a strong awareness of and commitment to the ideas and principles most frequently associated with community care at an international level. For example, official literature describes the Swedish Social Services Act in terms of 'the holistic view, normalisation, continuity, flexibility and a local focus' (National Board of Health and Welfare 1992: 27).

COLLABORATION IN THE UK

We do not propose to describe the British situation in detail. It has been exhaustively documented elsewhere. As British researchers familiar with this system, however, we took with us a certain assumption about the nature of collaborative problems and solutions which in retrospect can be seen as only one of the realignments of grid/group relations made possible by the collapse of institutional welfare.

There is a widespread concern about the problem of collaboration in the UK. One interesting feature of the debate has been that, on the whole, in so far as solutions have been proposed, they have been structural solutions – ways of organizing relationships around tasks and outcomes. The problem is often seen as one of imposing order onto chaos. The collaborative space, in other words, is most frequently seen as one which needs to be rationalized and organized (Trevillion 1996b: 11–14). All this seems to be linked to a tendency to assume that collaborative problems are best dealt with in 'structural' ways. Implicitly, this defines the problem of working together as a problem of social order and it defines collaborative solutions in terms of strategies for imposing social order. This, in turn, reveals a tendency to resurrect institutionalized control systems in an attempt to solve the problem of collaboration.

Our own research with social workers in London emphasized to us the way in which collaborative initiatives had often failed to generate communities at a team level. This, in our view, is closely connected with the highly fragmented and instrumental characteristics of British community care systems. While there are plenty of examples of individual good practice, in our experience many attempts at collaboration are located either in the bottom left-hand corner or the top right-hand corner of the community care quadrant.

We had found that in a context of scarce resources and demanding management, many British social workers had chosen not to invest in potentially difficult cross-boundary relationships or in the future of collaborative enterprises. Inevitably, we carried these thoughts and assumptions with us, even while we hoped to experience something different in Sweden.

EARLY CONTACTS

This project grew out of contacts made at the University of Stockholm and especially with Thomas Lindstein, Dean of the School of Social Work. Through him we were put in touch with the National Board of Health and Welfare and through them we made contact with a team of *kurators* or hospital social workers based in a large suburban hospital in Stockholm and specializing in the field of HIV. Without the enthusiasm of the *kurators* themselves, the project would never have begun, but the part played by others in enabling the key research relationships to be formed also needs to be recognized. It is probably true to say that the setting up of the project mirrored its subject matter in that it was, itself, a good example of networking and collaboration, in this case across national frontiers.

METHODS

To some extent, we have found that all qualitative research with professionals has to be seen as a form of action research, in that individuals and groups will only devote time and energy to projects which appear to them to have some practical benefit. Sometimes, the insistence on short-term practical outcomes can make exploratory research very difficult to negotiate. However, early on, we realized that the *kurators* valued the opportunity to reflect on their collaborative practices in an open-ended way, and so, although they were keen to make use of the research process, we did not find ourselves having to work to any agenda other than those of exploration and reflection.

Our fieldwork techniques had to be very intensive as we only had four sessions, spread over three days, in which to complete data collection. We were limited not only by financial constraints, and these were real enough, but also by the need to minimize the level of disruption to the lives of the busy professionals with whom we were working. For these reasons, long-term participant observation was never a realistic option. Instead, we decided to make use of a range of qualitative methods which would ensure that we made optimum use of the time available. We used a combination of network analysis (Scott 1991), case studies and semi-structured interviewing conducted with groups rather than individuals (Glaser and Strauss 1968). Most of the work was done on a face-to-face basis, but we asked the *kurators* beforehand to complete some simple forms detailing their interactions with others over a two-week period. This gave us important clues as to some of the characteristic patterns of interaction and informed the kind of questions we decided to ask on arrival in Stockholm.

The team we worked with consisted of three social work trained *kurators* who worked in a specialist HIV unit in a large hospital in Stockholm. Swedish *kurators* are medical social workers, frequently but not always based in hospital settings, employed by the *landsting* or county rather than the *kommun* or local authority (as would be the case in the UK). We worked with this team intensively over a period of four days, and what follows is an account both of our work and the encounter between British and Swedish perspectives on collaboration.

The fieldwork process began with a general and wide-ranging group interview with the *kurators*. This provided important data on attitudes, roles and practices. The second session was devoted to case studies presented by each member of the *kurators'* team. This enabled us to link general themes to specific practices, and to gain key insights into collaborative problems and dilemmas as well as successes.

The third session took the form of a network meeting which involved the *kurators* and a number of key individuals in their HIV community care networks. We used network analysis at the beginning of the sessions, asking participants to complete a simple record of interactions with others in the room and then developed this activity into a group discussion. One important feature of this interview was the way it directly addressed patterns and styles of collaboration. The final session consisted of a further group interview with the *kurators*, which sought clarification, contextualization and initial feedback.

PHILOSOPHY OF THE *KURATORS*

On our first day together we began by asking some basic questions about structures, systems and values. It was the discussion about 'values', however, which proved to be most interesting. 'Values' occupy a key place in professional thinking in the UK but in continental Europe the professional emphasis is frequently on 'theory' or 'knowledge'. The Swedish *kurators* saw 'values' as so general as to be meaningless. They did, however, recognize that a general 'philosophy' of care was important and so we eventually settled on the idea of working on a 'statement of philosophy' instead of a list of 'values'. This 'statement of philosophy' contained many clues as to the way in which collaboration was conceived.

1 Helping people to help themselves

The *kurators* described this in terms of helping people 'to fish', but that 'instead of one doing it for them, they do it for themselves. But then, of course, as they become sicker, we do more of the fishing for them.'

2 Respect for differences and respect for the uniqueness of individuals

For the *kurators*, 'respect' included both an awareness of the validity of different lifestyles ('having respect for each person's individuality') and an awareness of the inequality often underlying 'difference' ('that you can have very different resources in life and you try to react to that in the way you try to help').

3 Supporting and involving families and carers

It was important to the *kurators* that they tried to locate their clients in family networks even if these families were not especially supportive.

> We also have a strategy . . . to involve persons around the patient, the network, even if, maybe, it's a theoretical network; but talking about the family, trying to get the family to come together with the patient here at the hospital, talking to the doctor, talking to us.

4 Non-discriminatory practice

This was seen as a team or group responsibility, as well as an individual value: 'we know where the professional boundaries are and we have group pressure to keep those boundaries. If someone is slipping . . . there is always someone to step in'.

5 Normalization

This was defined both in terms of 'mainstreaming' or the idea that 'the ordinary type of organizations should be able to deal with HIV' and in terms of 'being included in society'. It was thus closely linked to another general principle – 'inclusiveness'.

6 Inclusiveness

This was seen in terms of enabling individuals with HIV to gain access to mainstream services, that they

> shouldn't be put out to specialized organizations. . . . You shouldn't have to travel from one side of the city to another, you should be able to use the school that is closest so that they [the children] can play with their friends.

7 Social education

This was both a value and an activity which struck us as quite distinctive. We felt that education was taken much more seriously as a professional responsibility than would have been the case in the UK:

> We often go out talking to different people . . . if we feel there is discrimination and our clients are being discriminated against, we talk to groups, bosses or whatever's necessary. At the moment we have a little premature baby at the children's ward and they have never had that and the mother now is going to go there . . . and so they have questions about the kinds of precautions they should take.

8 Overcoming isolation by building social support networks

The *kurators* saw themselves as working to locate individuals within society and specific support networks, 'to help people find people who they can talk to, family members, good friends, even at work, if that's possible. We don't help people to isolate themselves.'

9 Individualization of support initiatives

The principle that 'people are not the same – they have different backgrounds' and are in 'need of individual support' was important because it showed how seriously the *kurators* took the community care principle of flexibility, which in the UK would have been related to the concept of a 'needs-led' service.

STATE, SOCIETY AND COMMUNITY

As the *kurators* themselves tended not to prioritize any one of these statements over others, it is rather artificial for us to do so, and yet we were very struck by the strong commitment they felt to the principles of social inclusion. For them, these entailed both social support and the right to lead a life without experiencing prejudice and discrimination. If this is linked to the obvious importance attached to the question of choice and the negotiation of care needs on an individual basis, it is clear that this statement of philosophy places the *kurators'* model of practice firmly within the community care quadrant of our matrix, where little is imposed, much is negotiable, and yet there is a strong commitment to achieving a shared classification system.

Whilst most of these 'philosophical' principles were very familiar to us as 'values', it was noticeable that words such as 'community' and even 'citizenship', which would have been ubiquitous in the UK, were avoided. In fact, in the literal sense, there was no exact equivalent to the British concept of 'community care'. Rather the emphasis was on more specific ideas. This may have been because, in contrast to the British social workers, they did not see their work in this area as linked to a radical legal/policy shift, or even to a specific organizational or managerial objective.

There was also a more profound reluctance to adopt the idea of 'community' as something separate from the state or society as a whole. This is reflected in the Swedish language which likewise does not clearly distinguish between these ideas.

> This is how you use it [community] and they use it very much in the States as well. Everywhere 'community', 'community'. The thing is . . . we don't talk about that in that way here. We talk more about the *samhälle* in the bigger picture.

Samhälle was defined as 'the state or the political community'. 'It is too big in that way, but that's what we say,' said one *kurator*.

When talking about the local level the *kurators* preferred to talk in terms of local networks rather than local communities. This reminded us, as Britons, of the way we tend to define 'community' in opposition to 'the state' and how this split permeates social policy. When we put this to the *kurators* they made it very clear that this was alien to their way of thinking. 'I don't think that is something that is opposite – "community" as opposite to "the state". I don't think that we think like that', said one. 'We mix it all up. It's all the state in a way, the society', said another. One suggested

> That is typically Swedish really because we think of the state and society as the same word. We have a tradition in Sweden that the society is responsible for the individual and we don't always talk about the state. It's both the state and the other levels.

From this we drew a rather paradoxical conclusion. Whereas in the UK there is considerable talk about 'community' there is very little sense of any belief in specific communities of care either real or imaginary. On the other hand, in Sweden there is a reluctance to use the term 'community' because of its specific connotations. However, as we shall see more clearly later on, there is evidence of a considerable interest in 'communities', if these are defined as specific inter-agency or inter-professional groups or networks with which individuals closely identify, and which represent core professional meanings and aspirations. This preference for small-scale, flexible and interpersonal social relations over and above more generalized and abstract social constructs is, again, consistent with a form of practice which belongs in the community care quadrant.

SAMVERKA OR CO-OPERATION

The idea of 'collaboration' was recognized and they were obviously more comfortable with the term than with the concept of 'community', but the kurators nevertheless preferred to use the term 'co-operation' as a more accurate translation of the Swedish word samverka which literally means 'working together'. This preference for 'co-operation' rather than 'collaboration' turned out to be very significant.

'Co-operation' could only exist when certain, quite demanding, conditions were met. In particular, it seemed that where roles and philosophies diverged too much it was seen as preferable to abandon 'co-operation' rather than to continue simply because there might be some administrative advantage. This point seemed to be reached most frequently in relation to the tension between care and control. The kurators clearly experienced an internal conflict between the philosophy of social support and empowerment to which they were committed, and their more controlling roles especially in relation to 'contact tracing' and the enforcement of codes of responsible sexual behaviour. And yet, they seemed able to manage this except when they felt this delicate balance to be put under pressure by external forces such as their relationships with the Regional Medical Officers (RMOs) who had direct responsibility for the imprisonment of persistently sexually irresponsible individuals carrying the HIV virus. The relationships between kurators and RMOs seemed to constitute something of an outer limit for co-operation because sometimes the emphasis by the RMOs on the exercise of legal authority seemed to make continued co-operation impossible, and restricted the discussions *kurators* felt they could have.

In the UK, collaboration is not always seen in terms of a very close working relationship, let alone a meeting of minds. In the Swedish situation co-operation made more demands on those participating, especially in terms of what in the UK would be called 'core values'.

Some other co-operative relationships were also seen as very difficult to manage but for reasons associated less with values and more with money. For example, relationships with the *kommun* were seen as quite conflictual at times. The question of housing responsibility was identified as a potential flashpoint in the relationship between *kurators* and their *kommun* counterparts as well as in the relationship between officials of different *kommuns*.

> It's a struggle between the county (including the *kurators*) and the municipality (*kommun*) because of money. There is sometimes a struggle over who should pay. . . . If someone is ready to leave the hospital but can't go directly home . . . there can be a struggle about money. Stockholm's divided into different municipalities. . . . [One client] had his address in one but was going to move to the one next to it. So these two social welfare officers were bouncing back and forth with him, who was going to give him his money.

Nevertheless, co-operation with the *kommun* still survived. This may have been partly because the kind of market pressures so evident in the UK were not as evident in the Swedish situation. There seemed to be an important distinction in the minds of the *kurators* between problems which make co-operation difficult (such as arguments about financial responsibility) and problems which make it inappropriate (control versus care). We felt that *samverka* lay at the heart of the *kurators*' inter-agency and inter-professional practice. It epitomized both their commitment to developing close working relationships with others and a willingness to negotiate openly the terms of these relationships, provided that a common set of principles could be established. All of this indicated that *samverka* should be regarded as a strategy located firmly in the centre of the top left-hand, community care, quadrant.

CO-OPERATION WITH THE 'THIRD SECTOR'

Whereas much of the literature on Swedish social policy emphasizes the small role played by voluntary or 'third sector ' organizations, we were struck by the significant role played by some of these. An organization called Noah's Ark seemed to act as an umbrella group for the voluntary or third sector and constantly recurred in descriptions of co-operative working. The traditional complementary role of voluntary agencies seemed to be increasingly combined with a newer role of substituting for state services from the *kommun*.

This change was felt by the *kurators* to be forcing them to pay more attention to how they presented situations to external bodies, whereas in the past they would not have needed to do this. As one put it:

> Over the years, I have had to increase my skills in the sense of being nice, able to joke with people and making them like me in a way ... that has always been the social worker's role but over the last years I have found that I have had to put more emphasis on seducing them.

The fact that *samverka* was practised with the 'third sector' as well as with other more traditional state bodies added weight to our growing conviction that, at the philosophical level at least, the *kurators* were engaged in a process of community care.

THE ROLES OF THE *KURATORS*

When we spoke about roles, the *kurators* emphasized both social work and counselling. Although there was some ambiguity about the terms *kurator*, counsellor and social worker, there was considerable clarity about the part played by the team in the work of the unit. The *kurators* felt they provided continuity of care, and this emphasis on continuity and the long-term perspective was an important key to understanding the co-operative/collaborative model. 'With HIV patients you never lose responsibility, but that's a rather special situation in hospital care because usually you treat the patient ... and after that you let go. . . . With HIV patients we follow all the way.'

The *kurators* emphasized three key roles: psycho-social support, research and development work, and contact tracing. Whilst psycho-social support might be seen as synonymous with what in the UK is called 'care management', it did not involve purchasing and it did not imply a set of activities designed to set up a particular 'package of care'. It was a much more fluid and flexible way of conceptualizing support work and did not prioritize co-ordination over other issues or separate service delivery from assessment of need. It was also clear that this flexible supportive role was legitimated by legislation and current policy. It was also interesting to note the emphasis on research and development. 'Of course, besides, we do research. . . . We are always thinking about how we can improve our way of working. Mostly all social workers involved in HIV work have this research aspect in the Stockholm area.'

Few social workers we have spoken to in London attach any real significance to research and development. It was clear that what was meant by research in Sweden was less formal research and more reflecting on and improving practice. But even in this form it is difficult to find echoes of this in the British material. Individual British workers are, of course, committed to improving their practice but do not describe this as a major role. Again, the emphasis on long-term development in Sweden suggested a much longer time perspective than is usual in the

UK and was to constitute another clue as to the model of collaboration/co-operation.

This orientation to social education suggested that any tendency towards moral relativism or the privatization of meanings would be resisted by the *kurators*. They expressed commitment to establishing a strong common, if still negotiated, set of principles. This showed that they were not infinitely flexible in their philosophy and suggested that their community care practice should be located some distance from the bottom of the community care quadrant.

OUTCOMES AND PROCESSES

The *kurators* found it difficult to talk about their work in terms of precise goals. They sometimes emphasized prevention, but otherwise talked simply about the need to ensure that clients were 'satisfied' with services. One expressed their goals as being 'A combination, maybe, between psycho-social support of a high standard and the patient's confidence and satisfaction, because I think that they are really connected to each other. Without the confidence, it is very difficult to have good support.'

We were told that 'the prevention goal does not necessarily have anything to do with the patient being satisfied'. 'Satisfaction' seems to have much more to do with the way relationships are being conducted and the elusive quality of confidence than it does with the UK concept of consumerism, with its emphasis on service standards and specifications. This also suggested another difference. In the British situation roles have tended to become increasingly identified with specific service outcomes, such as assessment, construction of care packages, reviews, etc. Specific outcome 'talk' of this kind was not a feature of the *kurators'* discourse and they did not connect it with their roles.

The emphasis on process seemed to be at one with the strong value placed on negotiating the relationships underlying *samverka* and again seemed to indicate that the philosophy of the *kurators* was consistent with the kind of ideas which one might expect from a practice system located at the centre of the community care quadrant.

CASE STUDIES OF *SAMVERKA*

The case studies we looked at highlighted a number of new issues. They showed the extent to which questions of social exclusion were bound up not only with HIV but also with issues of race and culture, since most of them dealt with situations involving relatively marginalized and disadvantaged racial and cultural minorities. Therefore the co-operative and inclusive approaches adopted meant all had to address issues of trust and confidence.

One feature of the co-operative patterns described was that very few of them drew upon formal strategic links although, when asked, it was suggested that these had been created at an earlier stage. Rather, the links made tended to assume a context of co-operation which evidently stemmed from other factors. Moreover, most of the links made were created in partnership with service users. There was little sense of services being organized for people and so the relationships in question almost always included the client. They were always triangular, rarely dyadic.

Although support was a major aim it was rarely operationalized in terms of 'plugging' people into existing networks or services. The pattern was frequently of effecting introductions and then allowing clients to pace the way they engaged with new social contacts, as described in the following exchange:

KURATOR: I don't know how it happened but she started in a support group. I don't know when exactly . . . and it meant a lot to her seeing how other people behaved in these situations. It enabled her to inform her family and friends about being infected with HIV.

RESEARCHER: That sounds like a very important moment.

KURATOR: Definitely but I don't know how that happened really.

RESEARCHER: You didn't organize that.

KURATOR: No I didn't, but I was really happy about it. . . . It can can feel that you're talking to a wall for two years and suddenly they do something.

None of this would have been possible in a situation where services had to be purchased as there would have been a pressure for a much clearer definition of the support network at a much earlier stage, rather than just allowing it to develop at the pace of the client.

Another interesting contrast was in the use of network conferences. In the UK these are generally associated with reactive problem solving and constitute an extension of the co-ordinative role of the care manager. The Swedish *kurators*, on the other hand, spoke of this in terms of creating new possibilities for dialogue, and focused less on solving service delivery problems and more on enabling the client to benefit from a variety of perspectives. There was also an acceptance that a number of planned and unregulated interactive possibilities might emerge from such meetings, and that this might have a positive if unspecified impact on the client's situation. Again, we were struck by the open-ended and flexible approach adopted. For example, we heard about a conference being used in connection with some bereavement work:

> I really appreciate this, that the social welfare office (*kommun*), the woman [female social worker] there was sympathetic and really professional. She took the initiative to arrange a social network meeting where she invited the boy [son of the dead woman], the new family, the teacher, the child psychologist, the grandfather, people from the social welfare office, and me. So we were sitting all bunched, discussing what had happened and taped it. Her idea was that the son would have something to take with him. It [the conference] had the possibility of

explaining some things because they [the family] wanted to blame the Spanish man who had infected the woman. So I could really say that that was not how it was. And the boy was there. That was really a nice experience. It was a good way of finishing work with this family.

The *kurator* went on to emphasize that 'the motivation of the social worker was to give something to the boy, to show him how many people were engaged with him'.

In at least one case we heard about educational activities designed to reduce prejudice and discrimination. These activities were only possible because of the co-operation of key people but they were clearly of a challenging rather than collusive nature. They were however, clearly part of a co-operative stance designed to effect normalization. This suggested that some conflictual strategies were employed to further the co-operative approach. Although apparently para-doxical, this seemed to us to be quite consistent.

Almost all the collaborative interventions described were open-ended and oriented towards the long term. They could best be described as springing from an orientation to co-operative processes rather than collaborative structures. One *kurator* described an experience as useful 'because I learned to wait and not be in a hurry in the process. I think we have learned to step back for a while and let people find their own way. There isn't any other way, really.'

This was only possible because of the existence of a well-defined, established network of professionals, which had an enduring existence outside any formal pattern of meetings. We gained the impression of a co-operative stance linked less to problem solving than to a process of attempting the integration of indi-viduals within society. But clearly the existence of a network of professionals was very important to this goal. The question for us was: what was holding it together? We could find little evidence of formal links.

THE HIV NETWORK OR 'HIV WORLD'

The network members with whom we worked included psychologists, nurses, home care organizers and a representative of the 'third sector' from the Noah's Ark organization. Given that community care rests upon the ability of informal and negotiable social networks of all kinds not only to deliver services in a reli-able way but also to generate a shared set of classifications, we attached considerable importance to understanding the social glue that held *samverka* together.

While we could find little evidence of formal links, the fact that it was possible to meet with so many busy people occupying key positions was in itself a clue as to what held the network together – something which might best be described as generalized or *transferable trust*. We benefited enormously from this as researchers, and it was clearly a key component of the co-operative stance adopted by the network as a whole.

When asked to reflect on what it was that held their network together, its members identified a number of factors. These included: trust, reciprocity, familiarity and shared history/biography, opportunities for informal social interaction, which extended to socializing with one another outside the work context, and a strong sense of individual professional identity, which meant there was little confusion about who should take responsibility for what.

We explored these, in turn.

1 Trust

This was exemplified for us in two statements made by different members of the network:

> If I want something for my patient, how can I explain his situation? How colourful can I make the picture? If I know the person who is at the other end, I can make that picture colourful and if that person trusts me, he or she also knows that I tell the truth. I am not painting things up to get more things for him or her. I'm trusted as a person, so, of course, the fact that I know a person affects what my patient gets or doesn't get.

> I think there is some kind of ground trust to people in this room and to people in HIV care in Stockholm because I think we share a lot of common ideas about this type of care. Sometimes we may . . . not meet as much as we ought to do and maybe we have thoughts that we could do this in another way than that person is doing it, but I think there is a trust that people do the best they can and that they want the best for our common patients.

2 Reciprocity

This was linked to trust as in the belief and expectation that help offered would always be repaid.

PERSON 1: I think it's very good. I know that I can trust her (pointing). I know that if I want something then I always get it. And I hope that's reciprocated.
PERSON 2: Yes.

3 Shared history/biography

It was very obvious to us that the network had a shared history, as if the life courses of those involved had criss-crossed one another many times and influenced one another's development in certain ways.

Maybe it is because the world of HIV care in Stockholm is rather small. We are not so many persons. We really know each other rather well, at least the people I have spoken to over the years. I can understand that it is not very easy to come as a new person in this world because people know each other from many years back but I also think that you benefit from it, from just the fact that we know each other so well in the units and we know this trust is there.

This quotation also provides a very clear clue about the strong identification with an imagined community – the 'HIV world' of Stockholm. This is possibly linked to a wider identification with the global 'HIV world'.

4 Informal socializing

This was, in part, what kept alive the sense of shared history. One member of the network said:

There is specifically one woman . . . we have met over the years at conferences, different meetings, so when I meet her in the street we kind of hug each other, you know. We meet in private and we have this kind of contact.

Another member of the network added:

I think its because I meet B so often. So I have got to know her and her colleagues at Noah's Ark so well because I am there almost once a week with some patient or just to go up for a coffee and to have a talk.

5 Clarity about responsibility

The sense of mutual understanding was very strong but seemed to be promoted almost entirely by the depth of the relationship rather than any formal agreements about roles and responsibilities. In fact, they seemed mystified by the question.

PERSON 1: In the system, I think we know each other so well that we usually know who's responsible for what. If we don't know we have ways of finding out by talking to someone who knows.

PERSON 2: I wouldn't say that we have particular meetings just to discuss who is in charge of what, what is that person's function.

6 The view from the HIV world

When asked to reflect on what was shared in terms of professional philosophy, a number of orientations, or what in the British context would be called 'values', emerged characteristic of the whole network. Of these, the most striking was the holistic approach which valued the person. This was linked to a tendency to reject medical models in favour of social models and to see the person rather than the infection as their core interest. One quotation seems to sum this up:

> From my perspective, one very important 'value' is really to try to get people . . . to realize that people with HIV are human beings and more than a virus, and I think that is very much forgotten. . . . To understand people with HIV, I think that you have to understand the personality and the person's life history . . . not only respect but looking at the whole person.

In many respects this would have been very familiar to UK workers. However, the fact that these values were embodied in a network of people interacting with one another on a regular basis served to differentiate this situation from the British one.

The network then discussed recent changes in Swedish welfare and society, and it was acknowledged that UK-style conflict and confusion was growing in other fields but that HIV was to some extent still protected by its history, although we were also warned not to take away too rose-tinted a view.

> Sometimes I think that the organization or the institution has a big HIV infection . . . there's lots of fights, there's lots of struggle and a lot of killing – psychologically – and we behave just like the virus. I think it's also important that we bring forward that we do have problems.

Interestingly, it was also acknowledged that in some respects scarcity had generated more imaginative and innovative solutions to co-operation, with more opportunities for working together and a greater role for the 'third sector':

> because the security also made us a bit lazy and maybe we didn't use our heads in the way that we could, so what's happening is that we have to use our heads more, that we have to find other ways.

CO-OPERATION AND SOCIAL INCLUSION

A clear view about co-operation emerged out of our final discussions with the *kurators*. One feature of the collaborative/co-operative model developed by the Swedish network was that it was oriented to *process* rather than *structure*. The *kurators* saw co-operation not as a response to fragmentation or disintegration but rather as a way of making orderly but potentially unresponsive social institutions receptive to the needs of people with HIV. The whole orientation was towards social inclusion, the provision of choice and the creation of opportunities. This process of *opening up* the social structure was facilitated by a web of co-operative relationships through which these opportunities were created.

In contrast to the UK situation, with which we were familiar, the dynamism in these relationships sprang out of professional concerns rather than specific managerial initiatives. Management was important but collaborative initiatives were professional rather than managerial. The reason for this was clear. If the issue of 'co-operation' is seen in terms of the need to work with others across a range of organizational and sectoral boundaries to make services more responsive and flexible, standardized management-driven approaches of the kind dominant in the UK would not be considered relevant or appropriate to the nature of the issue. Underlying this was a much stronger belief in the role of the individual, and a much greater emphasis on the role of discretionary professional judgements, than is possible or acceptable in the UK.

Conversely, it might be argued that one of the weaknesses of the Swedish model of co-operation is that its strong reliance on a meeting of minds and the very existence of an imagined community or 'HIV world' makes it difficult to accommodate serious conflicts and philosophical differences.

CONCLUSION

We have argued that 'collaboration' emerges in anthropological terms as a reconfiguration and reinvention of the classificatory grid associated with a shift in power from the large-scale corporate group to smaller, informal groups and networks. We have looked in some detail at the way in which the model of 'co-operation' has been developed in one Swedish social work team, as a particular response to what is, arguably, a global cultural problem.

The Swedish model of co-operation is rooted in a concern with a shared philosophy and is not only strongly oriented to the importance of relationships but also premised on a specific concept, the 'HIV world', which constitutes both a tangible social network and an imaginary community, or point of reference, which allows the practice of *samverka* to be securely anchored in what would otherwise be a very difficult and conflict laden environment.

Finally, this comparative exploration of co-operation/collaboration shows the potential of anthropological models for illuminating some of the more complex socio-cultural areas of community care, in particular the ways in which collaboration culture is being constructed on a day-to-day basis through the interactions of those most closely involved in the definition of 'need' and the provision of services.

BIBLIOGRAPHY

Anderson, B. (1983) *Imagined Communities: Reflections on the Origin and Spread of Nationalism*, London: Verso.

Audit Commission (1992) *Community Care: Managing the Cascade of Change*, London: HMSO.

Benn, S. I. (1982) 'Individuality, autonomy and community', in E. Kamenka (ed.) *Community as a Social Ideal: Ideas and Ideologies*, London: Edward Arnold.

Bott, E. (1971) *Family and Social Networks: Roles, Norms and External Relationships in Ordinary Urban Families*, London: Tavistock.

Collins, J. (1989) 'Power and community care: implications of the Griffiths report', *British Association for Social Anthropology in Policy and Practice Newsletter* 4, 12.

Douglas, M. (1973) *Natural Symbols: Explorations in Cosmology*, Harmondsworth: Penguin.

Foucault, M. (1973) *Madness and Civilisation: A History of Insanity in the Age of Reason*, New York: Vintage Books.

Glaser, B. and Strauss, A. (1968) *The Discovery of Grounded Theory*, Chicago: Aldine.

Goffman, E. (1968) *Asylums: Essays on the Social Situation of Mental Patients and Other Inmates*, Harmondsworth: Pelican.

Griffiths, R. (1988) *Community Care: Agenda for Action*, London: HMSO.

Hudson, B. (1992) 'All dressed up. But nowhere to go', *The Health Services Journal*, 22 October, 23–4.

Leinhardt, G. (1966) *Social Anthropology*, Oxford: Oxford University Press.

National Board of Health and Welfare, Socialstyrelsen (1992) *Social Services in Sweden: a Part of the Social Welfare System*, Stockholm: National Board of Health and Welfare.

Orme, J. and Glastonbury, B. (1993) *Care Management*, Practical Social Work, British Association of Social Workers, Basingstoke: Macmillan.

Payne, M. (1986) 'Community connections through voluntary organisations: problems and issues', in G. Grant and M. McGrath (eds) *British Institute of Mental Handicap Conference Series*, 60–77.

Scott, J. (1991) *Social Network Analysis*, London: Sage.

Seed, P. and Kaye, G. (1994) *Handbook for Assessing and Managing Care in the Community*, London: Jessica Kingsley.

Trevillion, S. (1996a) 'Talking about collaboration', *Research Policy and Planning* 14, 96–101.

—— (1996b) 'Towards a comparative analysis of collaboration', *Social Work in Europe* 3, 1, 11–18.

Wagner, G. (1988) *Residential Care: A Positive Choice. Report of the Independent Review of Residential Care, National Institute for Social Work*, London: HMSO.

Chapter 7

Caring communities or effective networks?

Community care and people with learning difficulties in South Wales

Charlotte Aull Davies

INTRODUCTION

Care in the community no longer represents an innovation in the delivery of welfare services but has become the orthodoxy in service provision. 'Over the past thirty years community care has come to be almost universally espoused as a desirable objective for service providers and users and a central pillar of policy for governments and politicians of all persuasions' (Means and Smith 1994: 1). This virtually universal acceptance derives in part from its chameleon-like quality of being all things to all people. Practitioners working with people with learning disabilities argued for its implementation on the grounds that it best accomplishes the practical goal, derived from the philosophy of normalization, of enabling people to live ordinary lives (but cf. Dalley 1992). Planners, on the other hand, saw it as a way of cutting the costs involved in maintaining people in large institutions; their arguments for closing such institutions were strengthened by the exposure of malpractice and mistreatment of residents in many of them (e.g. Ryan with Thomas 1987). All these considerations combined with a growing political emphasis on self-help and privatization to make care in the community an ever more popular option for politicians and policy makers into the 1990s.

One of the most visible results of community care policies has been the drastic reductions in size, aiming towards eventual closures, of many large institutions providing care particularly for people with learning disabilities and mental illnesses, and the relocation of their residents in dispersed smaller scale facilities. Studies of adults with learning disabilities in the community have generally looked at the course of their lives subsequent to moving out of such institutions. The classic example, from an anthropological perspective, is Edgerton's (1967) ethnographic study of the effects of stigma in the lives of forty-eight people with 'mild mental retardation' relocated from a mental institution in California. These individuals all had some form of employment (as a condition of their release) and moved into private accommodation.

In contrast, recent studies in Britain look at people's moves into supervised accommodation, most commonly group homes, and attempt to assess their adjustment to more independent living and their quality of life in the broader community (e.g. Booth *et al.* 1990; Cambridge *et al.* 1994; Flynn 1989). Whereas most such studies judge the moves to be qualified successes, one anthropological study (McCourt Perring 1994) looks at the relationship between care and control in these new settings and suggests that many small group homes continue to accept underlying institutional and broader cultural assumptions that induce them to reproduce the attitudes and practices of control they were ostensibly designed to subvert. This suggests that an anthropological approach – that is, one which strives to adopt the perspective of those actually experiencing care in the community and which is relatively open to multiple interpretations and conflict – can provide valuable insight into the effects of such policies.

Another consequence of promoting care in the community, besides closing large institutions, has been to discourage entry to them in the first place (cf. Dalley 1991). In so far as people with learning disabilities are concerned, this largely means persuading parents to provide care for their children with learning disabilities at home. Clearly such an outcome is fairly easily accomplished by simply not providing many other options. It can, of course, be further facilitated by making support services more widely and readily available. This is an important aspect of community care provision, but one that has come in for considerable criticism as to the adequacy of the support services actually provided.

Community care policies have been subject to a more general critique by feminists who point out the gendered nature of the carers and the resulting exploitation of women (Dalley 1988; Brown and Smith 1989). One criticism advanced by feminists and others is that the concept of community on which these new forms of care rest is a very tenuous one indeed. In spite of the positive connotations of warm and supportive personal relationships, on which support for community care appears to have been built, particularly by politicians, the reality of 'community' is highly variable (cf. Means and Smith 1994: 5; Trevillion 1992: 8). Both perception and experience of community depend heavily on an individual's social position and roles. Community is not invariably supportive and may even be experienced as oppressive by some of its members (cf. Frazer and Lacey 1993; Young 1990). More recent theoretical treatments of community regard it as primarily an ongoing process of symbolic construction which individual members may interpret in varying ways to support their own personal identities (Cohen 1985). In this view community is not primarily a system of social support to ensure the material welfare of its members. In fact it could be argued that those most in need of such support in the form of material sorts of caring (e.g. elderly people; people with disabilities) are those who are most peripheral to this on-going process of symbolic construction.

Considerations such as these have led many of those concerned with evaluating the service delivery aspect of care in the community to promote the anthropological concept of personal networks (Mitchell 1969; Barnes 1954) as more relevant than the diffuse and poorly defined idea of community. Wenger (1991), for example, considers different types of personal networks of elderly people as an indication of how they relate to the community and then looks at their individual histories to explain how they develop such networks. Similarly for people with learning disabilities, Abraham (1989) suggests, 'if community care is to live up to its interpersonal promise then the "community" in which the person with a mental handicap is to live may need to be artificially created and maintained on a life-long basis' (1989: 127). Trevillion (1992) also argues that networking is the essential basis for care in the community and further notes that it does not simply happen, but must be planned and organized (also cf. Bulmer 1987). Thus efforts to develop forms of networking are often a primary concern of community care practitioners. One of the principal ways in which this goal has been pursued for people with learning disabilities is through the so-called 'Patch programmes' in which care workers attempt to utilize existing community facilities to develop a variety of activities, contacts and service provisions for their clients.

As already noted, community care has resulted in many more children with learning disabilities being cared for at home by their parents. These children have attended local schools, often sharing a building with non-disabled peers, and experiencing similar daily and weekly routines, and annual holidays. However, when they reach school-leaving age and in the subsequent years to full legal maturity, the gap between them and their non-disabled peers becomes wider and more difficult to bridge. Certainly parents can no longer take the major responsibility for their developing so-called normal adult lifestyles and the active role of community services is much more important. This transition to adulthood is particularly problematic for people with learning disabilities, both in terms of their achieving recognition as full social adults and (relatedly) their access to certain lifestyle changes normally associated with adulthood. These lifestyle changes – such as moving out of the parental home, developing social and financial independence, employment, sexual relationships, marriage, children – are closely linked to the questions of normalization and the provision of community care.

In this chapter I draw on research carried out with people with learning disabilities and their parents or carers as they worked through this transitional phase in order to discuss their perceptions of what care in the community means, and their experiences and evaluations of the forms it actually assumes. I also consider how various forms of community care affect their potential for developing supportive personal networks.

METHODS

Research was conducted during a three-year project supported by the Joseph Rowntree Foundation. The primary objective was a study of the transition to adulthood of people with learning disabilities.[1] I spent approximately eighteen months in the field, from March 1990 to October 1991, working with young people with learning disabilities, and their parents and other carers. Fieldwork was carried out in the former county of West Glamorgan in South Wales. West Glamorgan was among the first areas to be granted funding for its proposals under the All-Wales Strategy for the Development of Services for People with Mental Handicaps, established by the Welsh Office in 1983, and by the time of the research was very active in developing service provision based on a model of care in the community. Thus I investigated awareness and evaluation of these new forms of service provision, as well as understanding of the government's community care policy, particularly amongst parents.

Sixty young people, and the parents or carers of fifty-six of them, participated in the study. The research was a combination of semi-structured interviewing and participant-observation. Interviews were based on a questionnaire, but only as a memory aid for the interviewer. The order and wording of questions were varied to fit the circumstances and allow for clarification. Interviewees were encouraged to expand on a point, digress or introduce other topics. All interviews were recorded (except for one individual who declined the use of a tape recorder), transcribed and coded for analysis with *The Ethnograph*, a computer application package designed for use with qualitative data. Interviews with parents or carers were conducted in their homes and normally were completed in a single session lasting from one to four hours. The young people were each interviewed on several occasions, with the series extending over several weeks or months and informal contacts maintained throughout that period. They were interviewed mainly at the day centres they attended (Adult Training Centres, or ATCs;[2] special needs units in local colleges; other day centres such as training houses; and Patch-based centres).[3] A few interviews were carried out in other locations, for example, a workplace, café, club and residential centre.

Interviews were augmented by participant-observation at the various research sites. In a few cases, with people who had very poor communication skills, participant-observation was the major source of data; it was an important supplementary source with nearly everyone. While the findings deriving directly from participant-observation are less apparent in the material which follows than those that are verbally based, participant-observation was essential to the research. The relationships I established with the young people in these sites through my involvement in their everyday activities made the process of interviewing them much more effective and fruitful; in some cases, interviews would have been impossible without this prior involvement. Furthermore, participant-observation helped to contextualize the interview material, allowing me to interpret verbal explanations and comments in the light of lived experiences and behaviour.

The sample was not constructed to be statistically representative but I tried to ensure a relatively equal distribution by gender and class. It was also selected to include individuals from a variety of types of day centres plus a few who were not attending any such centre. I deliberately did not select people on the basis of their intellectual abilities or communication skills. Instead, at each site or with each service provider, I contacted all individuals in the age range of the study, that is, between eighteen and twenty-six, and invited them to participate. I eventually extended this range slightly at each end in response to the requests of three individuals to participate in the study. In the excerpts from interviews which follow, ... indicates a longer than usual pause, ... // ... material omitted. Names, and occasionally other minor personal details, have been changed to ensure anonymity for the participants.

COMMUNITY CARE AND THE LEARNING DISABLED – PERSPECTIVES, EXPERIENCES, VALUATIONS

I asked parents if they knew about the All-Wales Strategy and whether they thought it had made – or potentially would make – any difference in their lives. The fact that two-thirds of the parents interviewed responded affirmatively to the first part of this query no doubt reflected the relatively high profile and level of activity of the All-Wales Strategy in promoting a variety of organizations and activities under the impetus of the care in the community policy. Furthermore, among those parents who professed no knowledge of the Strategy were a few with sons or daughters who had in fact benefited from one of its initiatives, in particular, an employment agency and a Patch-based service. Certainly there was a greater awareness of local provision than national policy – somewhat less than half professed any knowledge of the government's care in the community policy. There was considerable variation in both the kinds of knowledge the affirmative responses represented and the overall opinions of the Strategy and its policy. Indeed there was a significant minority of opinion quite unfavourable to the All-Wales Strategy. One woman dismissed her husband's attempts to defend the Strategy, by pleading funding difficulties, for what they both regarded as a disappointing record, with the comment, 'It's all paper and no action with them.' Another pair of parents, of a 22-year-old man attending an Adult Training Centre daily, felt that all the emphasis had been on provisions for children, for example respite care, which had come too late for them.

LINDA RICHARDS: I can honestly say that it hasn't altered Gary's life not one bit.
CHARLOTTE AULL DAVIES: At all?
LINDA RICHARDS: Or ours. You know, we've had nothing ... // ... A lot of people doing a lot of jobs, but the likes of Gary not getting nothing out of it.

The majority of parents interviewed, in fact, appeared to interpret the Strategy, and community care in general, in terms of fairly conventional welfare provisions. For example, several parents regarded its most important function as one of ensuring that people were informed of the benefits – particularly Attendance Allowance – to which they were entitled. Several complained of having lost years of payments due to not being properly informed of their entitlements. These parents appear to view the policy of community care not as an innovative approach to providing for people with disabilities but simply as another term for welfare provision. Certainly, in a practical sense and from their perspective, care in the community was not new – their sons and daughters had always been cared for at home, hence in the community. None of these parents reported having seriously considered institutionalization as an option at any time in their child's life nor did they see it as a future option. However, they were all, in various degrees and ways, grappling with the changing relationship with community usually associated with the transition to adulthood. Their primary concern was with future living arrangements and associated forms of care for their sons and daughters. Another concern, not so important to parents but given much greater prominence by the young people themselves, was employment. Only a minority of the research group – nine out of sixty young people – were involved in a Patch form of day care but among this group of parents there was also an awareness of and concern about the nature of community per se. A consideration of each of these three areas – accommodation away from the parental home, day care (particularly Patch-based day care), and employment – and their relationship to personal networks will provide a much clearer picture of how these young people and their parents actually relate to the concept of care in the community.

The vast majority (87 per cent) of the young people in this study were living at home with their parents. Four moved from the parental home into group homes during the course of the research. When parents discussed the future living arrangements of their sons or daughters, a slight majority felt that they wanted them to live away from home in the not too distant future. It is indicative of the difficulties that parents face in attempting to promote such a 'normalizing' lifestyle that only two sets of parents saw this as something that would simply happen in the fullness of time without their taking any initiative. Each of these couples felt that their son or daughter would move out when they married and set up their own family; the daughter of one of the couples was in fact engaged. The other couple, whose son was nineteen, foresaw a scenario in which care to a degree would devolve onto a partner.

CHARLOTTE AULL DAVIES: What would you want for him in five years' time?

REG GRIFFITHS: Well, you know, settled, settled with his own family, probably. He'd be capable of providing for a family, by then, you know. . . . You just got to watch that he don't take on too much. You know, as long as he knows his limitations.

DELYTH GRIFFITHS: I don't think, I think it would be better if he had a healthy wife rather than a disabled one because, you know . . . // . . . What I'm saying is, if he does get married, if his wife was normal then they would have more of a chance of survival. At least there would be one normal one in the family.

Very many parents felt that their sons or daughters would much prefer to be at home, and to a degree viewed alternative living arrangements as rejection (cf. Richardson and Ritchie 1989). However, most recognized that a time might come when they were themselves no longer able to provide care. A few felt there were no acceptable alternatives and thus found this a very distressing issue. As the mother of a 19-year-old woman said, 'It's an awful thing to say but I do think, I hope that she goes before me. Cause I wouldn't like anybody else to look after her, cause they couldn't.' Several others were confident that siblings would assume the responsibilities of caring, including having their brother or sister move in with them: 'Our own children are very nice people, and if anything happened to us, I know that Catrin would be looked after. No question.' All of these parents had grown, married children, nearly always more than one, living in the same locality. Significantly, the one couple who did not fit this pattern but who looked to this extended family eventually to provide care for their daughter with learning disabilities, had moved to a new area away from their adult children on retirement. However, they were planning to return to their original home, mainly due to just these considerations. A few middle-class parents had also made some additional financial provisions for the son or daughter requiring care, usually planning to leave their disabled child the family home when they died. Thus this relatively small group of parents had fully accepted the individualistic emphasis in community care policy, which places greater responsibility on unpaid care provided by family members.

However, a larger group, parents of twenty-five of the young people in the study, definitely wanted them to live away from home some day and expected collectivist (welfare system) provision for them; indeed four young people in the study went through the process of moving into a group home during the course of the research. The preferred option in living arrangements for most of these parents was a group home, interpreted as a house with three or four people with learning disabilities and constant dependable support. Most were also concerned that the house should be physically close to them or other family members to facilitate regular visits as well as in a location that was familiar to the young person. The parents of a 21-year-old man, whose desire to be more independent of them was producing some considerable conflict, discussed the possibility as follows:

CHARLOTTE AULL DAVIES: If you could sort of imagine an ideal situation for him, say in five years' time, what, how would you like to see him?
SPENCER HIBBS: Well, I mean, home of his own, I mean with, he's got to have supervision, there's no question of it. As long as he's in a home of his own, call it his own, and happy, you have the supervision. I think that's about . . .
CHARLOTTE AULL DAVIES: That's what you mainly . . .
GLORIA HIBBS: Yes, just for him to feel independence, that's what I want.
SPENCER HIBBS: As independent as he can be, yes.
GLORIA HIBBS: I'd certainly like him living in [this] area because he's familiar

with everything, you know, and . . . he, it's his right to be in the community. That's how I look at it, there's no reason why he shouldn't be there. I mean, he could contribute to people and he can contribute to a little community, wherever, if he lived in a little road with other people. I mean he'd be the happiest, probably the happiest person there and he'd give a lot to his neighbours. It makes me a little bit annoyed when I think, see sometimes in the paper, people making objections to these houses being set up. Because these youngsters have got such a lot to give.

As this indicates, parents are well aware of the ambiguities in the concept of community: they know that it can be unwelcoming or even hostile and certainly do not assume that a diffuse community can be expected to provide a safety net in terms of support, but that this must come from elsewhere and be planned. Furthermore many parents indicated that the experience of community they desired for their sons and daughters was less a matter of their location than of their participation in or ability to create a network of friends and acquaintances. The parents of an 18-year-old man who had only recently moved into a group home, when asked about their hopes for his future, responded in terms of such a friendship network.

ALAN NORTHWOOD: I'd like him to be, ohhh, still in the group home, with a group of friends, that he's, he's not friends, who aren't officially people he knows through, because he belongs to Gateway or from Mencap or he's made in the college, but friends he's made.

SHEILA NORTHWOOD: Made. Even the pub next door.

ALAN NORTHWOOD: Of his own personality, in the pub, wherever, wherever the centre is, with friends that are friends because they want to be John's friend. And he wants to be friends with them.

Even parents who definitely opposed a move into the community in the form of a group home often defined the ability to develop a separate set of friends as their ideal for their child's future. One father had definitely rejected the idea of a group home for his 21-year-old daughter; instead he was planning to add a self-contained unit on to their house in order to give her some independence while still living at home. His ideal of how she might subsequently develop her life was to have

friendly relationships, you know. So that she can associate with somebody, like 'someone is going to call and see me on Thursday evening', or 'somebody's going to come and stay for the weekend'. So that she's got company, of her own kind, and own age group, then. That's what I'd like to see develop out of the project we're trying to get off the ground, where she gets an independent unit to herself. . . .

Another smaller group of parents held an ideal of community that was not in accord with the policy of care in the community but rather based on an ideal of an alternative community usually in a rural setting removed from what is seen as a competitive and cut-throat society. The mother of a 17-year-old recalled having seen a television programme about such a facility which she and her husband felt would be ideal:

> A group of handicapped people and they are all self-sufficient, and they are all working . . . // . . . Where they're like on a smallholding if you like, and each one has his own job to do. And each one takes part. And they have a communal table. Like a farm would be run then if you like – a family farm. Now that would be a good situation because they got their self-respect because they work and they're a part of what they're working for. And OK they may be shut off from towns and villages, but they still go to towns and villages and use the facilities there, the shops and the cinemas and things . . . // . . . Something like that would be ideal for Patrick, because he would then be able to choose what he wanted to do, and if he wanted to work on the land and the fields then that is what he would be able to do. You know, and still have the integration and the mixing with other people you know.

Such communities, based on alternative values and often run by religious foundations, do in fact exist, and three of the other young people in our study had spent some time in one such community. They had all eventually returned home for various reasons, including parental concerns about care and inadequate finances. Parents' evaluations of their experience were mixed. One father was very disillusioned: 'Because I thought to myself, "now this is the most wonderful place where my child can live for the rest of his life" . . . // . . . And I was completely deceived.' Both he and his wife came to believe that the young people in the community were not receiving adequate nourishment: 'But, now I found that, when I used to go up from here visiting and open days, we knew that there was a shortage of food up there. Plenty of food but the kids wasn't getting it.' They were particularly concerned about their son's weight loss while there, although the mother tended to attribute it to a lack of personal assertiveness rather than neglect. The parents of the other two young people who had spent time in this community were more positive about its effects on their daughters, both saying that the experience had brought them out, made them more self-confident. Although all three young people had been in residence for two or three years, parents reported that none wanted to return once they had moved back home.

CHARLOTTE AULL DAVIES: Was she happy there do you think?

LINDA BURKE: The first year she was. And most of the second year and then somebody was nasty with her and that finished it.

CHARLOTTE AULL DAVIES: Yes. She decided herself she wanted to come home?

LINDA BURKE: Oh yes, yes. And whatever she wants to do, we stick by. You know.

Certainly experiences such as these strike a note of caution about being too sanguine about the supportive framework available in any community, even those based in alternative values. However, this study did not include individuals who chose to remain in such a community and whose experiences may well have been more positive. Some analysts (Brown and Smith 1990) have pointed to advantages these arrangements may offer. In particular it has been suggested that the practice of placing people in small group homes in dispersed locations actually makes it more difficult for them to establish social networks and may leave them vulnerable to various forms of persecution. Furthermore, this sort of dispersal limits their ability to develop a consciousness of themselves as members of a group and makes it less likely they can activate forms of mutual support or organize for political action. On the other hand, it is suggested that alternative communities, while not in line with the prevailing orthodoxy of normalization and integration in community care, may provide an approach which does accord well 'with its goal of providing valued social roles for people with disabilities' (Brown and Smith 1990: 158).

One of the forms of day care most closely associated with the ideal of care in the community is that of Patch-based service provision. In this model social services assist people with learning disabilities to develop networks that make use of a variety of community facilities and services. There was a Patch-based service available to some of the young people in my research. It had been established under the auspices of the All-Wales Strategy and the parents of several of the young people who attended had been involved in setting it up. The experiences of the participants varied markedly. A few parents praised it very highly, for example the parents of 21-year-old Martin Hibbs.

CHARLOTTE AULL DAVIES: He's in Patch now four days a week. Do you think that's fairly valuable? How do you feel about that ?

GLORIA HIBBS: Yes, I think it's great. It gives choice; they vary things greatly and he loves it. And yes, I think he's very, very happy there, and Martin's the first one to let you know if he's not happy in a situation.

SPENCER HIBBS: Oh yes, it's a nice social mix and everything there. But what they're learning I don't know. If there's any sort of formal learning, I don't know.

Such reservations about the lack of structure, particularly in Patch-based day care, came out in parents' comments in several different ways. Hugh Edwards' mother, Lilian, complained that he was allowed to go without his glasses and hearing aid there, whereas when he attended a special needs unit in the local college 'if you seen photographs of him up on the wall in college, he's always got his glasses on and that's how it should be, but [in Patch] they're very easy-going, if he don't want them on, they don't bother'. Frances Kelly's parents complained that it did not offer the range of physical activities that she required and blamed Frances' recent excessive weight gain on that. Her mother said:

> She just does not do any exercise. Thursday afternoons they do a little very gentle exercise. But she needs more and choices are all right up to a point, but Frances, the people like Frances, need encouraging, you know. She was so agile at one time. But now she's eleven stone . . . // . . . It isn't all their fault. It's just, you know, fall through. So there's a lot of going shopping and looking around shops . . . // . . . [whereas at the Adult Training Centre she had previously attended] say every Wednesday morning would be swimming or running or whatever, so they'd do it.

The Kellys, along with a few other parents, also found the flexible hours, in particular what they felt was a tendency towards a very short day, nearly three hours shorter than at the ATC, problematic in terms of their own schedules. They were disappointed with the failure to follow through with plans to provide evening activities.

Frances herself was even more dissatisfied with Patch than were her parents. She consistently expressed a preference for a quiet and predictable lifestyle. One of her main complaints – whether about a family visit, a church service or one of the outings arranged by her day centre – was that things became 'a bit hectic'. She had been very unhappy about the move from the ATC to Patch and at the time of our interviews was making some headway in persuading her parents to arrange for her to spend more time in the ATC. As she explained, 'I prefer the ATC more better. More friends there . . . // . . . the staff's all right here [at Patch] but I still prefer the ATC. I'm more, I'm more comfy there.'

One of the most effective forms of service for the development of social networks is the provision of employment. Six of the young people I interviewed were in some kind of full-time (or near full-time) permanent supported employment; another twenty were either in full-time further education or job training. Thus just over 50 per cent were unemployed and not involved in any programme that was likely to lead to employment. The overwhelming majority said that they would like to have a job and most were able to specify what kind of job they wanted, some with very considerable realism as to their own capabilities, and others incorporating a degree of fantasy. A 23-year-old man who attended an ATC full-time discussed the question of employment with me:

CHARLOTTE AULL DAVIES: Have you ever had a job?
ANDREW LEGGITT: A proper job? Or?
CHARLOTTE AULL DAVIES: Any kind of job.

ANDREW LEGGITT: Only in the ATC now.

CHARLOTTE AULL DAVIES: Do you think you'd like to have another job, besides the ATC? . . . A proper job?

ANDREW LEGGITT: I might do.

CHARLOTTE AULL DAVIES: Do you know what kind of job you would like if you were going to have another job?

ANDREW LEGGITT: I wouldn't mind a woodwork job.

CHARLOTTE AULL DAVIES: Yes? . . . You said you did woodwork in the factory [on work experience], did you?

ANDREW LEGGITT: And I would like to do woodwork again, doing something woodwork.

A 21-year-old woman who also attended an ATC daily was equally clear about her desires, if somewhat less practical as to whether she could realize them.

CHARLOTTE AULL DAVIES: What kind of a job do you think you'd like to do?

ELLEN JAMES: Work in an office.

CHARLOTTE AULL DAVIES: Work in an office . . . Doing, what kind of things would you do, do you think?

ELLEN JAMES: Typewriting.

CHARLOTTE AULL DAVIES: Have you used a typewriter before?

ELLEN JAMES: No.

CHARLOTTE AULL DAVIES: Do you know how to type?

ELLEN JAMES: Yeah.

Parents were generally supportive of the idea that their sons or daughters should have a suitable job. However, they commonly expressed doubts about their capabilities and sometimes inadvertently belittled the kinds of things they could do. As Ellen James' mother commented, 'they wouldn't really be able to concentrate on a whole week's work. A simple job, you know, that they could do now and again, I think is good.' When asked whether being unemployed had an effect on their sons and daughters, most parents felt that their children were unaware of it, that they in fact considered they had a job because they referred to 'going to work' when they left for the ATC. However, as the case of Andrew Leggitt above illustrates, many in fact distinguished between the ATC and a 'proper' job. For example, the mother of a 21-year-old woman felt that a job 'would be a good thing, you know, it would give her another interest', but that her daughter was unlikely to get one because 'she's very lazy, very lazy. You've got to push her all the way to do anything. Could never see her keeping a job down to be honest. As I say she is terribly lazy.' Furthermore, she said, her daughter thought she was employed: 'to her she's not unemployed because she's in the Centre'. However, when the question of jobs was discussed with her daughter, Christine Lewis said she would like to have a job working in a supermarket and subsequently made a clear distinction between that and her work at the ATC:

CHARLOTTE AULL DAVIES: Why do you want a job?

[. . . // . . .]

CHRISTINE LEWIS: To earn money.

CHARLOTTE AULL DAVIES: Yes, that's a good reason . . . // . . . You don't have a job now?

CHRISTINE LEWIS: No.

CHARLOTTE AULL DAVIES: How do you feel about that?

CHRISTINE LEWIS: Awful.

CHARLOTTE AULL DAVIES: Do you? That's too bad . . . Why do you feel bad about it?

[. . . // . . .]

CHRISTINE LEWIS: Well, we don't get paid here anymore.

[. . . // . . .]

CHARLOTTE AULL DAVIES: So it's not a real job?

CHRISTINE LEWIS: No.

CHARLOTTE AULL DAVIES: Do you think it was a real job when you got paid?

CHRISTINE LEWIS: No.

All the young people were clear about their reasons for wanting a job; to earn money, to keep themselves busy, and, overwhelmingly, to meet other people. The importance of work for social contact was emphasized by very many of them. Ellen James said the main thing she would like about having a job was 'working with other people'. Nineteen-year-old Gaynor Jones, who was completing a college course, said she wanted a job 'just to get out of the house. I don't want to be stuck in a corner for the rest of my life, you know. I'm bad enough when I'm home from college.' The importance of the social aspects of work were also stressed by the handful of young people who were in work. Daniel Connor, twenty-three, explained:

CHARLOTTE AULL DAVIES: Do you like it there?

DANIEL CONNOR: I like it there. I blend in with the men, you know, but mostly I go for the women.

CHARLOTTE AULL DAVIES: Do you?

DANIEL CONNOR: Mm [laughing] I had to say that, didn't I?

[. . . // . . .]

CHARLOTTE AULL DAVIES: A lot of women work there, don't they?

DANIEL CONNOR: A lot of them!

CHARLOTTE AULL DAVIES: So that's why you like it, is it?

DANIEL CONNOR: Yeah. That's why I put my aftershave on.

And 24-year-old Katrin Daniels described the various tasks she fulfilled in her position as a general office helper and then compared it favourably to her other work experiences.

CHARLOTTE AULL DAVIES: So you like that best of all the jobs you've had?
KATRIN DANIELS: Yeah.
CHARLOTTE AULL DAVIES: Sounds like a good job.
KATRIN DANIELS: Nice people there as well.

Considerations such as these make it clear that one of the most valued aspects of a job is the social network it provides.

Certainly changes in patterns of socializing are among the first indications to parents of their children's approaching adulthood. Yet, aside from the handful of young people in this study who had some sort of employment, the social activities of the majority appeared to have altered very little since they were children. Their social lives typically consisted of weekly attendance at a Gateway Club (social clubs run by Mencap for people of all ages with learning disabilities) and outings with parents (such as meals out and weekly shopping trips). The only other opportunity for socializing was in their day care facility. Thus relationships with special boyfriends or girlfriends, one of the major lifestyle changes associated with the transition to adulthood, had to be constructed within these rather narrow parameters and were seldom able to develop beyond the sort of contact usually associated with 'school-days romances'. For example, Andrew Leggitt was twenty-three years old and had a long-standing relationship with a woman who attended the same ATC. However, in spite of his desire to broaden their relationship, it was highly controlled by both personal and institutional restrictions on their lives.

ANDREW LEGGITT: I met Caroline and we started talking and I said, 'Would you like to go out with me?' and she said 'Yes'.
CHARLOTTE AULL DAVIES: Do you go out very often?
ANDREW LEGGITT: Well, sometimes we take a walk down the shops.
CHARLOTTE AULL DAVIES: And you see her here every day?
ANDREW LEGGITT: I see her here every day except Monday, because I don't see her Monday. I'm not here Monday . . . // . . .
CHARLOTTE AULL DAVIES: Do you ever get to see her on weekends, on Saturday and Sunday?
ANDREW LEGGITT: Well I don't see her Saturday and Sunday because she's off with her, she can't come, her mother and father don't know the way to where I live. So she doesn't come there. . . . // . . . I wish I could get married to Caroline and have plenty of money . . . // . . . I could take her out then. To the pictures, or we could go on holidays together.

CONCLUSIONS

For the parents in this study – in common with very many other parents of children with learning disabilities born in Britain since the 1970s – the concept of care in the community is neither new nor particularly contentious in that they have cared for their children at home while they attended local schools, if not in their immediate neighbourhood, still certainly in the broader community. Nevertheless, as these children reach adulthood, the problems parents face in continuing to provide care increase in that the responsibilities for such care are not as readily contained within the usual expectations of what parents do for their children. Hence, during this transition, the tensions that are inherent to the concept of care in the community, such as those between individualist and collectivist responsibilities and solutions (cf. Dalley 1988), become much more apparent and pressing. My research has found that expectations and responses of both parents and their adult children to these inconsistencies and anomalies vary considerably. Differences are particularly apparent in expectations regarding future living arrangements, whether made in preparation for a time when parents would no longer be able to provide care or in order to promote a more 'normal' adult lifestyle for these young people. A relatively small number of parents essentially accepted the individualist assumptions hidden in much community care policy in that they were making their own independent arrangements for their son or daughter to continue to be cared for by other family members once they were no longer able to provide care themselves. It is note-worthy that all of these parents had access to considerable resources, both personal and economic: all had fairly large families with grown children who were economically, socially and geographically well placed; and they all had some personal financial resources to bequeath to the child requiring care. Even so, it must be noted that it was not possible in this study to interview these siblings and assess their feelings about this potential long-term obligation.

The majority of parents, however, did not have access to these sorts of resources and implicitly rejected such individualist assumptions about care in the community. Instead, most of them looked to welfare services to make available other forms of provision. These parents accepted fully that aspect of the 'care in the community' concept which assumed such provision would be in the localities where they, and their sons or daughters, lived, rather than in physically distant large institutions. However, none of them assumed that being in the community was in and of itself adequate to ensure effective care. Most wanted accommodation to be nearby so that they themselves or other family members could continue to provide some backup; and they generally agreed with Spencer Hibbs who, as noted above, fully sympathized with his son's desire to be independent but still insisted 'he's got to have supervision' in the form of paid professional staff.

The other principal way in which parents related to the concept of care in the community was in their concern with helping their sons and daughters to develop social networks. Parents were very aware of the restricted character of their sons' or daughters' social activities, particularly when they compared them with their siblings. A relatively small number had had the opportunity of trying a Patch day care service which was based to a degree on developing various forms of networking. The responses to Patch were mixed, with some parents and young people finding the variation and flexibility highly attractive, but others suggesting that the lack of structure was harmful to personal development and reflected more a lack of purposive activity than personal independence. Those young people who appeared to have the most satisfactory social contacts were the small number who were in some form of supported employment; for them, the workplace provided satisfactory social contact along with the status associated with productive activity and the financial rewards it also confers. A very small number of parents had looked to alternative communities as a way of combining just such a possibility for useful work with the security of long-term care. However, their actual experiences had not proven particularly successful.

The principal concerns of the young people in this study that relate to their position in the community were similar in some respects to their parents' but very different in others. For the most part, they too looked for continuing support in any independent living situation, and concern about the provision of material assistance – having their food prepared, receiving help with managing their money – was often at the root of any expressed resistance about leaving the parental home. They placed much greater emphasis on employment, for the reasons noted above, than did their parents, and were concerned with being able to develop their personal relationships more fully. Parents, in spite of their desire for improved opportunities for socializing for these young people, were often ambivalent about more adult forms of social activities, tending to be concerned about the perceived risks of more independent socializing. In particular, they were reluctant to condone, much less foster, the growth of more serious relationships with boyfriends or girlfriends.

Clearly the ambiguities that are inherent in the sociological concept of community, and which are reflected in the social policy of care in the community, are also apparent when the interpretations and expectations of those directly affected by its implementation are considered. My research indicated that although parents of young adults with learning disabilities relate in various ways to idealized notions of 'community' implicit in the community care policy, their experiences and evaluations – in common with those of their sons and daughters – of various forms of care are better understood in terms of social and personal networks rather than by reference to community.

NOTES

1 The grant holder and project director was Richard Jenkins. For further details see *Social Care Research Findings* no. 35 (June 1993), published by the Joseph Rowntree Foundation. Also see Davies and Jenkins (1997); Davies (1998).

2 Adult Training Centres are centralized facilities providing day care for people with learning disabilities. In the recent past they contracted to do unskilled work, such as packaging, for local industries. By the late 1980s, they were doing less of this kind of work and were beginning to provide other teaching and enrichment activities, both on site and through trips to nearby facilities.

3 Patch-based services provide locally based day care which makes use of a variety of services and facilities available in the community, such as leisure centres, shops and colleges.

BIBLIOGRAPHY

Abraham, C. (1989) 'Supporting people with a mental handicap in the community: a social psychological perspective', *Disability, Handicap and Society* 4, 2, 121–30.

Barnes, J. A. (1954) 'Class and committees in a Norwegian island parish', *Human Relations* 7, 39–58.

Booth, T., Simons, K. and Booth, W. (1990) *Outward Bound: Relocation and Community Care for People with Learning Difficulties*, Milton Keynes: Open University Press.

Brown, H. and Smith, H. (1989) 'Whose "ordinary" life is it anyway? – a feminist critique of the normalisation principle', *Disability, Handicap and Society* 4, 2, 105–19.

—— (1990) 'Assertion, not assimilation: a feminist perspective on the normalisation principle', in H. Brown and H. Smith (eds) *Normalisation: A Reader for the Nineties*, London: Routledge.

Bulmer, M. (1987) *The Social Basis of Community Care*, London: Allen and Unwin.

Cambridge, P., Hayes, L. and Knapp, M., with Gould, E. and Fenyo, A. (1994) *Care in the Community: Five Years On. Life in the Community for People with Learning Disabilities*, Aldershot: Arena.

Cohen, A. P. (1985) *The Symbolic Construction of Community*, London: Routledge.

Dalley, G. (1988) *Ideologies of Caring: Rethinking Community and Collectivism*, Basingstoke: Macmillan.

—— (1991) 'Beliefs and behaviour: professionals and the policy process', *Journal of Aging Studies* 5, 2, 163–80.

—— (1992) 'Social welfare ideologies and normalisation: links and conflicts', in H. Brown and H. Smith (eds) *Normalisation: A Reader for the Nineties*, London: Routledge.

Davies, C. A. (1998) 'Constructing other selves: incompetences and the category of learning difficulties', in R. Jenkins (ed.) *Questions of Competence: Comparative Perspectives*, Cambridge: Cambridge University Press.

Davies, C. A. and Jenkins, R. (1997) '"She has different fits to me": how people with learning difficulties see themselves', *Disability and Society* 12, 1, 95–109.

Edgerton, R. B. (1967) *The Cloak of Competence: Stigma in the Lives of the Mentally Retarded*, Berkeley: University of California Press.

Flynn, M. (1989) *Independent Living for Adults with Mental Handicap*, London: Cassell.

Frazer, E. and Lacey, N. (1993) *The Politics of Community: A Feminist Critique of the Liberal-Communitarian Debate*, Hemel Hempstead: Harvester Wheatsheaf.

McCourt Perring, C. (1994) 'Community care as de-institutionalization? Continuity and change in the transition from hospital to community-based care', in S. Wright (ed.) *Anthropology of Organizations*, London: Routledge.

Means, R. and Smith, R. (1994) *Community Care: Policy and Practice*, Basingstoke: Macmillan.

Mitchell, J. C. (1969) 'The concept and use of social networks', in J. C. Mitchell (ed.) *Social Networks in Urban Situations*, Manchester: Manchester University Press.

Richardson, A. and Ritchie, J. (1989) *Letting Go: Dilemmas for Parents whose Son or Daughter has a Mental Handicap*, Milton Keynes: Open University.

Ryan, J. with Thomas, F. (1987) *The Politics of Mental Handicap*, (rev. edn), London: Free Association Books.

Trevillion, S. (1992) *Caring in the Community: A Networking Approach to Community Partnership*, Harlow: Longman.

Wenger, G. C. (1991) 'A network typology: from theory to practice', *Journal of Aging Studies* 5, 2, 147–62.

Young, I. M. (1990) 'The ideal of community and the politics of difference', in L. J. Nicholson (ed.) *Feminism/Postmodernism*, London: Routledge.

Chapter 8

Staff models and practice

Managing 'trouble' in a community-based programme for chronically mentally ill adults in the USA

Dana M. Baldwin

INTRODUCTION

During and after World War II, the need for psychiatric services in the United States increased significantly. Day treatment, half-way houses and therapeutic communities all came into their own in the postwar years. The 1960s brought the deinstitutionalization movement in which large psychiatric institutions reduced their resident populations and some closed their doors. The impetus behind this movement sprang from different quarters: politicians who wanted to reduce state budgets, mental health advocates who wished to remedy or prevent 'social breakdown syndrome' or 'institutionalism' (Goffman 1961; Gruenberg *et al.* 1962; Wing and Brown 1970), as well as the development of antipsychotic medication and the therapeutic community. The end result was that many of the chronically mentally ill were returned to the community. Although the 1963 Community Mental Health Centers Act established community mental health centres (CMHCs), they were so broadly defined that they were criticized for treating the 'worried well' and ignoring the more pressing needs of the chronically mentally ill (Talbott 1978; Chacko 1985; Foley and Sharfstein 1983). In response to these critiques, CMHCs began to mobilize and redirect some of their resources. A number of CMHCs established psychosocial treatment programmes geared towards treating a chronically mentally ill population (Thompson 1994). Harbor House,[1] a psychosocial programme for the chronically mentally ill described in this chapter, is a product of this initiative.

As in treatment programmes of all kinds, the staff of Harbor House must contend with the fact that certain kinds of 'trouble' occur over and over again, especially among certain clients. While the staff of these programmes may have ideas as to why particular clients are more difficult than others, staff generally tend to view these problems as residing in the client, rather than being a product of the way the programme is organized and structured, or the wider culture. The research discussed in this chapter describes a treatment programme which employs two partially conflicting treatment models. These models are not simply ideological or cognitive, but also have tangible structural and organizational manifestations. It is because of these two models, and their structural and organizational expressions, that 'trouble' becomes unavoidable and compelling. I will examine how the two treatment models, together with staff conceptions of two general diagnostic types – Borderline Personality Disorder (BPD) and schizophrenia – are inextricably involved with how 'trouble' is defined and handled.

This research draws upon the cultural insights of a 'meaning-centred' medical anthropology, a constructivist approach which focuses on the interpretive activities through which health care practitioners formulate or constitute the world to which clinical knowledge refers (Kleinman 1980; Good 1994). This study is in line with ethnopsychiatric research conducted in western mental health settings which recognizes the culturally constructed nature of professional psychiatry. In this view, the knowledge and practice base of professional 'scientific' psychiatry is put on the same epistemological footing as informal, 'folk' psychiatries (Gaines 1992a, 1992b; Nuckolls 1992; Good 1996).

This study also addresses one major critique of the constructivist approach by demonstrating the importance of incorporating structure and organization into the analysis (van Velsen 1967; Lazarus 1988; Pappas 1990; Wright and Morgan 1990). Most research by 'meaning-centred' investigators has been primarily concerned with describing the health beliefs and 'explanatory models' of the various individuals involved in the clinical encounter (Gaines 1982, 1992c; Good and Good 1982; Good et al. 1985; Hahn and Gaines 1985; Nations 1985). These accounts often fail to incorporate power, social structure and social control into the analysis. The present movement in critical medical anthropology seeks to address this failing (Morsy 1979; Morgan 1987; Frankenburg 1988; Baldwin 1990; Singer 1990, 1995; Scheper-Hughes 1990), though what it often leaves out is equally valuable – active human agency (Ortner 1984) and an intermediate level linking the patient and practitioner with the wider political economy.

Lazarus (1988) has argued that studies of the clinical relationship must expand on the explanatory models approach to focus on the institutional level between the medical system and the doctor-patient relationship. As Lazarus points out, 'without incorporating social organisation at the institutional level into theory, we cannot fully understand the social contexts of relationships and consequently why they work the way they do' (1988: 54).

THE THERAPEUTIC COMMUNITY AND PSYCHOSOCIAL REHABILITATION

The history of treatment of the mentally ill is a long and mostly undistinguished one in Euroamerican societies. Two bright points stand out, however: moral treatment in the eighteenth century (Rothman 1971) and the experience of the city of Gheel in Belgium (Roosens 1979). Both of these movements represented efforts to utilize aspects of the social environment for the humane treatment of the mentally ill. Both therapeutic communities and psychosocial rehabilitation can trace their lineage to these efforts.

Although Tom Main coined the term 'therapeutic community' in 1946, the main person to develop the concept was Maxwell Jones who worked at Belmont Hospital in the UK. Here he founded what he called a 'therapeutic community' for 'personality disorders' or 'working class psychopaths' (Jones 1953). At the same time, on the other side of the Atlantic, psychiatric rehabilitation was in its infancy. It had its origins in the late 1940s in New York when a group of former state mental hospital patients called 'We are Not Alone' began meeting on the steps of the New York Public Library to seek companionship after their release. A small group of concerned women learned of their situation and began what they called Fountain House, a social club for former mental patients (Dincin 1975: 131). Fountain House is the progenitor of psychosocial rehabilitation (also known as the Clubhouse model) and Harbor House, the subject of this study.[2]

Psychosocial rehabilitation is a general orientation which emphasizes clients' strengths and assets. Anthony and Nemec contrast psychiatric or psychosocial rehabilitation[3] with the medical model:

> Medical and psychiatric thinking tends to conceptualize health in terms of the absence of pathology. In the 'medical model,' a decrease in symptomatology (such as may be achieved through drug therapy) equals an improvement in health. Both physical and psychiatric rehabilitation view health in positive terms, such as competence and coping. In the rehabilitation model, an increase in skills and abilities enabling a person to cope better with his/her environment equals an improvement in health. Traditional psychiatric treatment aims for symptom reduction; psychiatric rehabilitation has health induction as its goal.
>
> (Anthony and Nemec 1984: 376)

More specifically, the Clubhouse model conveys four important messages to all members:

1 The [Clubhouse] is a club and, as in all clubs, it belongs to those who participate in it and who make it come alive . . .
2 All members are made to feel on a daily basis, that their presence is expected, that someone actually anticipates their coming to the program each morning and that their coming makes a difference . . . to everyone in the program . . .
3 All program elements are constructed in such a way as to ensure that each member feels wanted as a contributor to the program . . .
4 Following from the conscious design of the program to make each member feel *wanted* as a contributor is the intention to make every member feel *needed* in the program.

> (Beard *et al.* 1982: 47, emphasis in the original)

Harbor House, like other psychosocial rehabilitation programmes modelled after Fountain House, contains elements of the therapeutic community. Much like psychosocial rehabilitation, the therapeutic community is not a clearly defined entity. Jones (1968), Bloor (1986) and others point to the diversity of practices which characterize the therapeutic community. Rapoport's 1960 study of Maxwell Jones' therapeutic community identified four main themes: democratization (each member of the community has a voice), permissiveness (members should tolerate from each other a wide range of behaviour), communalism (functioning of the therapeutic community should be characterized by tight-knit inter-communicative and intimate sets of relationships), and reality confrontation (patients should be continuously presented with interpretations of their behaviour as seen by most others). Other investigators have identified features such as the following:

- Some degree of patient government (Jeffrey *et al.* 1976; Rossi and Filstead 1973);
- Distribution of responsibility and decision-making power (Rapoport and Rapoport 1957; Gunderson 1978);
- Multiple role possibilities for both patient and staff (Jeffrey 1985);
- Flattening of hierarchy of staff and patients (Rossi and Filstead 1973; Schimmel 1997);
- Open communication among both staff and patients (Rossi and Filstead 1973; Jeffrey 1985; Schimmel 1997);
- Work programmes as a form of therapy (Karasu *et al.* 1977);
- Programme must resemble real world as much as possible (Rossi and Filstead 1973).

Clearly, the Clubhouse model shares points in common with the therapeutic community. Included among them are: 1) distribution of responsibility and decision-making power; 2) multiple role opportunities for both clients and staff; 3) flattening of the staff-client hierarchy; 4) the notion that the programme should resemble the real world as much as possible; and 5) the importance of work.

THE CLUBHOUSE AND TREATMENT MODELS

Harbor House is structured and guided by two partially conflicting models: the Clubhouse model and the Treatment model. The programme is explicitly founded on a type of psychosocial rehabilitation called the Clubhouse model. Psychosocial rehabilitation is a general orientation which emphasizes clients' strengths and assets. The Clubhouse model is a multi-faceted behavioural approach which emphasizes the healing qualities of the community in the form of prevocational work units, member involvement and recreational activities (Dincin 1981; Beard *et al.* 1982; Fountain House n.d.; Smith *et al.* 1984; Woodside 1985). This model influences how Harbor House is organized, what clients do during the day, how staff relate to clients, even what clients are called ('members').[4] In contrast, the Treatment model stresses medication, psychotherapy and the adoption of a psychodynamic (versus behavioural) orientation. The Treatment model, as it is used here, has much in common with the 'medical model', a term which staff use as freely and frequently as the term 'Clubhouse model'. 'Treatment model' is used here rather than 'medical model' because of possible misunderstandings stemming from the latter's long and varied history of usage. The Treatment model is taken to be a multi-faceted concept characterized by dyadic and hierarchical relationships in which staff assume a 'one up' relationship to clients. Very generally, the Clubhouse model provides for the structure of Harbor House and is best seen in group or 'membership' activities, while the Treatment model is more 'behind the scenes' and can be observed on a case-by-case or situational basis.

Differences between the two models can be illustrated by examining different types of daily social interaction. Clubhouse model interactions typically occur over group activities such as prevocational work activities, member government and other committee meetings, and recreational events such as volleyball and outings. While Clubhouse activities are usually group activities, they can also be dyadic ones in the sense that a client interacts with another client or a staff member informally or over some sort of task in one of the prevocational work units. In contrast to these Clubhouse model activities, Treatment model interactions are dyadic, usually between staff and client, and are characterized by a staff member addressing a client's problem, be it medication non-compliance or psychological distress. Treatment model interactions between clients also occur, though less frequently (see Table 1).

Table 1 Features of the Clubhouse and Treatment models

Clubhouse	Treatment
Informal normalizing atmosphere. 'A community'	A 'clinic' removed from the everyday world
Staff role: 'generalist'/advocate	Staff role: limited (milieu worker or therapist)
Flattening of staff-client hierarchy (members have a voice)	Staff-patient hierarchy
'Members'	'Clients' or 'patients'
Emphasizes assets and strengths (rehabilitation)	Emphasizes deficits and symptoms
Behavioural orientation	Psychodynamic orientation
Sociotherapy	Psychotherapy
Community organization	Individual dyads (therapist–patient)
Community as healer	Individual as healer
Good of the community	Good of the individual

In many ways Clubhouse and Treatment models are complementary, allowing staff a flexibility of approach which they believe is necessary when trying to treat a range of psychiatric disorders. In other ways, however, the models are contradictory or conflicting in that they may call for different courses of action. For instance, contradictions are built into the programme at the very broadest level. In order for the programme to survive, staff must contend with two potentially conflicting requirements which can be traced back to the demands of the two models: 1) as a treatment facility, they must attract and keep a large number of clients with a wide range of disorders; and 2) as a Clubhouse, they have to make sure Harbor House remains a safe place for everyone. It is in this sense that 'model conflict' or 'model muddle' becomes a much more compelling concept than is conventionally thought (see, for instance, Siegler and Osmond 1974). That is, the kinds of cases that staff consider particularly troublesome, as well as the inter-personal difficulties that arise between and among them because of troublesome behaviour, can be viewed to some extent as the products of ideological and structural contradictions and ambiguities in the programme. As in Rhodes' study of a psychiatric emergency room, contradictions in context are inextricably linked with contradictions in practice (Rhodes 1993: 131).

The first part of the chapter describes the research methods, the setting, its staff and clients, as well as some of the tensions and ambiguities that arise in the programme as a result of the two models. In the second part, I examine how psychiatric diagnoses are constructed, and how these, together with the structure and organization of the programme, impact on the nature of 'trouble' in Harbor House.

METHODS

I conducted ethnographic research at Harbor House over the course of two and a half years, though intensive data collection did not take place until the last eleven months. I observed, participated in and documented weekly staff meetings as well as a range of formal and informal daily activities involving both clients and staff. In addition to these activities, I conducted extensive semi-structured, open-ended interviews with staff. Informal interviews were conducted intermittently to clarify emerging questions and themes.

As the research progressed, I became woven into the Harbor House network of relationships, established a comfortable rapport with both staff and clients, and became able to observe relatively unobtrusively. The importance I attached to maintaining good rapport and a low profile was reflected in how I collected the data. I confined use of a tape recorder to formal interviews. I felt that using a tape recorder outside this context was both inappropriate and reactive, especially since many of the remarks made to me by staff and clients were off the cuff and addressed more to me as a friend than as a researcher. Other than the formal interviews, which were audiotaped and transcribed, data derives from narrative fieldnotes of staff meetings and daily Harbor House events. Data analysis entailed conducting a thematic analysis of all fieldnotes and interview transcripts.

THE SETTING, STAFF AND CLIENTS

Harbor House is located in the Los Angeles area of California. Situated half a block from the more clinical-looking CMHC, Harbor House leases the spacious top floor of a large, two-storey red brick building. After passing a small flower garden and climbing two sets of old wooden stairs, one enters the main room, a large airy space with comfortable but worn furniture. As with other clubhouses, an attempt has been made to make the interior informal and home-like, while still making room for prevocational and recreational activities.

Harbor House has morning and afternoon programmes. The morning is designed as a Clubhouse programme, with three prevocational work units (a Clerical Unit, a Kitchen Unit and a Maintenance Unit), informal socializing and other member-involvement activities. The afternoon programme is more like a traditional day treatment programme in that it is more structured, there is no informal socializing, and members are expected to participate in groups ranging from art therapy to closed group therapy. Because of the increased programme structure, troublesome incidents occur less often in the afternoon than in the morning. The analyses of the two models presented in this chapter are primarily based on what occurs during the morning Clubhouse programme.

Harbor House is staffed by people with either bachelors or masters degrees. Two staff members have clinical counselling licences, and none of the staff have doctoral or medical degrees. Many of these staff have been with the programme for a number of years. Of the nine staff members present during the research period, six had been with Harbor House since it was founded five years earlier and the others had been with Harbor House for a year or less.

Harbor House membership fluctuates between 110 and 120 clients, though on any given day only about half that number might attend. The membership is quite heterogeneous in terms of diagnosis:[5] 56 per cent of the clients have primary diagnoses of 'schizophrenic disorders' and 'psychotic disorders not elsewhere classified'; 21 per cent have diagnoses of 'affective disorders'; 16 per cent have primary diagnoses of 'personality disorders', and the rest have miscellaneous mental disorders.[6]

CONTRADICTIONS WITHIN THE CLUBHOUSE

Psychiatric rehabilitation proponents generally argue that work and recreation activities are designed to enhance clients' strengths and assets. Ms Drake, the programme director and a rehabilitation advocate, takes this a step further and implies that rehabilitation *is* therapy; she contends that these activities not only enhance clients' strengths but also manage and contain their symptoms. In her view, the programme structure rather than individual staff members should be the primary change agent. Ms Drake explained that the programme treats clients – that is, 'contains' their symptoms – in the following ways:

> We provide structure, we provide tasks that may be soothing or stimu-lating or may reduce their preoccupation with their crazy thoughts. We may dyad them . . . which requires them to say something. Some people think that hearing voices is subvocalizing, so we do something that makes them talk, so it interrupts that. So we are intervening on the symptoms with the structure of the programme.

As this quotation indicates, Ms Drake is firmly in line with the behavioural orien-tation of most Clubhouse practitioners. As such, individual psychotherapy is not for the most part condoned on the premises, especially in the morning.

Yet, as a treatment facility, staff frequently need to deal with symptomatic clients on an individual basis. The programme has attempted to deal with this need by creating two types of staff roles: advocate and milieu worker. The role of advocate epitomizes the ideal of the 'generalist', a person who does everything from supervising the prevocational work units to giving support and advice or serving as buddy on recreational outings. The role of milieu worker is more limited. Ms Vahn and Ms Simpson, the two licensed clinical staff who serve in this role, act as crisis managers and are responsible for monitoring and inter-vening with symptomatic clients.

The role of milieu worker contains within it an inherent contradiction. On the one hand, the Clubhouse model as espoused by the programme director postulates that the work-oriented milieu will treat the client. On the other hand, the milieu worker, whose job is to treat 'symptomatic' clients, has to intervene and deal with these clients on a one-to-one basis. Intervention can mean different things; it can entail encouraging medication compliance, asking about symptoms, or making brief psychotherapeutic interventions.

Psychotherapy is a Treatment model intervention which exists uneasily within a Clubhouse environment, especially given the director's stance that these kinds of interventions should not be part of on-going Clubhouse activities in the morning. Ms Vahn told me that one of the worst aspects of her job is how Ms Drake does not like her to spend any time alone in her office during the morning, since that means that when clients want or need individual psychother-apeutic attention, she is unable to give it to them.

THE THERAPEUTIC IMPERATIVE

Harbor House has few firm rules. Ms Drake characterizes Harbor House as a low expectation, highly individualized programme in which 'there aren't many bottom-line rules that we live with'. Only in cases which involve violence or weapons, when the safety of the community is directly threatened, do rules get strictly applied. Other than that, rules become so flexible that they are better called expectations. There is wide variability in the degree to which these rules or expectations are applied and advocates are given a great deal of autonomy in dealing with their clients.

The flexibility of 'rules' is complicated by the fact that advocates have the option of allowing their clients to break rules, especially when there is a 'therapeutic' reason involved. In an often-used analogy comparing advocates to parents, Ms Drake stated the rationale for this: 'It's like a family. My Mom will let me do something and your Mom won't let you.'

In the end, the *therapeutic imperative*, the requirement that staff absolve symptomatic members of responsibility and treat their symptoms, overrides the egalitarian ideals put forth by the Clubhouse model. Given the Clubhouse model, which postulates that members work 'side by side' with other members and staff, staff attempt to treat all their clients equally, at least to the extent that clients' abilities allow for it. The therapeutic imperative cuts through this egalitarian ideal by explicitly recognizing that each client must be dealt with on an individual basis.

The therapeutic imperative is most clearly seen when a client is psychotic. According to Ms Simpson, 'I don't believe that if someone is psychotic, that I should sit by and let them make decisions for themselves.' It is in this respect that the Clubhouse model and the Treatment model complement each other. Ms Simpson describes this complementarity the best:

> For me how I kind of conceive of meshing the two models is that it's a psychosocial rehabilitation programme as long as someone is capable of making decisions for themselves. When they are not capable of making decisions for themselves, I then treat them. That kind of goes on a continuum too, but if somebody is actively psychotic, we intervene with that person, which isn't really psychosocial rehabilitation because in psychosocial rehabilitation it's kind of letting the members decide what they want to do and staff in the purest sense would not intervene at all.

DIAGNOSIS IN THE CLUBHOUSE

Staff understandings of client diagnoses

Most of the long-term staff at Harbor House have developed strong opinions and feelings about what to expect from clients with different diagnoses, as well as ideas about how they personally react to these different types. These impressions and feelings cannot be traced back in any direct way to textbook descriptions of psychiatric diagnoses (Lock 1985). Similarly, these diagnostic impressions and feelings are influenced by a number of non-clinical factors (cf. Helman 1985; Gaines 1979, 1992c; Light 1980; Pill 1987; Brown 1987; Stein 1986).

Most of the staff had little trouble articulating what diagnosis means to them.

When asked about diagnosis in an open-ended manner, most staff singled out two diagnostic types for comment: Borderline Personality Disorder (BPD) and schizophrenia. References to 'borderlines'[7] were common; these types of clients were brought up frequently in the staff meetings, largely because staff found them among the most difficult to treat.[8]

While BPD and schizophrenia were the two diagnoses most commonly mentioned by staff, depression was much less frequently mentioned. This no doubt stems from the fact that there were relatively few depressed people (specifically, depressed people without other psychiatric problems) and these were the least likely to cause problems in the programme. According to Ms Drake, they were also the most easily and effectively treated in the programme.

It must be stressed that staff discussions about diagnosis, particularly BPD, were often intended as an impressionistic and shorthand way of communicating with other staff about a particular facet of a client's personality or behaviour. Light (1980), in his work with psychiatric residents, made much the same point. He argued that American Psychiatric Association diagnoses were 'an essential, telegraphic vocabulary' which provided organizational and legal labels and facilitated easy communication (1980: 44).

More than any other type of personality disorder, staff conceptions of BPD were stereotyped and carried a strong negative emotional charge. Rather than intending their use of this diagnostic label to be clinically valid, diagnosis was used as a heuristic means of organizing and communicating thoughts about clients. The following excerpts are observations about BPD taken from interviews with staff:

> [A] diagnosis that sets off flags is borderline personality. It means to me that they are going to be manipulative, personally intrusive and attacking towards me – those are the ones who come and say, 'What degree do you have?', 'How long have you been working here?', 'You're not a doctor, huh?' I get bristly; I get ready to do battle when I have a borderline coming in. Also, I set real firm limits; I'm not going to give them free rein to do what they want. When I get them in here, though, that kind of goes.

> A borderline is going to be intensely labile, they are going to be really down low and really highly excited. The borderline is going to be much more intense in their relationship attractions. They are not going to have a steady relationship situation like with the staff. They are going to really pull and avoid, push and avoid, and they are going to most often pull out either the need to protect and nurture or to punish and hurt. Those are the feelings that I would have internally about these people. They are going to pull for me for a bizarre feelings, they are going to make me feel . . . overconsumed.

When I'm told someone has a borderline personality disorder, my reaction is to put my guard up. . . . I have the strongest reaction to the word 'borderline'.

[With] the borderline I feel like I am on trial. I feel like everything I say can and will be held against me so that makes me guarded.

Contrast these comments about BPD with those that staff made about clients with schizophrenia:

'Paranoid schiz' sends off some flags for me; make sure that you give this person some room. That's the paranoid schiz chair over there [in the corner]. If anybody sits there, I'm pretty clear on the diagnosis. If that was a neurotic, depressed, shy person who was sitting there, my move would be to sit next to them. If it's a paranoid schiz, then I'm going to stay here.

I have the least reaction to schizophrenic diagnosis. It doesn't mean much to me except that I may have to hear some crazy thinking. If we have someone paranoid, I figure we'll have to deal with some hostility and some 'looks'.

When I'm in the room with a schizophrenic-type person, I feel like this . . . a blank [laughter]. No, really. There's a feeling that there's a vacancy, there's a connection missing.

A schizophrenic is really flat or really kind of consistent. Look at the demeanour, the carriage, see over an extended period of time, they are going to be impoverished and flat. . . . I would take more 'care' of someone, or assist them in their functioning if they were really perceptually screwy – like schizophrenia . . . whereas with a borderline person I would not. I would be more neutral. . . . A schizophrenic is burned out, their whole existence is a kind of burn out or steady state of craziness.

The above quotes show that staff conceive of borderline clients to be, among other things, 'manipulative' (or what they also sometimes call 'gamey' or 'attention-getting') 'personally intrusive', and 'intensely labile'. In reaction to these qualities, staff 'get bristly', and feel like they are 'on trial' and need to put their 'guard up'. Staff reactions to schizophrenics are quite different. With the exception of paranoid schizophrenics, from whom they expect some 'hostility' and 'looks', staff feel that there is a great deal of variability among schizophrenics. Nevertheless, they also describe schizophrenics as being 'blank', 'vacant' and 'flat'.

As the preceding quotations suggest, borderlines have the ability to trigger aversive emotional responses in staff. This is reflected in the fact that staff sometimes assess the characters and even the moral worth of borderline clients and find them lacking. Ms Drake, for instance, said that one client is 'not a nice man' and called another male client 'yukky'. Ms Simpson alluded to similar feelings when she said the following about a new client: 'My instinct is to stay away from her which means she may very well be borderline. My intuition is usually right.' In the latter case, Ms Simpson used her 'intuition,' namely her aversion to the client, as a diagnostic indicator.[9]

Staff beliefs about treatment

When staff were asked to talk about the treatment that they provide clients, they invariably answered this question by talking about schizophrenia and the importance of neuroleptic medications. These responses are understandable in part because the majority of clients at Harbor House are diagnosed with schizophrenia, and in part because rehabilitation programmes such as Harbor House are designed, albeit implicitly, to work with major mental disorders, mainly individuals with schizophrenia. Yet staff tend to think of schizophrenia as having a biological base and personality disorders as not having one.[10] For this reason, neuroleptic medications are thought to be the most important means of reducing the psychotic symptoms characteristic of schizophrenia, but not of personality disorders. The belief that patients with schizophrenia respond to antipsychotic medication and borderline patients do not informs both staff understandings and practice.[11]

Similarly, in cases where Harbor House staff were not sure about the extent to which a client had a major mental disorder such as schizophrenia or a personality disorder such as BPD, they sometimes made tentative differential diagnoses on the basis of clients' responses to antipsychotic medications. For example, in discussing an incident in which a client, Denton, almost got into a fight with another client at the pool table, Ms Drake asked in the staff meeting, 'Is Denton on medication?' Mr Bundy replied that he did not think so; he believed that Denton has 'more of a character thing'. Likewise, in trying to determine the diagnosis of a new client, Gerald, Ms Simpson noted that his chart indicated he was not taking antipsychotics. 'Why would someone who is psychotic not be on antipsychotics?' asked Mr Bundy. In an interview later, Mr Bundy had this to say:

> The medication regimen – he's not on psychotropic medications right now. . . . He refuses to take them and they haven't had much of an effect. When he flips out, it's more brief, reactive-type psychotic episodes. There's a strong affective component to his behaviour. . . . I think it's just real characterological.

More on the therapeutic imperative

The therapeutic imperative states that when a client is psychotic and not capable of making sound decisions, staff must intervene and treat the client. The key issue here is how staff judge whether a client is psychotic or not. While this judgement may be fairly clear-cut in most cases, in others it is not. When asked to tell me how they can tell that someone is psychotic, most of the staff fumbled and said the usual things about bizarre statements and behaviour. Underlying all statements about psychosis was the notion that a psychotic person is 'out of control'.[12] Yet there was another meaning to being 'out of control': manipulation. When I asked Ms Vahn if a person who is out of control is psychotic, she replied, 'It certainly would be a sign . . . [but] he might just be being manipulative. There again it's according to the individual. . . . You go incident by incident.' The idea that being 'out of control' is either a result of psychosis or manipulation came up over and over again. Yet when asked how one can tell whether a client is psychotic or manipulative, staff generally replied that it is 'intuitive' and each case has to be considered individually.

The notion that 'out of control' can mean either psychotic or manipulative behaviour is an important one, one which has major ramifications for how staff respond to clients' untoward behaviour. Since staff believe that they need to intervene with psychotic behaviour, but not always with manipulative behaviour, staff judgements as to what kind of behaviour a client is exhibiting are critical.

Underlying all evaluations of clients as 'in control' or 'out of control' are notions about who is and is not responsible for their actions. While one of the goals of Harbor House is to make clients as responsible for their actions as possible, this means different things when applied to clients with BPD and schizophrenia.

Staff evaluations and treatment of BPD clients

Individuals with BPD and other personality disorders tend to be some of the 'highest functioning' clients in the programme. They are the most capable of assuming responsibility in the Clubhouse, and the most able to actualize the Clubhouse ideal of member involvement. Yet because they are often involved in 'member government' and other membership activities, these clients are also often able to evade expectations made of other clients. Both staff and other clients recognize that special rules sometimes apply to them. As a group, they are the hardest for the Clubhouse to deal with because there is less staff consensus about what is expected of them. This lack of consensus frequently results in strong disagreements among the staff. By itself, lack of consensus is not enough to cause dissent among staff. However, when coupled with the kinds of aversive emotions that borderline clients are capable of evoking, the recipe for conflict is complete. There was not one instance of strong staff disagreement involving a person with a schizophrenic disorder, whereas this happened in several cases involving personality disorders.

The most visible expression of client responsibility for the programme is the Clubhouse expectation that all clients work in a prevocational work unit for at least half an hour in the morning. This expectation repeatedly gave rise to problems between and among staff. On the one hand, there is the Clubhouse expectation that all clients will be treated similarly – individual differences are minimized. The Treatment model, on the other hand, emphasizes individual differences and maintains that clients must be treated on a case-by-case and situational basis (see Table 1, above).

There were those borderline clients who were expected to work but did not. Vinnie, for instance, became the subject of heated discussion when Ms Drake and Mr Bundy argued over whether and how much he should work. In this case, Mr Bundy offered a psychodynamic reason for why he did not push Vinnie to work on the unit. Ms Drake, on the other hand, demanded that staff be consistent in their expectations that everyone work, so that even if Vinnie really did not work he must *act* as if he did. That is, Vinnie's behaviour must be consistent with the Clubhouse expectation that all clients do some work in the morning. Ms Drake and Mr Bundy debated this in the staff meeting as follows:

MS DRAKE: [*asking Mr Bundy*] Does he work in the kitchen?

MR BUNDY: Sometimes. He works on talking.

MS SIMPSON: He gives a running commentary on how people are doing.

MS DRAKE: [*not satisfied with the answer*] Does he participate on the work unit?

MR BUNDY: Sometimes. He's probably involved to his capacity right now.

MS DRAKE: [*not really caring whether he's involved to his capacity right now; she just wants to know whether he does anything. The tension rises*] Should he come in the morning? Members may see him as getting specialness. It's risky to let him have that kind of leeway when everyone else is expected to work. There must be some evidence that he is contributing to the work unit. . . . Even George, at first, did his half hour, or at least he would act like it. He shouldn't appear like he's not contributing.

MR BUNDY: [*standing his ground*] I think he is involved.

MS VAHN: [*pitching in for Mr Bundy*] If Mr Bundy is in the kitchen, he will come in. If I'm in the kitchen, he makes some excuse, like his arm is hurting. He does make contact with Mr Bundy when he's there.

MS SIMPSON: When I ask him to help me, he will if he has some choices. For instance, if I say he can chop tomatoes or grate cheese. [*Ms Simpson interprets this as Vinnie's need to be 'one-up'*]

MS DRAKE: He seems to be at the pool table all the time.

This case points up the differences between the Clubhouse model behavioural orientation and the Treatment model psychodynamic orientation. The fact that Ms Drake insists that clients at least *look* like they are working is consistent with her focus on the milieu. In contrast, Mr Bundy's belief that Vinnie is doing as much as he is capable of given his psychological state is consistent with his emphasis on the individual. 'Capable' is the key word here. From a cognitive point of view, Vinnie was 'capable' of working. This is precisely what Ms Drake was responding to. From a psychodynamic perspective, though, Vinnie resisted because he had not worked through certain issues germane to authority figures and their attitude to work.

This case also demonstrates how rules, such as expectations that people work, are enforced most strongly in cases where clients are perceived as defiantly breaking them or acting passive-aggressive – that is, where clients deliberately choose not to comply. These expectations are waived in cases where staff do not view the clients as deliberately trying to break the rules. These clients are generally less 'functional' and more symptomatic. Ms Koller makes this point when she describes how she decides whether or not someone should work: 'If they are symptomatic then that's OK, as long as they are here . . . but if they are just being real resistant, it's almost like they are taking control of a boundary that they have decided to intrude upon.'

Staff evaluations and treatment of clients with schizophrenia

Clients with schizophrenia also go 'out of control', though the meaning attributed to this is very different than with borderline clients. In general, clients with schizophrenia who are 'out of control' are thought to be psychotic, not manipulative. The idea of losing control is one that is employed by staff and clients alike. The following excerpts are comments made in the Confusion Group[13] by Ms Simpson, the facilitator, and group members:

> When Claudio spoke about feeling 'confused' at the shopping mall, Ms Simpson asked him if he felt like he would go out of control.

> Derek said about Claudio, who was evincing uncontrollable laughter, 'I don't think that Claudio has much control over his laughter.' When Claudio decompensated even further, Ms Simpson intervened and told him 'You're losing control, Claudio. You need to be in a safe place.'

> When Rafael asked Billy what he meant by 'insanity', Billy replied, 'not being able to control yourself'.

Clients with schizophrenia who are experiencing psychotic symptoms are relieved of responsibility, including the expectation that they work. Since their behaviour is not viewed as volitional and hence manipulative, as is the case with borderline clients, no moral judgement is made and no sanctions are applied. For instance, when one young man diagnosed with schizophrenia became very symptomatic and 'flaked out' on his job running the snack bar, he was not criticized or blamed.

Since clients with schizophrenia are not viewed as manipulative, and because their actions do not usually carry a negative emotional charge, staff are generally more willing to accommodate their wishes. Changing work units is a good example. When clients with diagnoses of schizophrenia want to switch work units, their requests are routinely granted. Such is not the case with borderline clients. Their requests to change work units generally entail a good deal of discussion and are not always granted.

Of the two diagnostic types dealt with here – schizophrenia and BPD – the behaviourist orientation of the Clubhouse appears best suited for individuals with schizophrenia, and not so well suited for borderlines. More specifically, it appears that the Clubhouse, especially when combined with neuroleptic medications, works best for individuals with stabilized schizophrenia, of whom there are a number at Harbor House. Clients with schizophrenia whose symptoms are controlled usually cause few problems for the Clubhouse, and are allowed all the responsibility that they want and can tolerate.

Staff consider medication compliance to be a valuable adjunct of the Clubhouse milieu. While actively psychotic clients may be difficult to deal with because they are, for example, medication non-compliant, disruptive, or self-destructive, staff generally agree on the course of action to follow. Staff actions are guided by the therapeutic imperative which states that if a client is psychotic and not capable of making sound decisions, staff must intervene and treat the individual. One-on-one therapeutic intervention takes clear priority over the milieu therapy espoused by the Clubhouse model. The therapeutic imperative is thus most clearly seen with regard to clients with schizophrenia who are actively psychotic.

For instance, James was constantly in and out of the hospital because of psychotic episodes and suicide attempts. Staff believed that the main cause of James' deterioration was his medication non-compliance. In part, James did not take his medication because he did not like the side-effects. More importantly, though, he usually did not take his medication because he refused to accept that he had schizophrenia. James told me on one occasion, 'I do not believe in schizophrenia. Anyone who says you're insane is insane themselves.' When I asked him whether the medication makes his thinking clearer, he flatly stated 'no'. He claimed that the medication did not help his thinking at all; it just helped him to sleep.

Staff believe that understanding the psychodynamic reasons why James denies his illness and has trouble with medication compliance is to miss the point. The bottom line is that he has these problems and they are jeopardizing his life. Staff tell him as clearly and unambiguously as possible that he has to take his medication; if he does not, then he has to pay the consequences. Ms Simpson explained that,

> With James, we've more taken the stance, 'James, bring in your medication.' I can remember when James jumped out of the window and just destroyed himself. But when he comes back and says, 'Ms Simpson, I

want to get back in the programme,' I'll say, 'James, look at what happens when you don't take your medication. We're going to lose you one of these days!' Be real clear with him that that's what I see as the connectors. With James, we've taken more the approach, 'You want to be in this family, you take your medication.' . . . It's a constant battle for him.

Dual diagnosis and diagnostic uncertainty

The notion that clients with schizophrenia who are 'out of control' are generally thought to be psychotic, whereas 'out of control' borderline clients are manipulative, is not always clear-cut. Even borderlines can have psychotic episodes, though staff tend to see this behaviour as manipulative in nature. In much the same way, the meaning of 'out of control' is complicated in cases where clients are thought to have both schizophrenia and BPD.

The case of Ellen, a woman with diagnoses of both schizophrenia and BPD, points up the different meanings that 'out of control' has for how clients are treated in the Harbor House Clubhouse. During Ellen's first two weeks at Harbor House, she cut her wrists twice. Although these cuts were very superficial and not life-threatening, they were quite conspicuous and frightening to other clients. As her advocate pointed out:

> She was cutting herself. We're not a facility that is equipped to search her for anything that she's using to cut herself, we're not a facility equipped to rush her to the hospital in case she cuts too deep. . . . The first week she got blood on the rug and on the chair. . . . I remember one of the clients mentioning [that] it scared him. We're not equipped for that kind of thing. We're mostly socialization.

Staff managed to get Ellen to quit cutting at Harbor House by firmly telling her that if she cut herself again on the premises then she would have to leave for the day. She never cut herself again at Harbor House.

More difficult to deal with were two dramatic episodes of hysteria. In both of these incidents, staff didn't give Ellen the amount of attention they thought she was seeking and she didn't have another hysterical episode.

Staff considered Ellen's outbursts to be both psychotic and attention-seeking (i.e. manipulative). This was reflected in Ms Drake's comment that Ellen may have schizophrenia, but 'it's the borderline that we have to manage'. Staff believed that Ellen's psychosis could best be treated by medication, while the manipulative behaviour indicative of her BPD diagnosis was considered more difficult to deal with because it affected the therapeutic milieu. Not only was her cutting upsetting to other clients, but as Ms Drake stated about her behaviour in general: 'She's frightening to other members. She puts up a big wall, and then acts like she really needs people. Other clients then feel like we're not taking care of her. It's tough in a milieu setting.' Thus, it was the 'borderline' behaviour, not the psychotic behaviour per se, that staff found most difficult to deal with in the Clubhouse.

The distinction between psychotic and manipulative behaviour that is high-lighted in Ellen's case has another implication for the Clubhouse as well. There were no clear-cut guidelines about how to intervene in her disruptive behaviour. When Ms Vahn commented, 'it's hard to sort out what is psychotic process and what is just manipulative', she was expressing frustration over how to under-stand, and thus best treat, Ellen's psychiatric problems. Staff believe that if a behaviour is psychotic, then they need explicitly to tell the client what is going on (i.e. what is real and what is not) and emphasize the importance of medication. If the behaviour is viewed as manipulative, then staff believe that they should set firm limits and try not to reinforce the attention-seeking behaviour by attending to it, something that is hard to do when a client is crying out hysterically. As Ms Vahn put it, 'how do you not reinforce the behaviour when the behaviour requires attending to?'

DISCUSSION AND CONCLUSION

This chapter has sought to demonstrate the importance of taking analytical account of the institutional or organizational level of analysis when examining staff-client interactions. I have focused specifically on staff understandings of diagnosis, how these understandings interface with the Clubhouse and Treatment models, and how these render some clientele more problematic than others.

Treatment and rehabilitation

Not only do Clubhouse staff attempt to treat clients' symptoms and deficits, they also aim to rehabilitate them by engaging them in a normalizing non-medical environment. Productive work activities are emphasized and self-determination is encouraged. This can cause some uncertainty among staff because of contra-dictory directives: What is the place of work in the programme? What are grounds for exempting different kinds of clients from work expectations? How much responsibility does one give members? When does one give it and when does one absolve members of it?

This can sometimes become an exercise in tightrope walking. The general problem of exactly how much power and authority staff have, and how much of it is passed on to members is never resolved. The issue of where the power lies is constantly changing; the answer depends on such things as the exact nature of the problem, the specific clients and staff involved, staff availability, the number of other clients needing attention and the overall 'state' of the community. As Rhodes (1993) similarly noted in her study of a psychiatric emergency room, the situational nature of practice cannot be avoided when there are internal contra-dictions in the programme. The fact that the solution is an emergent one can sometimes lead to problems. By not clearly distinguishing between the Clubhouse and Treatment models and thus becoming aware of the areas in which conflict is bound to arise, staff continue to experience similar problems.

Structure and explanatory models

Staff interactions with clients, including problem cases, have been analysed in terms of the way that staff conceptualize psychopathology and treatment, and how these conceptions are influenced by the organizational context in which they work. Staff explanatory models include ideas about the Clubhouse and Treatment models, ideas about how they emotionally react to clients with different kinds of diagnoses, ideas about the kinds of problems these clients typically have with other clients and in the Clubhouse milieu, and ideas about medication-responsiveness and treatment. These notions, and the actions to which they give rise, are shaped by the demands of a specific organization with specific characteristics: a low staff-client ratio, few firm rules, relative lack of structure and the expectation that clients assume some responsibility for the programme.

The Clubhouse and client heterogeneity

Harbor House staff have had to struggle with the issue of how to maintain the Clubhouse framework while at the same time making sure that clients with a range of different psychiatric disorders receive treatment appropriate to their needs. It is unrealistic to rely exclusively on the healing qualities of the milieu with such a wide range of psychiatric disorders.

The rehabilitation aims of the Clubhouse appear best suited to the needs of individuals whose schizophrenia has stabilized, not individuals with personality disorders (including 'borderlines'). The therapeutic imperative as applied to persons with schizophrenia provides relatively clear guidelines to action: it sanctions one-to-one intervention in the form of checking for medication compliance and implementing behavioural interventions (such as relieving work expectations). Such is not the case with one-to-one psychotherapeutic interventions aimed at borderlines which sometimes clash with the behavioural emphasis of the Clubhouse milieu.

The fact that borderline clients are difficult to treat in a milieu setting may not come as a surprise to clinicians, since the psychiatric literature largely presents explanations in psychodynamic terms that highlight patients' psychopathology (e.g. talk of 'splitting staff' and transference and countertransference), the staff, setting and broader cultural values and attitudes are much less frequently considered.

A constructivist approach sensitizes us to the fact that staff have certain biases which are reflected in such pejorative descriptors as 'yukky' and 'intrusive'. Though only borderline personality disorder has been dealt with in this chapter, staff attitudes toward borderline patients are not unique. Other personality disorders such as 'antisocial' and 'histrionic' personality disorders are also burdened by value judgements about patients' moral worth (Nuckolls 1992). Fabrega has argued that psychiatric diagnoses are 'commentaries on and of the self' (1993: 167). I would modify this statement to say that diagnoses of BPD, particularly, are commentaries on and of one's *essential* self.

Stein (1986), in a study of a family medicine clinic, described the 'splitting of affect' on the part of residents toward 'sick people' and 'trolls'. 'Sick people' constitute those patients who have a bona fide biomedical diagnosis and who are not held responsible for the control, if not cure, of that disease. In contrast, 'trolls' are a generally disdained group of patients who may or may not have a bona fide biomedical diagnosis and who are held responsible for the control of their disease. Stein goes on to say, 'the patient-typing diagnostic distinction between "sick people" and "trolls", together with the emotions associated with each, pervades medical practice and to a considerable degree competes with if not supersedes the official biomedical model' (1986: 225). The parallel between 'sick people' and 'trolls' and individuals with schizophrenia and BPD should be clear. By dichotomizing one's feelings between 'deserving' patients (those with schizophrenia) and 'undeserving' ones (those with BPD), the latter carry all the bad affect, thereby colouring whatever value resides in 'impartial' and 'objective' diagnostic categories. In fact, this study and that of Brown (1987) indicate that some practitioners rely heavily on these negative emotional reactions when determining whether or not an individual has BPD. Staff conceptions of diagnosis are thus far from impartial. In the case of clients with BPD, diagnosis is frequently laden with emotion and moral overtones.

Because there was little staff consensus about what was expected of borderline clients in the context of the Clubhouse, staff often disagreed over how to deal with them. These disagreements often arose because of the staff's aversive emotional reactions towards borderline clients, coupled with unresolved tensions over the place of work in the programme. These disagreements exposed latent tensions or cleavages in the programme's ideology and structure.

In sum, my purpose has not been to say that one model is superior to the other, or that both models should not be used simultaneously. Mentally ill persons living in the community face a myriad of challenges, from dealing with exacerbations of their illnesses, dealing with family members and neighbours, to maintaining housing and managing finances. No one model of mental illness and its treatment can effectively address all these potential problem areas. Care providers must necessarily have flexibility in their choice of therapeutic approaches. Both the Clubhouse and the Treatment models described in this chapter are useful, though staff should be made aware of the areas in which the two models conflict as well as of their biases and how these affect clients.

NOTES

1 The name of the programme as well as all other identifiers and personal names have been changed.

2 The therapeutic community movement as espoused by Maxwell Jones became popular in the United States as well. This chapter is concerned with only one variant of it, psychosocial rehabilitation.

3 Psychosocial rehabilitation is sometimes used interchangeably in the literature with the terms social rehabilitation and psychiatric rehabilitation. While there is some fuzziness in how these terms are used, in general, psychiatric rehabilitation is the broadest and most general category.

4 In practice, staff regularly refer to 'clients' in staff meetings whereas they almost always use the term 'member' when speaking with members. I will use both terms in this chapter and let the context dictate which term is employed.

5 Diagnosis was determined according to the Diagnostic and Statistical Manual III-R (DSM-III-R) (1987).

6 The programme included clients with a number of other diagnoses, among them bipolar disorder, personality disorders other than BPD and a few cases of mild mental retardation.

7 I realize that to refer to clients as 'borderlines', borderline personalities or schizophrenics rather than as people *with* these diagnoses is tantamount to implying that these individuals *are* their illnesses. Clearly, one's identity is more than one's diagnosis. With this caveat in mind, I will for the sake of convenience sometimes refer to 'borderlines' in the following, as this was the categorization used by staff themselves.

8 Significantly, schizophrenia and BPD are also the two main diagnoses dealt with in the psychiatric literature on therapeutic milieus (e.g. Adler 1973; Simon 1986; Van Putten 1973; Jeffrey, Kleban and Papernik 1976; Pardes *et al.* 1972).

9 In Brown's (1987) fieldwork at a CMHC, one of his informants, a clinical supervisor, said much the same thing. The clinical supervisor admitted to being sceptical of the BPD diagnosis, and observed,

> borderline is a countertransference diagnosis. It tells you more about the therapist than about the patient. We give the diagnosis to people we don't like. It tells you nothing about what to do. Other diagnoses tell you what to do, what to look for. It's more a sociological diagnosis than a psychiatric one, since it involves people doing things against the law or which upset people.
>
> (Brown 1987: 41–42)

10 Clients can have both schizophrenia and BPD, and even borderline patients can experience brief psychotic episodes, for which antipsychotic drugs are useful (Simon 1986: 570).

11 Brown (1987) also observed this in his work in a CMHC, leading him to propose a category of 'drug-related diagnoses'. 'In this type, patients are diagnosed according to past, present, or future responses to medication. The nature of their response is used to support or not support the diagnosis of a specific condition' (1987: 45).

12 In his deconstruction of the American professional psychiatric classification system, Gaines (1992b) has suggested that a central ethnopsychological aspect of the idealized self is the sense of 'self-control' and its absence.

13 The Confusion Group is a group for individuals with schizophrenia which meets in the afternoon.

BIBLIOGRAPHY

Adler, G. (1973) 'Hospital treatment of borderline patients', *American Journal of Psychiatry* 130, 32–6.

Anthony, W. A. and Nemec, P. B. (1984) 'Psychiatric rehabilitation', in A. S. Bellack (ed.) *Schizophrenia: Treatment, Management, and Rehabilitation*, New York: Grune and Stratton.

Baldwin, D. M. (1990) 'Meeting production: the economics of contracting mental illness', *Social Science and Medicine* 30, 9, 961–8.

Beard, J. H., Propst, R. N. and Malamud, T. J. (1982) 'The Fountain House model of psychiatric rehabilitation', *Psychosocial Rehabilitation Journal* 5, 1, 47–53.

Bloor, M. J. (1986) 'Social control in the therapeutic community: re-examination of a critical case', *Sociology of Health and Illness* 8, 4, 305–24.

Brown, P. (1987) 'Diagnostic conflict and contradiction in psychiatry', *Journal of Health and Social Behavior* 28, 37–50.

Chacko, R. C. (1985) *The Chronic Mental Patient in a Community Context*, Washington DC: American Psychiatric Press.

Dincin, J. (1975) 'Psychiatric rehabilitation', *Schizophrenia Bulletin* 13, 131–47.

—— (1981) 'A community agency model', in J. A. Talbot (ed.) *The Chronic Mentally Ill*, New York: Human Sciences Press.

Fabrega, H. (1993) 'Biomedical psychiatry as an object for a critical medical anthropology', in S. Lindenbaum and M. Lock (eds) *Knowledge, Power, and Practice*, Berkeley: University of California Press.

Foley, H. A. and Sharfstein, S. S. (1983) *Madness and Government: Who Cares for the Mentally Ill?*, Washington DC: American Psychiatric Press.

Fountain House (n.d.) *Concept Paper*, New York: Fountain House.

Frankenburg, R. (1988) 'Gramsci, culture, and medical anthropology: Kundry and Parsifal? Or rat's tail to sea serpent?', *Medical Anthropology Quarterly* 2, 4, 324–37.

Gaines, A. D. (1979) 'Definitions and diagnoses: cultural implications of psychiatric help-seeking and psychiatrists' definitions of the situation in psychiatric emergencies', *Culture, Medicine, and Psychiatry* 3, 381–418.

—— (1982) 'Knowledge and practice: anthropological ideas and psychiatric practice', in N. J. Chrisman and T. W. Maretzki (eds) *Clinically Applied Anthropology: Anthropologists in Health Science Settings*, Dordrecht: D. Reidel.

—— (1992a) 'Ethnopsychiatry: the cultural construction of psychiatries', in A. D. Gaines (ed.) *Ethnopsychiatry. The Cultural Construction of Professional and Folk Psychiatries*, Albany NY: State University of New York Press.

—— (1992b) 'From DSM-I to III-R: voices of self, mastery, and other: a cultural constructivist reading of U.S. psychiatric classification', *Social Science and Medicine* 35, 1: 3–24.

—— (ed.) (1992c) *Ethnopsychiatry. The Cultural Construction of Professional and Folk Psychiatries*, Albany NY: State University of New York Press.

Goffman, E. (1961) *Asylums: Essays on the Social Situation of Mental Patients and Other Inmates*, Garden City NY: Doubleday.

Good, B. J. (1994) *Medicine, Rationality, and Experience*, Cambridge: Cambridge University Press.

—— (1996) 'Culture and DSM-IV: diagnosis, knowledge, and power', *Culture, Medicine, and Psychiatry* 20, 2, 127–32.

Good, B. J. and Delvecchio Good, M. (1982) 'Toward a meaning-centered analysis of popular illness categories: "fright illness" and "heart distress" in Iran', in A. J. Marsella and G. M. White (eds) *Cultural Conceptions of Mental Health and Therapy*, Boston: D. Reidel.

Good, B. J., Herrera, H., Delvecchio Good, M. and Cooper, J. (1985) 'Reflexivity, countertransference and clinical ethnography: a case from a psychiatric cultural consultation clinic', in R. A. Hahn and A. D. Gaines (eds) *Physicians of Western Medicine*, Boston: D. Reidel.

Gruenberg, E. M., Kasius, R. V. and Huxley, M. (1962) 'Objective appraisal of deterioration in a group of long-stay hospital patients', *Milbank Memorial Fund Quarterly* 40, 90–100.

Gunderson, J. G. (1978) 'Defining the therapeutic processes in psychiatric milieus', *Psychiatry* 41, 327–35.

Hahn, R. A. and Gaines, A. D. (eds) (1985) *Physicians of Western Medicine*, Boston: D. Reidel.

Helman, C. G. (1985) 'Disease and pseudo-disease: a case history of pseudo-angina', in R. A. Hahn and A. D. Gaines (eds) *Physicians of Western Medicine*, Boston: D. Reidel.

Jeffrey, W. D. (1985) 'Pathology enhancement in the therapeutic community', *International Journal of Social Psychiatry* 31, 2, 110–18.

Jeffrey, W. D., Kleban, C. H. and Papernik, D. S. (1976) 'Schizophrenia. Treatment in therapeutic community', *New York Journal of Medicine* 76, 3, 384–90.

Jones, M. (1953) *The Therapeutic Community*, New York: Basic Books.

—— (1968) *Beyond the Therapeutic Community*, New Haven: Yale University Press.

Karasu, T. B., Plutchik, R., Conte, H. R., Siegel, B. and Hertzman, M. (1977) 'The therapeutic community in theory and practice', *Hospital and Community Psychiatry*, 28, 6, 436–40.

Kleinman, A. (1980) *Patients and Healers in the Context of Culture*, Berkeley: University of California Press.

Lazarus, E. S. (1988) 'Theoretical considerations for the study of the doctor-patient relationship', *Medical Anthropology Quarterly* 2, 1, 34–58.

Light, D. (1980) *Becoming Psychiatrists*, New York: W. W. Norton and Company.

Lock, M. (1985) 'Models and practice in medicine: menopause as syndrome or life transition?', in R. A. Hahn and A. D. Gaines (eds) *Physicians of Western Medicine*, Boston: D. Reidel.

Morgan, L. M. (1987) 'Dependency theory in the political economy of health: an anthropological critique', *Medical Anthropology Quarterly* 1, 2, 131–54.

Morsy, S. (1979) 'The missing link in medical anthropology: the political economy of health', *Reviews in Anthropology* 6, 3, 349–63.

Nations, M. K. (1985) '"Hidden" popular illnesses in primary care: residents' recognition and clinical implications', *Culture, Medicine and Psychiatry* 9, 3, 223–40.

Nuckolls, C. W. (1992) 'Toward a cultural history of the personality disorders', *Social Science and Medicine* 35, 1, 37–47.

Ortner, S. B. (1984) 'Theory in anthropology since the sixties', *Society for Comparative Study of Society and History* 26, 126–66.

Pappas, G. (1990) 'Some implications for the study of the doctor-patient interaction: power, structure, and agency in the works of Howard Waitzkin and Arthur Kleinman', *Social Science and Medicine* 30, 2, 199–204.

Pardes, H., Bjork, D., Van Putten, T. and Kaufman, M. (1972) 'Failures on a therapeutic milieu', *Psychiatric Quarterly* 46, 29–48.

Pill, R. (1987) 'Models and management: the case of "cystitis" in women', *Sociology of Health and Illness* 9, 3, 265–84.

Rapoport, R. N. (1960) *Community as Doctor*, London: Tavistock.

Rapoport, R. N. and Rapoport, R. S. (1957) '"Democratization" and authority in a therapeutic community', *Behavioral Science* 2, 128–33.

Rhodes, L. A. (1993) 'The shape of action: practice in public psychiatry', in S. Lindenbaum and M. Lock (eds) *Knowledge, Power, and Practice*, Berkeley: University of California Press.

Roosens, E. (1979) *Mental Patients in Town Life: Gheel – Europe's Therapeutic Community*, Beverly Hills CA: Sage.

Rossi, J. J. and Filstead, W. J. (1973) *The Therapeutic Community*, New York: Behavioral Publications.

Rothman, D. J. (1971) *The Discovery of the Asylum*, Boston: Little, Brown, and Company.

Scheper-Hughes, N. (1990) 'Three propositions for a critically applied medical anthropology', *Social Science and Medicine* 30, 2, 189–97.

Schimmel, P. (1997) 'Swimming against the tide? A review of the therapeutic community', *Australian and New Zealand Journal of Psychiatry* 31, 120–7.

Siegler, M. and Osmond, H. (1974) *Models of Madness, Models of Medicine*, New York: Macmillan.

Simon, J. I. (1986) 'Day hospital treatment for borderline adolescents', *Adolescence* 21, 83: 561–72.

Singer, M. (1990) 'Reinventing medical anthropology: toward a critical realignment', *Social Science and Medicine* 30, 2, 179–87.

—— (1995) 'Beyond the ivory tower: critical praxis in medical anthropology', *Medical Anthropology Quarterly* 9, 1, 80–106.

Smith, M. K., Brown, D., Gibbs, L., Sanders, H., and Cremer, K. (1984) 'Client involvement in psychosocial rehabilitation', *Psychosocial Rehabilitation Journal* 8, 35–43.

Stein, H. F. (1986) '"Sick people" and "trolls": a contribution to the understanding of the dynamics of physician explanatory models', *Culture, Medicine, and Psychiatry* 10, 221–9.

Talbott, J. A. (1978) *The Chronic Mental Patient: Problems, Solutions, and Recommendations for Public Policy*, Washington DC: American Psychiatric Association.

Thompson, J. W. (1994) 'Trends in the development of psychiatric services, 1844–1994', *Hospital and Community Psychiatry* 45, 10, 987–92.

van Putten, T. (1973) 'Milieu therapy: contradictions?', *Archives of General Psychiatry* 29, 640–3.

van Velsen, J. (1967) 'The extended-case method and situational analysis', in A. L. Epstein (ed.) *The Craft of Social Anthropology*, New York: Tavistock.

Wing, J. K. and Brown, G. W. (1970) *Institutionalism and Schizophrenia*, New York: Cambridge University Press.

Woodside, H. (1985) 'The day center and its role as a social network', *Hospital and Community Psychiatry* 36, 2, 177–80.

Wright, A. L. and Morgan, W. J. (1990) 'On the creation of "problem" patients', *Social Science and Medicine* 30, 9, 951–9.

Chapter 9

A local anthropology of exclusion

John Given

> One knows intimately a local history, a social and psychic geography with its fault lines and upthrusts, just as one knows the landscape through which one moves daily. Such knowledge is particular and narrative in nature: it is just like – indeed it often is – gossip.
>
> (Carrithers 1992)

INTRODUCTION

This chapter reflects on the experience of a number of action research projects on 'problem estates' in the north east of England. The estates are viewed as 'landscapes of power' on which are inscribed and enacted the narratives of the powerful and the powerless. The boundaries between 'respectable' local culture and the 'dreadful enclosures' (Damer 1974; Walter 1977) are examined in terms of these narratives. Themes for the development of such narratives are located in local political, economic and social geographies, and elaborated in the routine interactions between the agents and agencies of 'local authority' and the residents of the estates. Following Layder's (1993) 'new strategies in social research', I attempt to describe and interpret the stories, reputations and narratives that evolved in and around the estate at the levels of context, setting, social situation and self.

I begin with a few comments about the context in which I found myself involved in these issues. In 1976 I got a job as a research associate in the social work department of what was then Newcastle Polytechnic in the north east of England. The job description included a remit to design and develop community-based action research projects. For four years previously I had worked voluntarily with a variety of community groups, focusing mostly on housing and welfare rights issues in some of the most disadvantaged parts of the city's West End. Inspired by a mixture of Freirean, Marxist and libertarian ideas, we developed pressure groups, campaigned on various issues and put up independent candidates in local elections. 'We' were all local residents, but while most were born and bred 'Geordies', some of us were students, or ex-students, and so regarded by the locals with considerable suspicion and some disdain. As a recent graduate in sociology, I fell into this category and was always aware, no matter how close to people or issues I became, that I had options – I could always walk away, I had an 'out'.

Having grown up in a 'rough' steel town and coming from a working-class Irish immigrant family, I didn't feel too out of place. I made some good friends in the West End, and spent a lot of time drinking and playing darts in various local bars, where outsiders were few and mostly unwelcome. My dad had been a champion darts player and so I could play a bit, an accomplishment that opened some interesting doors. I thought of myself more as an 'activist' than an anthropologist or sociologist and considered that the important issue was how people could have more say in, and more control over, decisions that affected their lives. Our style was confrontational and direct, most of the action took place in slum areas in west Newcastle (the 'Wild West') in the Civic Centre (Dan Smith's castle – sometimes also known as Newcastle PLD – the palace of lies and deceit), or in the offices of the local Department of Health and Social Security (the 'Broo').

These observations are intended to give the reader some idea of my orientation towards social and urban issues at the time. Like many activists, I found that there was a market for those with experiences like mine. I joined the growing ranks of the new professionals of deprivation.

The first project I became involved with was set up through a colleague who was a well-known independent councillor in South Tyneside. Through his contacts within the controlling political group, known locally as the 'Jarrow Mafia', we negotiated an action research role in relation to the Deans estate, an estate that had the worst reputation in the borough and which was about to be scheduled for demolition. The agreement we arrived at was that, from a base on the estate provided by the local authority (LA), we would research the estate, produce action plans in relation to identified issues, and pilot some of these. We were allowed access to a range of LA records including those of the housing and social work departments. A parallel negotiation within the Polytechnic produced an agreement to use the base as a fieldwork centre for social work students looking for experience of community-based action research. We undertook to staff the base three days a week and after some months of preparation, we 'set up shop' in a disused betting office on the edge of the estate, scrounged some furniture and fittings, had a phone installed and opened for business.

The day book records three visitors in the first afternoon. One complained that 'the old couple' were having their windows repeatedly broken and their rubbish bins kicked over. The second complained about riff-raff, the burglaries and the constant aggravation. The third wanted something done about her neighbours who were always drunk and shouting. In the first year over 500 visits to the shop were logged, a liaison role with LA departments was established, a social survey carried out, and a considerable amount of housing and welfare rights casework undertaken. The project lasted two years during which time the estate was demolished, and the population dispersed throughout the borough. Other projects on other estates followed, and over the next six years we had a unique opportunity to look at what was happening on and around such places.

Layder claims that his research strategy attempts to bridge the gap between macro- and micro-social analysis, and allows the researcher more fully to 'convey the "textured" or interwoven nature of different levels and dimensions of social reality' (Layder 1993). According to Layder, this approach has two general advantages. First, it allows the researcher to concentrate on the organic links between macro- and micro-levels of social analysis. Second, it views 'society or social reality as a series of independent layers each with its own distinctive characteristics', an approach which 'enables the researcher to be sensitive to the different units and timescales that are involved in social processes and social change' (Layder 1993). This strategy is summarized in Table 9.1, what Layder calls a 'resource map for research'. It is this that I shall apply to my account of the Deans estate.

I intend to apply this approach retrospectively to the study of the stories, reputations and narratives that evolved in and around the Deans estate, beginning at the level of context.

CONTEXT

Walter (1977) has argued that public housing schemes are 'a great domain of urban myths . . . [which] . . . in the manner of all mythology, are based on projections, social and psychological, which are all efforts of the mind, concealed from awareness, to externalise something that originates within'. I wish to consider whether the stories and reputations that surrounded the Deans could be regarded as forms of urban myth and if so, what kind of local narratives were being elaborated and what sort of 'projections' they incorporate. As Maines

Table 9.1 Resource map for research

	Research Element	Research focus
H	CONTEXT	Macro-social forms (e.g. class, gender, ethnic relations)
I		
S	SETTING	Immediate environment of social activity (schools, family, factory)
T		
O	SITUATED ACTIVITY	Dynamics of face-to-face interaction
R		
Y	SELF	Biographical experience and social involvements

Source: From Layder 1993

(1993) puts it, 'the most complex contexts are routinely understood and negotiated in local, personal, particular, and narrative ways'. I will begin with two 'contexting narratives' that were offered by senior LA officers in an early meeting.

Eighty per cent of those families are problem families.

That was a model estate that those animals have wrecked.

These two beliefs provided the essential elements of the dominant local 'Deans narrative', which featured a golden age finally destroyed by the arrival of the 'problem families'. It rapidly became apparent that these beliefs, or versions of them, were shared by officers, politicians and tenants, not all at once, and not all together, but enough of the time when the subject was under discussion for this to form the dominant local context within which the Deans had come to be understood.

To say that you were working on the Deans estate was enough to produce a flow of horror stories and prophecies of doom. Although I was used to this as a general reaction by non-residents of such areas, I was struck by the degree to which such ideas were embedded in the LA agencies which, perhaps somewhat naively, I had expected to take a more detached and professional view of things.

In our early meetings with the LA, it emerged that there was a debate in progress about whether to demolish the estate or attempt to renovate it. An openly expressed fear was that demolition would provoke a crisis as the movement of people from the Deans to other areas would spark off protests from the existing tenants and begin a cycle of decline in these new areas. Offering decent accommodation to such people was often commented on as a folly, with the fate of 'the model estate' often cited in support of such views. At times it felt like a local moral panic was threatening – the idea of a social 'contagion' was in the air. Looking at the Deans it was hard to believe it had ever been a 'model estate'. I was aware of examples of better quality working-class estates from the same period, having grown up on one, and also that better houses had been built at an earlier period in South Shields. In order to properly assess the model estate claim, it is first necessary to locate its construction in the relevant historical context.

Housing conditions in South Shields were among the worst in the country, and had been so since the latter part of the nineteenth century. The population of the town doubled in the twenty years between 1881 and 1900 and house building in no way kept pace, resulting in thousands of people being crammed into multiply occupied houses in conditions which, even by the standards of the day, were appalling. As the Tyne reaches north before curving east to empty into the North Sea, it helps to create a site for the town, effectively bounded on three sides by water, a site the town had now outgrown. Some sense of what things were like can be gained from the Medical Officer of Health's (MOH) report for

1891. When speaking of one slum area it said, quite simply, 'all such property should undoubtedly be closed as unfit for habitation'. In the following twenty years the borough used such housing acts as there were only to close or demolish the very worst properties and to clear up after the occasional spontaneous collapse.

By 1928 in the Thames Street/North Street area there were 1,735 inhabitants, of whom 676 lived in 212 one-roomed tenements, with only fifty-four containing less than three people, while the remaining 158 contained families of up to nine. What life was like in these slums can be gleaned from contemporary accounts and by looking at an example of a typical tenement in the riverside area of South Shields. This case is of particular interest, as it was from places like this that many of the Deans estate's first tenants moved. Any ideas they may have had about 'model estates' would have been developed against such backdrops.

Price (1982) details how in November 1928 a tenant, Mr Ishmail, complained about the state of the range in the one-room tenement he rented from a Mr Finn. When lit, it belched smoke into the room and windows had to be thrown open to let out the fumes. One of the borough's sanitary inspectors visited the property and then wrote to Mr Finn advising that either suitable repairs be undertaken or that a closure order would be made. The borough engineer had stated that in his opinion a heavy fall of snow would bring the property down! There then ensued a three-year tussle between Mr Finn and the council about what constituted repairs sufficient to make the house habitable. Mr Finn's attempts at repairs were halting and unconvincing to say the least, and the case took an even more Dickensian turn when, two years later he was arguing for a further postponement of the closure order on the grounds that 'it was not desired to disturb the tenants at Christmas' (Price 1982).

In common with many of the riverside properties in that area of town, the house had been cut into the ballast hills, mounds accumulated along the riverbank as ships had dumped their ballast over the years prior to taking on their cargoes of coal. In the absence of a damp proof course, the basement of 21 Rekendyke Lane was described as 'wet rather than damp', daylight could be seen through the ceiling of an upstairs bedroom and, as a result of the demolition of an adjacent property, one of its external walls was only four inches thick.

In 1933 a housing inspector listed the tenants, two of whom, Ismail and Ahmed, were probably part of the small community of Yemeni seamen who had been a feature of life in Shields since before World War I (Table 9.2).

In this one slum property, thirty-five people lived and shared one outside toilet and one tap in the yard. The rooms occupied by Oates and Foster were in fact semi-basement rooms, Foster's measuring 10 feet by 14 feet and housing nine people.

If there was misery in the slums there was money too. Mr Finn had bought the house in 1923, and clearance records show that he owned at least twenty others. He paid £95 for it and collected rents totalling £2 a week for ten years, a

Table 9.2 Tenants in 21 Rekendyke Lane/8 Barrow Street

Room	Tenant	Rent	Family size
Ground floor front	Oates	7/6	5
Ground floor front	Foster	5/9	9
First floor front	Watson	6/6	5
First floor back	Watson		
First floor front	Elliott	5/1	2
First floor back			
Second floor front	Ahmed	8/9	6
Second floor back			
Second floor front	Brennan	6/-	6
Ground floor	Ismail	6/-	2

Source: From Price 1982

profit approaching 1,000 per cent, and, if his other twenty recorded slum properties yielded a similar return, the basis for a small fortune in those days.

Mr Finn finally went to court in April 1933 to oppose the closure order for which the council had applied. Mr Finn was part of a powerful property owners' protection association who supported him in his case, which they rightly viewed as liable to set an important local precedent. Fortunes were clearly being made in these slums and several firms in business on Tyneside today can trace their origins back to the slums of prewar South Shields. Other large-scale landlords in the slum districts included the University of Durham and the Ecclesiastical Commissioners, which latter body was in 1930 asking £700 an acre for derelict land from the council in order 'to compensate themselves for ground rents lost because of the demolition of unfit properties' (Price 1982).

Mr Finn finally lost his case, but only on the grounds that the cost of repairs exceeded the value of the property and so would 'deprive the owner of the whole value of his property'. The judge also pointed to the availability of modern accommodation provided by the LA at lower rents than those now being paid by Mr Finn's tenants, on the newly completed Deans estate. One story we were told had Mr Finn dying in a local asylum, so obsessed had he become with demanding rents even when none were due that he was eventually committed. He apparently spent his last days wandering the wards demanding rent from other inmates.

One thing is clear: from these contemporary accounts, the first residents of the Deans estate came from some of the worst slums in the country. What kind of a place were they going to?

SETTINGS

In his discussion of intermediate levels of social organization, Layder (1993) suggests a number of questions about how the nature of the setting might intrude on, or influence, the action: 'is it enclosed or dispersed for instance, what forms of attachment and commitment do individuals have in these settings, what are the characteristic forms of power and authority and to what extent do conflict and tension characterise the setting?' Other writers have emphasized the close interrelationship between elements of situated activities and the settings in which everyday life takes place. Writers such as Sibley (1995) have recently talked about 'geographies of exclusion' and have begun to treat socio-spatial issues as being 'concerned particularly with symbol, ritual and myth, taking cues from social anthropology and psychoanalysis'. Earlier writers (Jacobs 1961; Newman 1972; Coleman 1985) took a rather narrower approach that pointed to the importance of design and organization of space as influences on social behaviour, particularly in relation to public housing schemes. How did the setting of the Deans estate come to influence the lives of those who lived there and the stories that were told about them?

In 1931, with South Shields the only municipality in the north to have done nothing about the slums, with one baby in five dying within a year of birth in the Thames street area, with local engineering firms needing to expand into the slum areas, and under the threat of penalties from central government, something was finally done. The council purchased land at Deans farm in spite of last-ditch objections by one Labour member to the purchase of this 'cheap and nasty land'. He declared:

> If . . . the ghost of Keir Hardy or Karl Marx could traverse it, it would say 'What have I done that my followers should send poor people to this land?' Why should the poor and needy be banished to the end of the borough facing Jarrow slake?
>
> (Price 1982)

The Deans was built in 1932. Two years earlier the local MOH had estimated that there was an immediate need for 4,236 new working-class houses to be built in the next three years alone. The effects of council house building schemes to date were summed up by one local councillor:

> There is one section of the community that is always forgotten and that is the slum dweller. We have not built a single house under any of our schemes which will provide suitable accommodation for one of those people who are forced to dwell in the slums.
>
> (*ibid.*)

In the absence of new houses, the slums simply had to be tolerated, and tolerated they were, in many cases until after World War II.

Photographs from the local history archive show that the site of the estate at Deans farm was liable to flooding. One of the first tenants I visited during the course of conducting a social survey lifted some floorboards in his living room to show stagnant water lying under them, which, he claimed, rose and fell with the tide on the nearby River Tyne! The site lay in the fork between two embanked railway lines which stood ten feet or more above the general level of the estate. The long triangular shape of the estate was defined by the two streets of Tyne and Thames Lanes that diverged from each other as they paralleled the railway lines until they ran into Deans Crescent, which fed, at each of its points, into a busy main road that defined the estate to the East. Two hundred and forty-eight flats were crammed onto this site, looking like redbrick terraces and semi-detached houses, although they were in fact a cheap variation on a local style known as 'Tyneside flats'. In the first twenty years of the century thousands of these flats had been constructed by speculative builders for the skilled working classes, and they remain a popular form of accommodation on Tyneside today. Those built on the Deans however suffer by comparison. Bedrooms had no fireplaces, and thus no heating, while the upstairs flats had only one entrance, with the kitchen between the rest of the accommodation and the staircase, thus rendering them potential fire traps.

Access to the estate was possible only from the east through either entrance to Deans Crescent, or by illegally crossing one of the railway lines. Well-worn tracks up the embankments showed that this was a routine procedure for many residents, especially the children and young men, who wished to avoid walking all the way down out of the estate, and back around to pubs and shops situated only yards from their houses by the more direct route. This practice, not to mention the obvious dangers involved, set up a running battle of wits between the responsible authorities and the estate's residents. Both these lines had been closed since the mid-1960s, but up to that time passing steam trains and the soot that drifted across the estate proved a curse when trying to wash and dry clothes without the benefit of washing machines, an irritation commented upon by several women who had lived on the estate at that time. Perhaps the main point to make about the site was that, as it was enclosed, no-one without business there would ever be liable just to pass through.

One rationale advanced for using sites like the Deans at the time of building was in relation to transport costs faced by workers being relocated to peripheral green field sites. In relation to the Deans development it was further argued that:

> The necessity of housing a population such as yours engaged in casual work at the docks within call of their employment is essential, and this can only be achieved by the building of flats of two storeys or more in height, to a density of twenty to the acre.
>
> (*ibid.*)

The casual work in question was hard to come by and entailed standing in 'the pen' twice a day and hoping to be one of the few chosen by the foreman. Failure to get work meant standing in a queue, again twice a day, to sign on the dole. For many men this meant a daily routine of standing in some form of queue for up to six hours.

In May 1931 the borough engineer had come up with a scheme which he described as 'the cheapest in the country', so cheap that in the first instance even the Ministry of Housing turned them down. A letter from the local Trades Council to the Minister of Housing later put on record the reservations of those tradesmen who actually built the flats. The letter commented both on the poor quality of materials being used, which they feared would lead to permanent dampness of the walls, and to poor aspects of the design, namely hot water pipes running through the larders, rendering them unsuitable for the storage of food.

In some respects decline was inevitable, a decline accelerated by the onset of World War II, which effectively suspended routine maintenance, rationed domestic fuel supplies, and severely disrupted social and family life. The physical fabric of the flats suffered as did the back gardens from the installation of Anderson air-raid shelters. The location of the estate so close to the docks and ship repair yards rendered it acutely vulnerable to the effects of German air raids and some houses were destroyed or damaged, luckily without loss of life. Elsewhere in South Shields, however, a total of 125 people were killed as a result of bomber raids, many in one incident when a communal shelter took a direct hit.

One tenant, whose family had lived on the estate since 1933, visited the project office and offered another theory of how the war years had played their part in the estate's decline. He said that in the war friends would often sign up on the same merchant vessel, which meant that if the ship were lost, the pattern of casualties was often highly localized, something which by his account had directly affected several Deans families. The place, he said, was never the same again.

Removal of the shelters did not take place until long after the war and was poorly executed, leaving many of the concrete foundations in place, inhibiting productive use of the gardens and doing nothing to enhance the look of the estate. In later years the poor condition of many of the gardens was often attributed to the 'couldn't care less' attitude of some of the tenants.

With the renewal of central government subsidy under Macmillan's government in the 1950s, the focus swung back to the building of good standard modern houses on green field sites. The Deans increasingly began to suffer by comparison and, although what was now perceived as its relatively central site continued to hold attractions for some, after this period few people without prior connections would voluntarily accept a house on the estate. As the estate became labelled as difficult to let, a conscious strategy of dumping problem tenants was adopted, in part as a way of letting empty properties, and in part as a way of trying to exercise some local social control. The Deans was now on its way to becoming what Damer (1974) and Walter (1977) have classically described as ' a dreadful enclosure'.

The evidence shows that the Deans estate was badly designed and cheaply built, on a poor site, with poor quality materials, for tenants who were deemed able to afford, or deserve, no better, and who had previously occupied some of the worst slums in the country. How was it possible that the Deans was being represented as a model estate, when it had clearly never been one?

One source of the myth can be seen to have sprung from the contrast between the conditions in the old riverside slums and those on the Deans. Tenants from the former probably did feel that they were moving into a model estate even if the Deans was well below the best contemporary standards of the day. Ironically, the original tenants and their children, who would form the bulk of the estate's population throughout the war and on into the 1950s, became in part responsible for the origin of the myth which would so complicate their lives in later years. Writers such as Denzin (1989) have talked about 'epiphanies' as interactional moments and experiences which leave marks on people's lives: 'they alter the fundamental meaning structures in a person's life'. Furthermore, 'the meanings of these experiences are always given retrospectively, as they are relived and re-experienced in the stories persons tell about what has happened to them' (*ibid.*). Moving from the riverside slums to the Deans was often described by the older tenants in such terms. One such resident told us that the living room in their tenement had no windows, and the only illumination was often from the candles that burnt beneath enlarged photographs of family members lost in World War I. His memory of moving as a young boy to a new flat on the Deans, he told us, was of 'moving to heaven'.

This account of why, for whom, where and how the Deans was built, goes some way towards explaining why it eventually became a 'dump estate', and goes a long way towards exposing the 'myth of the model estate'. If it was a model, it was only in comparison with the worst housing in the land, or as an example of how to replace one set of slums with another.

> A myth is, of course, not a fairy story. It is a presentation of facts belonging to one category in the idioms appropriate to another. To explode a myth is accordingly not to deny the facts but to re-allocate them.
>
> (Ryle 1949)

SITUATED ACTIVITIES

When Layder refers to situated activities, he is referring to face-to-face activity which takes place in a particular context and setting. The focus is on emergent meanings, understandings and definitions, as these are mediated both by the local language of context and setting, and the unique psycho-biography of the participating individuals. For our purposes we will look at how the activities situated on or around the Deans are interpreted in a series of competing narratives through which 'local authority' is constructed and maintained or resisted and challenged. The contextual narrative mentioned earlier had two main parts: the myth of the model estate, and the 'animal theory' used to describe the residents and to explain the estate's decline. I will look more closely at how and why such language could openly be used to describe a group of tenants, and what it tells us about the culture of 'local authority'.

> By revealing the stereotypes that shape the myths about life in housing projects I do not mean to romanticize or to deny the severity or bitterness. Everyone knows how harsh life can be there, but not everyone knows that it is not all bad.
>
> (Walter 1977)

Living on the Deans in the last few years of its existence was not an easy business but, as Walter's comment implies, not everyone thought it was all bad. A survey we conducted showed that roughly a third of the residents would stay if the houses were modernized, a third would consider staying, while a third wanted out at any cost. In an early meeting senior officers admitted that 'previously there was a definite policy of dumping the problem families together in South Shields and the Deans estate was one of the dumping grounds'. In the same meeting a senior officer claimed that 80 per cent of the Deans' residents were 'problem families'. The same survey also showed that 28 per cent of the tenants had lived there for more than fifteen years, 15 per cent for more than ten years, 37 per cent between two and ten years, and 20 per cent for less than two. A high proportion of households showed gross overcrowding; there was a high concentration of single-parent families, large numbers of young children, a high proportion of elderly and handicapped, and a very high level of unemployment and welfare dependency. The overall picture was one of extreme deprivation and dereliction. The records of the local authority showed that 11 per cent of the residents were 'known' to social services, 16 per cent to the housing department, and 25 per cent of families with children had at least one child known to the education department for truancy. Detailed analysis of these referrals showed that ideas about 'tangles of pathology' could only be entertained in relation to about five families on the estate. The overwhelming issue on the Deans was that of deep-rooted poverty compounded by the appalling housing environment. None of the agencies involved had any real solutions to these kind of problems. There were no welfare rights agencies in the borough, no community-based social work or housing management projects, and no active tenants' groups advocating for, or agitating about, places like the Deans.

Perhaps it was because nobody wanted to know about the Deans that an outside agency such as ourselves was invited in. The pressure to do something about the Deans only became pressing with the decision to demolish, and the pressure came from the local forces of respectability who did not want the 'problem families' moved anywhere near them. Local councillors cultivated their role as gatekeeper to a range of local services as part of a system of patronage that helped cement their local power base. This produced a tension between local professional and political rationales or narratives, a tension that was acknowledged in routine accounts from residents who sought to demonstrate that what mattered was 'who you knew'. Policy initiatives that were seen as eroding the ability of the local councillors to personally solve an individual's problem, or which were seen to challenge the traditional structures of 'local authority' were unwelcome. For the most part, the Deans residents were not, at an individual or family level, connected to such systems of local power and influence, and collectively had not developed an effective voice. I will return later to the issue of the local political culture but want first to look in more detail at how the Deans narrative was negotiated and elaborated by the tenants, the officers and the councillors.

Obviously those tenants with memories of better days on the estate were not wholly negative, remembering organized bus trips and gardens that had won prizes. More recent and reluctant arrivals would often feel they had little to look forward to but trouble. We came to think of residents as either Pioneers, Settlers or Refugees, largely in terms of when they, or their family, had arrived on the estate. One thing all the tenants had in common was the need to find a way of 'managing' their identity when residence on the estate was locally regarded as such a stigma.

There was a broad consensus among most people we talked to about what was wrong on the Deans, and that was the presence of 'the problem families'. This explanation had the merit that all groups could buy into the story while in the process of telling it attempting to buy themselves, and often those listening, out of the category 'problem family'. The Refugees, for instance, would be well aware of the estate's reputation through lurid coverage in the local press or word-of-mouth accounts. If they were not local, then their housing careers to date, the initial impression of the poor physical conditions on the estate, or the 'warning stories' with which they would quickly be acquainted, would have left little doubt that they had entered a 'dreadful enclosure'.

They could still, however, subjectively exclude themselves from the problem family category by reference to the fact that they had no choice about coming to, and did not intend to stay long on, the estate. This was a strategy that had its risks and was usually short lived. A fine line had to be negotiated between defining yourself as quite unlike other residents, and yet still retaining the capacity to make friends and get on with the neighbours. One way to do this is to attempt to form tactical alliances with some tenants based on the understanding that both can identify what constitutes a problem family and explicitly exclude themselves from that category. Such alliances were often accomplished through the exchange of 'horror stories' about other tenants which, at one level may simply be regarded as gossip, but at another as the day-by-day reinforcement, examination or construction of reputations. The exchange and elaboration of these narratives was a primary means of day-to-day sociability on the estate.

While this strategy would begin by minimizing contact between the newcomer, their family and existing residents, this was not easy to sustain. Keeping young children indoors, especially in the often overcrowded flats, would probably do little to endear such families to their neighbours, particularly if they lived underneath. As several pairs of flats had been knocked through to create four- or five-bedroom units for families with many children, this could be a real problem at times.

These dynamics were reversed, of course, when looked at from the point of view of the existing tenants. New arrivals on the estate had to be 'problem families' by definition and were best avoided or treated with caution. The mobile nature of the category has been commented on by Damer (1974), who talked about the reputation 'buzzing about within the estate like a bee in a bottle'. Pioneer families naturally excluded themselves from the category while often being the most vehement about who should be regarded as the 'problem'. The Settlers, not having such an investment in the 'golden age' story, could distinguish themselves from either of the former groups as the occasion demanded.

This consensus about the nature of the problem guaranteed a ready audience for stories or accounts that seemed to confirm this view of things. The narrative of the 'problem family' suited almost everybody because it was almost always about someone else. Part of the audience for the horror stories were the officers of the housing department who had contact with the Deans residents, although contact was generally limited to weekly visits by tenants to the housing office to pay their rent, or the occasional visit of a repair man to the estate. Complaints, requests for repairs, housing transfers or interviews about arrears were usually conducted in the housing department's office in the middle of town. Housing officers for the most part avoided visiting the estate as the backlog of requests for repairs or transfers was so great that, once spotted on the estate, escape could prove difficult, as various anxious tenants cornered them to press some case or other. It was in the interests of some tenants to convey their case through horror stories, the function of which was often to demonstrate to the listener that the teller was 'misplaced' among the 'animals' on the Deans. These stories would then do the rounds of the local authorities' offices and agencies, being 'improved' and embellished as they went.

An example of this was a chip-pan fire incident which was transformed into a 'psycho-killer on the Deans' horror story. I was on the estate when a fire engine was called to an incident involving a burning chip pan. The fire had been extinguished by neighbours by the time the fire brigade arrived, leaving an embarrassed and relieved young mother to deal with some minor damage from both smoke and local comment on her mothering abilities. Within the week I heard an account of this incident related by a housing department officer which had an unknown 'psycho' deliberately upturning the chip pan, while the tenant had been borrowing some milk from her neighbour. The chilling punchline was that young children were playing in the flat, the 'psycho' must have heard them and, to have been in and out of the flat unobserved in the minute or two available, must have been a 'local'.

Stories and accounts like these formed a pervasive backdrop whenever the estate was being discussed, often being used to demonstrate the pointlessness of trying to do anything on the estate and to defuse potential criticism of the local authority. In other words, these accounts were highly functional in different ways for the different groups engaged in the Deans narrative. Narrative flows in the stream of power, and narratives can be adopted or adapted to reflect the interests of those involved.

To establish the belief, or myth, that the 'model estate' had been wrecked by the 'animals' simultaneously identifies the council as benefactor and proceeds to 'blame the victim'. This may be a crude strategy, but in the absence, or with the silencing, of dissenting accounts, a highly effective one. Potential conflicts between council departments, especially between social services and housing, almost inevitably occurred when the boundary of responsibility became blurred in particular cases, as it often did on an estate such as the Deans. Evicting a family with children, for instance, who would have to be taken expensively into care, for rent arrears, did not make economic sense. In disputes of this kind the Housing Department seemed to exercise the most power. This is a matter to which I will return when discussing the political culture of South Tyneside. The conflicts routinely revealed on the Deans between departments were often routinely mitigated by an exchange of horror stories which, while establishing 'street credibility', did so by reinforcing the essential differentness of the Deans tenants. Such conflicts could then be resolved on a one-off basis which did not threaten the local balance of power between departments, did not prevent something similar happening again, but left the participants feeling that the immediate problem had been resolved.

One formal arena in which the issue of 'problem families' and rent arrears was discussed was the curiously named Inter-Liaison Committee. This committee comprised representatives from the various LA departments and was intended to ensure that they took a co-ordinated approach to families who posed problems for more than one department. The atmosphere in the meetings I attended sometimes verged on the 'knockabout', and were often characterized by a lively trade in horror stories. Cases discussed revealed that being on the agenda did not always work out to a tenant's advantage and clearly illustrated the potential conflicts referred to above.

In one case a young housing officer described the amazed reaction in the office when the 14-year-old daughter of a tenant with one of the highest rent arrears in the borough turned up with over £1100 in a plastic carrier bag. The officer explained that he'd taken all the money, £400 more than the arrears, and had marked the rent book paid up for some months in advance. When the girl asked 'are you going to take all the money, mister?', he told the committee that he felt sorry for her and so gave her £100 back. The education representative commented that the tenant would not have held on to that for long because the department had taken him to court for the daughter's non-attendance at school and he'd been fined. The tenant in question had three other younger children, and following the death of his wife two years before, had found it difficult to cope with the domestic responsibilities while still in full-time work. His eldest daughter had been thrust into the role of surrogate mother and her visit to the rent office had been made possible only by her father's redundancy payment.

The estate also had a number of other useful functions for the authority. By always having empty property available, statutory responsibilities for homeless families could be discharged without making any special provision. Tenants causing problems for the department could be threatened with rehousing on the Deans. Large families were a 'problem' for the authority simply because they did not build many houses with more than three bedrooms. Knocking empty adjacent flats together provided a cheap solution for the housing department. From the point of view of a housing manager, whose efficiency might be judged, for instance, by the level of rent arrears, or the number of complaints from tenants about levels of service, establishing a local hegemony based on stories emphasizing the essential 'differentness' of the residents was highly functional. Some local councillors took a punitive view of various marginalized groups, and as these groups did not form part of their local power base, buying in to such a discourse had its attractions.

Variations on the horror story were provided by other cautionary tales dealing with 'fiddles'. Within the culture of the housing department stories emphasizing the streetwise and hard-nosed attributes of its members were highly valued, and often used to distinguish themselves from what they saw as the 'do-gooding' and gullible approach of social workers. One officer explained 'we're not interested in what goes on within those four walls, that's their business. We're interested in them paying the rent, not bothering the neighbours, and looking after the property.' These kinds of distinctions were typically emphasized in accounts that revealed the housing officer confronted by a tenant's story which he did not believe. The punchline usually demonstrated the officer's insight into the fiddle being attempted. Tenants had their own views on fiddles and, as one of them put it, housing allocation policy was more a question of the 'pints' than the 'points' system!

The policy of dumping tenants with 'problems' on the estate meant that a majority of households were dependent on welfare benefits and were living on very low incomes. Unemployment levels in South Shields were, and remain, among the highest in the country. Historically, male employment had relied heavily on the ship-building and ship-repair yards which went into a steady decline from the late 1960s onwards. Some work which used casual labour was dirty, dangerous, poorly paid and on the margins of legality. Several families on the estate had members who were involved in jobs like defouling ships' hulls or cleaning ships' tanks. Labour was organized on a subcontracted basis, with workers being offered a fixed price for the job, often on a cash-in-hand basis.

If payment from the subcontract work was declared, as required by law, the amount earned was divided by the local average unskilled weekly wage and benefit payments would be suspended for the appropriate number of weeks. As gangs employed on such work tended to work sixteen-hour shifts, or longer if a particular ship had to be turned round quickly and bonus payments were on offer, the cash paid could be accounted as several weeks' income. While this obviously provided a strong incentive not to declare such earnings, it also fed into a local culture that was already somewhat geared to a 'boom or bust' philosophy. This derived in part from the seagoing traditions of the town which ensured that 'when the boat came in' celebrations were in order.

Francie Nichol was a Deans resident in 1933 'and we were quite content there. In fact those were the happiest days we ever had'. Her son was a merchant seaman and

> after a voyage he'd be dafter than ever. When his ship docked in the Tyne, he would come home with at least a dozen of his shipmates . . . Night after night was the same thing, and usually the same crowd . . . After the pubs had closed, they would all troop in singin' and laughing, bangin' and fallin' about. Joe thought there was nothin' I liked better. When he came in he always took the place over.
>
> (Robinson 1975)

This pattern of behaviour, widely acknowledged to be a characteristic of 'sailor towns', was often a feature of the stories that went the rounds of local authority offices. Damer talks about the weekend singing and drinking parties which 'would degenerate into a soulful shambles around two or three in the morning', and which were a characteristic of 'Wine Alley'. This sort of behaviour was something of a feature of life on the Deans, and was often used by officers to illustrate the 'fecklessness' of the Deans tenants.

There was a wider issue here which related to ideas of acceptable or even desirable male behaviour and the changing social economic structures. The image of the big-drinking, anti-authoritarian 'hard man', relatively free from career or domestic obligations, has a place in the culture, and a particular place in the local culture, of the north east. Stories which ended with the punchline 'so I told him where to stick his job!' were common and highly valued as exemplars of a rugged and independent masculinity.

The culture of the local authority departments was very masculine: lunch was usually in the pub over a couple of pints and a game of darts. The local authority had in this period become one of the biggest employers, and had generated large numbers of clerical and administrative jobs. Against the local backdrop of high unemployment and dirty work, such a job was widely regarded as a 'cushy number' and a job for life. It was also a widely held local belief that access to such jobs was heavily dependent on either party membership or patronage. If such jobs were safe, they were not highly paid, and did not enjoy the status of 'real work' in the yards or down the pit which had been traditionally so important in local culture. Concepts of respectability embraced the idea of the skilled man who was also the backbone of party and union organization. Many of the people taking up lower-tier clerical and administrative jobs were the first in their families to have made the transition from manual to non-manual work, from 'dirty' to 'clean' work. They also tended to be the group that had most face-to-face contact with the Deans tenants and I often wondered if the enthusiasm with which horror stories were traded was in some way to do with their insecurity in these new job roles.

Emphasizing the negative qualities of the tenants was a way of displaying one's own respectability and projecting threatening or uncomfortable feelings elsewhere. Sibley (1995) refers to 'abjection' as the process by which 'the urge to make separations, between clean and dirty, ordered and disordered, "us" and "them", that is, to expel the abject, is encouraged in western cultures, creating feelings of anxiety because such separations can never be finally achieved'.

While these 'separations' may be considered to operate at a largely subjective and informal level they can also find expression within more formal processes. Most local authority housing departments will 'grade' their tenants, although some are more open about this than others, and at the point of slum clearance whole estates will be formally graded. In this critical process of grading, the Slum Clearance Officer (SCO) was responsible for visiting each house on the estate, ostensibly to determine the tenants' housing preferences, but at the same time surreptitiously to grade the tenants. This officer obviously occupied a relatively powerful position as a gatekeeper to a scarce and valued resource. In the process of negotiation with each tenant about the kind of house and area to which the tenant might move, the SCO usually held most of the cards.

When the LA decided to demolish the Deans, I accompanied the SCO on his rounds as he assessed the housing needs and status of the tenants. Naturally I was interested to know what kind of criteria he would use to locate each tenant into one of the four available grades of A, B, C or D. The officer in question was disarmingly frank.

> Category A tenants, well I doubt if there would be any on this estate. You'd have to spend a fortune on Formica, substantially improve the property to be category A. I wouldn't call myself category A, I'm in category B, that's people from good families, who look after and maintain their homes. Category C are people who might try to maintain these standards but can't quite manage, or don't try and don't care much. Category D are the 'no-hopers'. You can usually smell them from the end of the path.

An 'A' grading allowed access to new housing, and a grading of 'B' to good quality housing or the first let of a newly revitalized house. Category C would be offered poorer quality, often prewar housing, while category D were destined for 'acquired' property – houses bought up by the council during the course of other slum clearance schemes, and usually of very poor quality. Tenants allocated such properties could of course find themselves in another slum environment. The cumulative stress, expense and disruption of such experiences could only be extremely damaging to families who, fairly or unfairly, had already been labelled as having 'problems'.

The grading process was, of course, prone to all kinds of subjective judgements and the SCO was in any case required to make some very difficult judgements about the domestic circumstances of the families he encountered. Some people, especially those who were never reconciled to being on the Deans long term, and more generally those who had been aware of the estate's impending demolition, might well not have invested money and effort in decorating, preferring to save the money to help make a new start elsewhere. The material condition of the property was, however, one of the prime factors involved in the officer's judgements about the tenant. Others, often children or relatives lodging with the official tenants, would find themselves graded as part of the household even though they might consider their own standards to be higher.

In the case of such multi-occupied properties the officer had to decide if the situation was genuine or an attempted 'fiddle'. Had the new household moved in purely to better its chances of rehousing, in effect to jump the queue, since slum clearance tenants had the highest priority, or as a result of a genuine housing emergency? In order to deter this kind of move another rule decreed that anyone moving in less than six months before the clearance was announced would not be treated as a legitimate case, would only be offered category C or D and, as the SCO put it, 'they were lucky to get that'.

Other pressures operated on the SCO, not least those from within the organization when, for instance, as was observed on a number of occasions, colleagues from the same department would attempt informally to intervene in order to prevent 'any of those families' being moved near to them. Some tenants were better able to advocate for themselves than others and it would be difficult to say to what extent these informal pressures actually affected the kind of offers made in particular cases. As mentioned earlier, most people on the Deans were not connected to the mechanisms of local power either through trade union or party affiliation, but when they were, this was often openly acknowledged and dealt with accordingly.

We found that the local political culture was such that space in which a 'professional identity' might be developed was restricted by the intrusion of local political considerations into almost all areas of agency activities. Because of the jobs for life idea, and the local tendency to 'look after our own', those people who joined the organization from outside this local culture were in a minority and could be vulnerable because of their lack of local knowledge.

This manifested itself in a variety of ways. As such an outsider I would find myself stumbling into networks which introduced family and political loyalties into what I had imagined were professional arenas. There was much local speculation, sometimes surfacing in the local press, but more commonly featuring as grist in the local gossip mills, that Labour party membership was a very useful, if not necessary, qualification for a post with the local authority. Trying to establish the extent to which this was true would obviously not be easy, but the extent to which people believed it was true was routinely apparent in the way such topics were discussed or, just as significantly, avoided.

Because of the density of such local knowledge, and its diffusion within the structures of local government, outsiders found advancement within these organizations problematic. Career moves would tend to be 'out' in order to be 'up', not only diluting the pool of potentially new 'culture carriers', but leaving behind in the organization a series of cautionary tales about what could happen if policy were challenged on professional or on any other grounds. Decisions, even about very minor things, had a 'provisional' feel about them, rules were subject to reinterpretation, cases could be reviewed and, unless you knew the inside story, unless you knew what 'political interest' had been infringed, it could be difficult to make sense of what was going on.

Recently the full extent of the dangerously eroded boundaries between the professional and the political have become apparent. Internal party documents claim to detail how senior officers have been victimized for disagreeing with the ruling group over spending allocations. The same documents claim that in the absence of a list of members' interests, crude conflicts of interest go unchecked. Officers who are party members report that they have been visited at home and threatened with their job being 'deleted' in the next review if they don't vote the right way at party selection meetings. In one notorious incident the deputy leader of the council was found guilty in court of physically assaulting his principal rival in the town hall. In spite of being asked by the national executive to 'consider his position', he was re-elected as deputy leader and now serves at Westminster as MP for Jarrow. One leading councillor recently commented in the national press 'The whole thing, rooted in old Labour big boss politics, stinks and has to be sorted out once and for all – even if the national executive is forced to suspend the local party' (Guardian 20 June 1997).

SELF

> The notion of a history or narrative seems to be necessary in order to make sense of the notion of the 'self'; for we make sense – or fail to make sense – of our lives by the kind of story we can – or cannot – tell about it.
>
> (Dunne 1996)

When Layder deals with the level of the self, he refers to the way in which the unique psycho-biography of the individual interacts with particular contexts, settings and situated activities. He suggests operationalizing this level by thinking about the 'subjective career of the self', citing the general approach of writers such as Goffman (1961) and Stebbins (1970). I have emphasized in the above the way in which the ongoing process of narrative construction and exchange can illuminate the dynamics of situated activities, context and setting.

While that phase of narrative construction can be considered as interactive, albeit with selected audiences, we can also think about a subjective moment of narrative construction. This moment is present for instance in the individual's subjective attempts to reconcile different, and potentially conflicting, narratives, that they may have presented to different audiences. Thus the individual inhabits and is inhabited by a repertoire of narrative themes which function as 'sense making devices' (Gergen 1988). The repertoire of themes from which the self can be constructed has often been represented as limited and limiting in the literature describing life on the margins. Sibley (1995) highlights the way in which the concept of 'abjection' may be used to suggest how narratives might be structured at the level of the unconscious in such situations. Damage to self-esteem flowing from life in 'the dreadful enclosures' is widely commented on in the literature both internationally (Sibley 1995) and locally (Barke and Turnbull 1992; Coffield et al. 1986).

This damage is often illustrated through stories that emphasize hopelessness or helplessness. They portray situations that are bad and likely to get worse, accounts described by Gergen (1988) as 'regressive narratives'. On the Deans, progressive narratives (Gergen 1988) were just as common, perhaps because the impending demolition held out the prospect of better days to come while, unsurprisingly, narratives of stability were few and far between. Dramatic narratives dealing with the management of crisis abound in places such as the Deans, and welfare workers will often comment on the ability of families and individuals to sustain some form of identity in the face of almost constant crisis.

CONCLUSION

A narrative approach seeks to identify accounts that exemplify experience. In any study of marginalized groups within the ghetto, particular attention should be directed to those accounts which have been overlooked or discounted by the prevailing culture of local authority. Accounts which sustain the marginalization of certain groups need also to be examined in terms of their utility for those that use them. Interventions in such situations can be interpreted as attempts to reframe or reinterpret narratives which are considered damaging at an individual, group or community level.

At the same time those intervening in such situations need to examine how their personal or professional rationales or narratives will collide with or contribute to the power dynamics of the situation in question. That discussion is pursued by writers like Thompson (1997) in relation to social work practice and Humphries and Truman (1994) in relation to social research.

Our involvement on the Deans was overtaken at an early stage by the decision to demolish the estate. We redefined our immediate priorities and focused on the need to ensure that the residents got the best deal possible in the circumstances. This meant opposing the pressure to dump the residents in the next worst available properties and so create another slum estate. We attempted to use our status as relatively privileged outsiders to ask awkward questions and highlight unjust practices. We attempted to act as witnesses and advocates for individual tenants through our presence on the estate. We tried in this way to function, at very local level, as 'interruptors of the social relations of dominance' (Lather 1991). The ethical, professional and political dilemmas generated by this stance were numerous and beyond the bounds of this paper to explore.

Prior to conducting our survey of the Deans, the Housing Department had supplied us with the names of residents of each flat, according to their records. One of the first tenants I interviewed was an elderly woman who was recorded as sharing the house with her husband and six sons. The interview was in part aimed at updating the information we had been given, which, it was acknowledged, was out of date. In response to the question 'Who is living here at the moment?', the woman replied that she was a widow and lived there alone. I asked if any of her sons lived nearby to which she replied, 'No hinney, they're all dead.' She went on to explain how they had all died from illness, accident, or in the war. She said she felt her life had been a cruel waste and that she was now just waiting to die and put an end to the whole sad story. I did not handle the situation very well, stumbled through a series of increasingly grotesque questions about desired improvements to the flats and the estate, and got out of there as fast as I decently could.

I had found myself in a situation I had not anticipated and for which I was not prepared. It has occurred to me since that this was a situation that many local authority officers would often have found themselves in when dealing with residents on the estate.

> All that I have asked of narrative understanding is that it enables humans to interact with complexity. They need only agree and understand each other to the extent that they work more or less reliably together, to keep the social flow of things moving all the more energetically.
>
> (Carrithers 1992)

BIBLIOGRAPHY

Barke, M. and Turnbull, G. (1992) *Meadowell: The Biography of an 'Estate with Problems'*, Aldershot: Avebury.

Carrithers, M. (1992) *Why Humans Have Cultures*, Oxford: Oxford University Press.

Coffield, F., Borrill, C. and Marshall, S. (1986) *Growing Up at the Margins*, Milton Keynes: Open University Press.

Coleman, A. (1985) *Utopia on Trial*, London: Hilary Shipman.

Damer, S. (1974) 'Wine Alley: the sociology of a dreadful enclosure', *The Sociological Review* 22, 221–48.

Denzin, N. K. (1989) *Interpretative Biography*, London: Sage.

Dunne, J. (1996) 'Beyond sovereignty and deconstruction: the storied self', in R. Kearney (ed.) *Paul Ricoeur: The Hermeneutics of Action*, London: Sage.

Gergen, M. M. (1988) 'Narrative structures in social explanations', in C. Antaki (ed.) *Analysing Everyday Explanations: A Casebook of Methods*, London: Sage.

Goffman, I. (1961) *Encounters*, New York: Bobbs-Merrill.

Humphries, B. and Truman, C. (eds) (1994) *Rethinking Social Research*, Aldershot: Avebury.

Jacobs, J. (1961) *The Death and Life of Great American Cities*, New York: Vintage Books.

Lather, P. (1991) 'Deconstructing/deconstructive inquiry: the politics of knowing and being known', *Education Theory* 41, 2, 157.

Layder, D. (1993) *New Strategies in Social Research*, Cambridge: Polity Press.

Maines, D. R. (1993) 'Narrative's moment and sociology's phenomena: toward a narrative sociology' *The Sociological Quarterly* 34, 1, 21.

Newman, O. (1972) *Defensible Space*, London: Macmillan.

Price, D. (1982) *Fighting like Tigers: the Rise and Fall of Council Housing in South Shields 1914–1932*, Newcastle: North East Centre for Community Studies.

Robinson, F. (1975) *The Life and Times of Francie Nichol of South Shields*, London: George Allen and Unwin.

Ryle, G. (1949) *The Concept of Mind*, London: Hutchinson.

Sibley, D. (1995) *Geographies of Exclusion*, London: Routledge.

Stebbins, R. (1970) 'Career: the subjective approach', *The Sociological Quarterly* 11, 32–49.

Thompson, N. (1997) *Anti-Oppressive Practice*, London: Macmillan.

Walter, E. V. (1977) 'Dreadful enclosures: detoxifying an urban myth', *Archive European Sociologie* 18, 151–9.

Chapter 10

Considering the culture of community care

Anthropological accounts of the experiences of frontline carers, older people and a researcher

Lorna Warren

INTRODUCTION

This chapter draws on my research into social care for older people living in their own homes in two northern cities. Its aim is to illustrate the various ways in which anthropological approaches have helped both to inform my understanding and to shape my accounts of this aspect of community care and to reflect, from that, on key features that might be central to researchers in the practice of welfare anthropology.

BACKGROUND: AN EMERGING APPLIED ANTHROPOLOGY AND AN EMERGING APPLIED ANTHROPOLOGIST

When I first set out into the field as a researcher in the early 1980s, anthropologists in Britain were generally perceived as having failed to specialize in the way that they had in the United States. This was primarily because of the small scale of the discipline and the chronic shortage of funds (Gowler and Clarke 1983). However, another reason was the association of the term 'anthropologist' with colonialism which, according to Jackson (1987), made the idea of anthropologists, especially those doing research at home, 'so unwelcome'. Misplaced as the connection may have been, it was sociology which had traditionally been linked to notions of social welfare and progress, the label 'sociologist' denoting a scientific examination of one's own society *for its own good* (Jackson 1987: 7).

Nevertheless, the picture was beginning to change, partly because sociologists were failing to explain their own societies while anthropologists were discovering large areas of ignorance about them (Jackson 1987). Important contributions were being made to the theory and practice of managerial control (Gowler and Clarke 1983) and to the illumination of the interests of 'invisible' or 'problematic' subgroups (Ballard 1983; Okely 1983, 1987) which were aiding the development of a practical public image.

Such studies helped to illuminate the usefulness of social anthropology which, driven by the goal to provide answers to the questions of how and why people live as they do, offered insight into 'practice' as a topic in its own right and not just as a means of finding out about policy. Methods of direct observation and recording of information were brought to play at the level of the relation of what people said to what they actually did (Gowler and Clarke 1983). Also highlighted was the role of the longitudinal approach (Tambiah 1985) and of concrete qualitative information which could not be easily discredited in the way that statistics could be manipulated or massaged (Okely 1987). In other words, applied anthropology was offering a challenge to the orthodoxy of the classic model of evaluation and policy-related research.

Since then, there have been an increasing number of publications on the issue of welfare and, specifically, on the topic of community care. For example, Cecil (1989) has explored the topic of 'Care and the Community in a Northern Irish Town'. In 1992, *Anthropology in Action*, the journal of the British Association for Social Anthropology in Policy and Practice (BASAPP), published an issue which focused on the topic of Community Care and Social Policy.[1] Included were articles on resettlement schemes for people with learning disabilities (Collins 1992); on people with MS and their supporters (Monks 1992); and on psychiatric hospital closure and resettlement (McCourt-Perring 1992, 1993, 1994). Brian Gearing and Peter Coleman (1996) have described how, when flexibly used, a biographical approach can prove to be a valuable tool in the assessment of the health and social care needs of older people living in the community. More recently still, Twigg (1997) has, through her analysis of the 'social bath', raised questions about some of the traditional ways in which community care has been constructed. Of particular interest is her exploration of the aspects of being and of social exchange which bathing entails and which are typically left out of the disembodied approach to community care adopted within the rationalistic and bureaucratic world of policy makers.

Postmodernists have furthered the challenge to what they see as over-deterministic, structuralist analyses. Gubrium and Silverman (1989) have described the deconstruction of the familiar polarities of theory/practice, fact/value, reason/emotion, science/ideology, and society/individual, as having discomfiting, as well as potentially anaesthetizing, implications for research, through its challenge to the idea of an onward march of progress and the status of intellectuals to promote change for others. However, this may be an overly pessimistic reading of postmodernism which, as others have sought to show, retains a concern with the politics of the social world. Fox's (1995) exploration of postmodern perspectives on care traces developments in the professionalization of caring which have led to care as 'vigil' or a technology of surveillance. However, he argues that it is possible to recognize an alternative caring which is about love, generosity and a celebration of otherness. 'This "gift" of care seeks to enable the cared-for person, and resists the discourses of the vigil' (Fox 1995: 107).

Such alternative approaches to traditional positivistic research influenced, and continue to play a part in framing, my research into social care. I entered into research having won a postgraduate Social Science Research Council (now Economic and Social Research Council) CASS award. The full title of the award, 'Collaborative Award in the Social Sciences', indicated that I was to work with another organization in carrying out my doctoral study. In this case, Salford social services department had planned to carry out an extensive survey of domiciliary services for older people to determine the efficiency of services in meeting needs. My brief was to supplement this data with 'intensive field studies of values and expectations concerning older people as well as their own values and expectations'. However, blocked by the unions, the department was forced to shelve the scheme and I found my involvement 'in the field' to be much more immediate, intense, prolonged and isolated than I had anticipated.[2]

It was clearly not the case that I perceived the situation as a simple dilemma of objective versus subjective, causal versus interpretative, quantitative versus qualitative, or organization versus humanitarian perspectives (Guba and Lincoln 1987). The original plan was to have involved me in bringing together 'hard' and 'soft' areas of research, connecting the bit of the iceberg that 'sticks up above the water' (Stanley 1986: 46) with the bit below. Given the increasingly monetarist context of the British academic contribution, I did not wish to take the kind of postmodern, relativist approach likely to be perceived as blind antagonism (Strong and Dingwall 1989). Along with other organizations, Salford social services were still facing the challenge of how their limited resources might be best allocated. And finally, those whom I was researching – and not just government funding bodies – rightfully expected a return from my activities. I did not want to 'loot without reciprocity' (Tambiah 1985: 17).

So, I determined to offer a (complementary) alternative to the typical quantitative study of home care services in the form of a detailed qualitative picture of the work of home helps, and the lives and circumstances of older users of services, and to reflect from this on the adequacy of service organization in meeting people's needs. The process became one whereby I showed the organizationally tentative nature of experiential realities while engaging with policy 'in the short term'.

Since then, I have undertaken projects which are explicitly concerned with the evaluation of systems of care and service innovation. The second major study – which I use as a source of illustrative material in this account – was an evaluation of the Neighbourhood Support Units (NSUs) innovation in Sheffield. The scheme was conceived of by Sheffield Family and Community Services (F&CS) in response to the critique of residential care and the development of family-based community care, but born into the Griffiths era of an increasingly mixed economy of welfare and residualized local authority social services. It aimed to replace the traditional tripartite division of services for older people – domiciliary, day and residential care – with a more integrated and flexible deployment of resources. The objective of the research project was to assess the impact of the NSU innovation on older people and their informal carers. It is an illustration of the way in which my engagement with policy has become more long-term, though sharing my findings and providing 'enlightenment' (Cecil 1989) are still central aims.

METHODOLOGY

Responsive research

If a driving goal has been the desire to make research relevant to the world in more responsive ways than has been done before (Tambiah 1985: 17), how has this shaped my choice of methods? It has been suggested that people within the 'caring professions' tend to find qualitative studies more appealing than quantitative research: the small-scale, case-study approach is 'accessible, understandable and appropriate' when people and their social and health problems are under focus (Cecil 1989: 118). I wanted, at the outset, to avoid the narrow confines of social surveys, but I also did not want to risk fragmenting aspects of social processes which should be analysed as a whole (Weiss 1986). It has been important to me to respect the importance of contextualizing key concepts such as old age, dependency and care (Warren and Walker 1992).

Community care may take many forms and approaches. Considering the issue of user involvement, Grant (1992) has argued that researchers should, perhaps, be embracing the entire gamut of research designs, including longitudinal case studies and experimental design studies, if the impact of the many and varied empowerment strategies on both service quality and the quality of users' lives is to be teased out. In general (and with the qualification that I have already been resident in the area where my studies were set), I have made use of a typical 'anthropological blend' of methods (Cecil 1989), seeing it as the model most suited to an attempt to satisfy the concerns which I have noted. Of what has that blend consisted?

Home care for older people in Salford

The core of the fieldwork for my doctoral thesis was carried out from November 1983 to February 1985, in the ten patches within Salford local authority boundaries. I conducted interviews in fifty households, involving a total of sixty-one older people. Interviews were typically semi-structured and in-depth, though home helps acted as proxies and/or translators for a handful of older people. A small group of eight key informants were visited a third or fourth time.

Home helps were observed at work in the homes of older people and in the patch offices. I also conducted group interviews in each of the patches in which a total of fifty-four home helps participated. Likewise, I combined participant observation studies of home help organizers with more formal interviews though, in this case, the latter were held on an individual basis. (For a more detailed discussion of methods used, see Warren 1988 and 1990a.)

Neighbourhood Support Units

The NSU evaluation was based on the Manor Neighbourhood Centre and employed a triangulation of methods to obtain data from a number of key groups (Walker and Warren 1996).

A survey took the form of a comparative study of ninety-six older people getting NSU services and a group of eighty-four in receipt of more traditional home care in a comparable area in Sheffield – Southey Green. Follow-up interviews were conducted some twelve to sixteen months after the first round of the survey, and the extent to which the NSU had shifted away from traditional service provision was measured through matching fifty-three pairs of older people. Eighteen case studies of older people in Manor and their carers were also put together, in order to explore the objective of user involvement in more detail. These were based on informal, unstructured interviews, supplemented by notes from users' records as well as observational data .

Support workers (thirty-two women and two men, out of a possible forty workers) talked about their jobs, in semi-structured or focused group interviews. They were also observed at work in the homes of older people. Comparative data was drawn from four diaries kept by workers from the NSU and three by members of the home care service in Southey Green.

As well as interviewing higher managerial staff to obtain details of the policy development process, researchers spoke to managers and other staff involved in the day-to-day operation of the NSU. These included the current and previous managers of the Manor NSU, three team leaders, the clerk and senior clerk, the current and previous senior nurses on the Manor project, and the manager of the Ecclesfield NSU.[3]

In addition to the separate methods used for each of the groups above, information was gathered through the general observation of the day-to-day activities of the NSU – including team, user group and resource panel meetings, administrative and managerial operations, day centres and events such as the launch of the new assessment form and the Christmas show. Team leaders were also accompanied on assessment visits to new referrals.

So far I have set out how my studies have been influenced by anthropological principles and methods. But I have also tapped anthropology for theoretical perspectives in making sense of my subsequent findings. The intention of the next section is to illustrate these elements, singly and in combination, through exploration of accounts of the experiences of frontline carers in providing services to older people, and of the attempts to make such services (as well as research into them) more user-oriented.

FRONTLINE WORKERS IN COMMUNITY CARE

Surprisingly, there has been relatively little research about the experiences of the personal social services workforce, despite its central role in the organization and delivery of care. Wright has noted the lack of ethnographic analyses connecting the structure and practices of an organization's management to the ways in which frontline workers relate to clients (Wright 1992, 1994). By examining the activities and experiences of frontline workers, it becomes clear that policy is not always analysed in terms of how it works in practice. It is often caught by 'symbolic associations with ideals' (McCourt-Perring 1992). The failure to recognize these associations leads to institutions supposedly undergoing reform still retaining traditional patterns of working, and basic structures of power and control. Yet frontline workers are rarely given the chance to analyse their roles (Warren 1990a, 1990b): it may not be regarded as important, or even as suitable activity for 'ordinary' workers (McCourt-Perring 1992: 11). Both my doctoral thesis and, subsequently, the NSU evaluation set out to place workers at the heart of the respective studies, to examine how they experienced their roles as carers of older people and how they translated care philosophies into practice.

Home helps

Individuals – in this instance, all were women – became home helps due to a mix of material and ideological factors: wanting to help or meet people; the necessity of paid employment; convenient hours to fit in with family responsibilities; and because it required no formal training. With limited knowledge of what was involved in domiciliary services, most drew on skills and experiences accrued as housewives and mothers and, where relevant, paid employees in their anticipation of their roles. The process of recruitment did little to challenge this perspective. Organizers commonly stressed general social traits of flexibility and reliability, sympathy and compassion, domesticity, and common sense rather than formal skills or educational qualifications as the qualities they looked for in home helps, while departmental descriptions of duties defined activities very loosely as 'all the *usual* [my emphasis] household duties' and talked of achieving a 'good standard of cleanliness'. Guidelines appeared to distinguish between 'general care' – which translated widely as the maintenance of users' welfare or 'well-being' – and 'domestic duties' – part and parcel of general care, which involved washing, shopping, cooking and cleaning. Duties forbidden to home helps mainly comprised outdoor activities on the house and garden, not conceived of as part of what is an essentially female home help model, and 'nursing duties', though exactly what such duties encompassed was not specified.

The criteria home helps used in organizing their work included distinctions between different areas of care – domestic, errand, personal and emotional – and the various categories of users which depended on duration of visits and the nature of the disability or circumstances of the person visited (Warren 1990b). The categorizations were useful for apprehending the activities encompassed by the job. However, they were not sufficient to understand the complexities of women's roles. As one of the 'human service industries'

(Stevenson 1976), the outstanding characteristic of home help work is the face-to-face relationship between workers and users (Soloman 1968). It was therefore by concentrating, in an interactionist sense, on the negotiations and transactions between women and older people that I could best capture the nature of domiciliary care.

I found interviewees' relationships with users to be individually (though usually covertly) negotiable, though within limits which were socially determined. Transactions were clearly very different from those which might take place between, for example, a cleaner and her employer, or a nurse and her patients. These are based respectively on public service and medical models of care. Instead, interviewees constructed models and rationales of their caring relationships based on the ideology of the good housewife and caring relative. The ideology of housewifery 'places a premium upon making do and mending, upon coping and budgeting, and upon managing within the resources available' (Bond 1980: 24), while that of the caring (female) relative places a premium on the handling of personal care tasks. These models were used to explain why interviewees found themselves, in their words, 'involved' with users to a degree they had not anticipated, and in a way which meant they shouldered large burdens of responsibility without public acknowledgement.

Evidence of home helps' involvement lay chiefly in their descriptions of what I have called their unofficial activities: 'favours' and rule-breaking activities which have been highlighted in other studies (cf. Egington 1983) (see Warren 1990b for full details). What I want to concentrate on here, however, is why workers became involved, particularly as this was just as likely to occur in respect of older people who had family as with those who did not.

Reasons for involvement lay chiefly in the nature of care and in the setting in which care was given. I turn first to the example of personal care tasks as illustration. Personal care tasks are those tasks that adults would normally do for themselves without assistance. They are characterized by such things as touching, nakedness, and contact with excreta. Drawing on the work of Mauss, Douglas and Elias, amongst others, Twigg has shown how these tasks are 'intimately connected with the bodily expressions of values of privacy, autonomy and adulthood' (1986: 15). For this reason, personal care is so often conceived of as a nursing activity, despite the fact that the skills required are not in any way medical. The medical model offers a means to negotiate these boundaries through the restructuring of the social body into the medical body.

The problem which home helps and older people alike faced was how to renegotiate these rules of intimacy without the aid of a medical model and the concomitant symbols of technical language, starched uniforms and rules and explanations of hygiene. Their solution was to fall back onto personal relationships, on 'particularistic rather than role-specific aspects' (Twigg 1986: 17). The favoured model seemed to be that of the caring relative: 'we treat them with a mum attitude'.

Older people clearly played a role in this process. In one instance, an older woman left fruit for the home help in her bag. On one level, the user's actions reminded the interviewee of things done for her by her mother when she was a child. On another, the action of gift-giving, and the notion of reciprocity central to it, suggested a process of renegotiation, particularly since reciprocity is usually taken to be a key principle in kin relations.

Gender was, of course, particularly significant in this context, since the skills regarded as necessary to carry out personal tasks are imbued with sex-role stereotyping. Women have a virtual monopoly in dealing with taboo aspects of tending, such as the management of human excreta and tasks involving touching and nakedness which, when carried out by men, appear to threaten rules of incest (Ungerson 1983). For this reason, home helps became involved with older people who had family, it usually being the case, here, that relatives were sons who drew the line at personal care. Some workers drew the line for them, while on other occasions, older people themselves preferred to turn to home helps rather than ask male relatives for help with personal care.

But how did home helps rationalize their involvement with older people not requiring such intimate personal care? Again, reasons were rooted in the nature of tasks performed by interviewees. Anthropologists have long recognized that in all societies the preparation and serving of food and drink have symbolic significance and may act as indicators of social relations (cf. Douglas and Nicod 1974). Often the provision of healthy, nutritious, filling meals lies at the heart of women's family caring role (Graham 1983). Amongst those home helps who were responsible for ensuring that older people received 'proper' meals, it was not surprising, then, that they conceived of their role in familial terms. The fact that these tasks were performed in older people's own homes was central to their interpretation. Neither the resources and power which reside in the territorial autonomy of hospitals (Twigg 1986), nor the anonymity which characterizes restaurants, cafes or canteens (Mars and Nicod 1984) are to be found in the setting of older people's own homes. However, what mattered ultimately was not so much the absence of models for public, social production but the strength of the pre-existing informal ones.

This, in part, explains why few interviewees saw themselves as nurses and cooks-cum-waitresses (with the concomitant detachment). Why, then, did they give themselves the label of caring relative? The majority of interviewees and older people were working-class people amongst whom the home remains largely the preserve of kin (Allan 1979). Non-kin are rarely entertained in this social setting. Home helps, as non-kin, were threatening these 'rules of relevance', in particular because of their intimate knowledge of older people's rooms. One way to negotiate the subsequent sense of dissonance felt by both parties was to conceive of each other as kin. Thus, in some cases, home helps who were carrying out domestic tasks alone described themselves and were described using kin terms. Their perspective and understanding of the ways in which older people's households functioned was quite different from that of the professional, whose focus is likely to be highly concentrated. Home helps saw older people in unguarded moments and had knowledge of how they managed their lives (Dexter and Harbert 1983: 35). Their relationship was more akin to that usually shared by primary kin, especially when conversation was relaxed and reciprocal, embracing home helps' own lives. Finally, at all levels of care there existed moral qualities which echoed qualities characterizing relationships between kin or 'true friends' (Allan 1979: 160). These were qualities of trust and loyalty. Home helps were sources of comfort and support in situations of personal crisis.

Workers did not necessarily see themselves as caring relatives. They also spoke of their role as being allied to that of a 'good housewife'. In this context, interviewees highlighted other features inherent in the wider setting of the local authority: chiefly, resources and responsibility. Home helps carried a heavy responsibility for the well-being of older people with little time to fulfil their caring duties, especially the less easily routinized activities of cooking and 'being with'. Thus, they explained their unofficial activities in terms of practical exigencies: unexpected queues at the supermarket led to women shopping in their own time or they stood on chairs to clean windows because stepladders were unavailable. Involvement arose from a sense of moral obligation: with responsibility came feelings of worry, guilt and concern.

Staff were not rotated, but the situation was exacerbated because the boundaries of tasks remained largely ill-defined. Ideas about the kind of activity housework is may differ quite significantly between individuals (Oakley 1974) and over time but 'caring is experienced as an unspecific and unspecifiable kind of labour, the contours of which shift constantly'. Since it aims 'to make cohesive what is often fragmentary and disintegrating', it is only visible when it is not done (Graham 1983: 26). In other words, women felt under pressure to prove that caring was being done but it was very difficult for home helps to judge where to draw the line and, even where it was drawn, it appeared easy to cross. Indeed, by organizers' own admissions, they 'turned a blind eye' to most unofficial activities and even privately condoned them, rationalizing and justifying them as evidence of women's caring nature.

Support workers

I was able to extend my study of frontline workers in community care through the evaluation of the NSU innovation in Sheffield. The organization of frontline staff, in fact, constituted the key departure of the NSU initiative from traditional practice. Under the NSU scheme, domiciliary staff – in this case home wardens and home helps, now known in Sheffield as home carers – were replaced by teams of support workers aiming to fulfil an expanded range of activities and to work collaboratively with community health personnel (for full details, see Walker and Warren 1996). There were, indeed, significant differences between the home help and the support worker services but, crucially, the NSU retained original patterns of working, some of the reasons for and implications of which I highlight below.

Interviewees came to work in the field of social care services for much the same push and pull factors as home helps in Salford, though they appeared less likely to be looking after school-age children and more likely to be caring for older relatives. The majority took up the post of support worker as a result of redeployment, either due to the opening of the centre or to the closure of residential homes. Only a handful had actively chosen the job of support worker: to move beyond the limited cleaning role in which, as home helps, they felt themselves to be confined, or to escape the 'conveyor belt' organization of residential care.

The key differences, for support workers, between the new NSU service and the home help services can be summarized as follows:

New activities   Tasks performed outside older people's homes which encompassed running day centres, providing transport, delivering Meals on Wheels, and organizing shopping trips, outings and other social events.

Increased responsibility   Ordering of day-to-day activities and involvement in the longer-term assessment and arrangement of support to older people.[4]

More flexible work schedule   Shift from cleaning to caring and increased range of 'medical' tasks.

Greater autonomy   Flexible timetabling of help; replacement of the 'two class' system of care with a combined support worker role and system of team working; move to work *with* users rather than giving help *to* them or working *for* them.

Stress   Limited availability of time and resources, 'more mental' nature of work, 'on-call' duties, and tensions and divisions within teams.

Despite their new activities and roles, however, other features of frontline workers roles remained the same. The idea that the notion of flexibility precluded the drawing up of detailed guidelines appeared implicit in the units. Again, there was a notable absence, aside from their basic job description, and health and safety regulations, of any specific policies or written guidelines spelling out support workers' duties. Expectations concerning the availability of staff to provide emergency cover were particularly hazy. At the same time, important, often demanding, elements of the support worker role which could not be defined easily and regimented as 'activities' per se – social and emotional support, advice, companionship, motivation/rehabilitation – were given little attention in training. The upshot was that issues of shortages of time combined with the need to be seen as caring were still not addressed. Workers followed 'traditional patterns' or simply used their 'common sense', and familial models of care continued to underpin workers' relationships with older people.

In general, support workers used a model of kinship to articulate their relationships with older people in much the same way that home helps in Salford had. In light of the aims of the Unit, some elements of their role were given greater emphasis. For example, particular stress was placed on the importance of older people remaining in their own homes, and on the practical and symbolic significance of those homes in terms of the preservation of autonomy, independence and motivation (Sixsmith 1990).

Conversely, support workers were much more likely than home helps to talk of relationships which were of a more formal nature. Some older people – typically requiring help of a purely practical kind, such as heavy cleaning – saw themselves as 'the boss' and set out very strict parameters for the conduct of activities. It may have been, in this instance, that interviewees were more sensitive to such behaviour because of the implied resistance to attempts to change workers' roles. In fact, few older people called staff by their new title of 'support worker', though this group of users not only used the former title of 'home help' but some had been known to refer to workers as cleaners, and in one case as a 'scrubber'. Whatever the explanation for the use of such labels, workers referred to in this way felt they were being 'taken for granted' or treated as 'skivvies'.

Insight into the significance of gender as a key factor in the culture and organization of community care was expanded through the NSU research as a result of the fact that two of the support workers, both of whom took part in group interviews, were men. What they helped to show was that caring roles were not simply perceived traditionally by most people as women's jobs. Caring was synonymous with femaleness (Graham 1983). Subsequently, when female support workers gave help to an older user which was of a personal nature, such as washing, it was 'natural' for them to perform this role (Ungerson 1983), and women, in turn, were able to rationalize it as an extension of their feminine/motherly role: 'Like caring for a child, you know.' This was not possible in the case of male support workers, since caring of this kind was not a feature of maleness. It required a level of intimacy which, instead, carried sexual undertones. Increasing numbers of men may have been entering the nursing profession but in the private setting of the user's own home the medical model was not appropriate and some older people – men as well as women – found it impossible to renegotiate rules of intimacy: 'When we're washing them they relate to us as like a nurse, whereas a man, they relate to it as sex, don't they?'

Attitudes to men doing domestic tasks were acknowledged to be changing, yet a number of female workers still believed it 'not a man's job' to provide personal care in a one-to-one situation. Male support workers themselves could do very little in response to older people's refusals to accept their help in this context. One commented that he understood and respected the reasons for their objections. He felt a greater sense of frustration regarding other assumptions made about him on the basis of his status, including the fact that he must be gay and that he would not be able to cook. Instances were cited where male support workers had taken over the care of older men because of persistent harassment of female staff, offering an alternative solution to women workers who typically dealt with sexual advances, at an individual and gendered level, as an occupational hazard. But the opinion that it might be better if violent or abusive male users were cared for by male workers threatened to further constrain men to a very limited caring role, in this case with a recognizably masculine profile.

Finally, given the collaborative element of the NSU initiative, details of how care arrangements were additionally shaped by relationships with managers and other professionals were much more prominent in the Sheffield study compared to the Salford study. (For discussion of support workers' relationships with informal carers, see Warren 1994b; Walker and Warren 1996.) In the same way that support workers were expected to work *with* users and carers, so the emphasis was on team leaders working *with* their respective teams in the organization of care. Certainly, in practical terms, the amount of contact between frontline workers and their supervisors had increased relative to their greater involvement in the organization of care. Symbolically, parties were on first-name terms and shared a staff room. But achieving supportive working relationships required a fine balance by team leaders between abandoning traditional disciplinarian practices – for example, covert monitoring of activities – but not leaving support workers to 'sort everything themselves'. Tellingly, the most successful management style was judged by the support workers as being one born of 'grass roots' understanding of the job and workers' capabilities.

Successful relationships with other outside professionals likewise depended on 'respect' for the work of staff, based on first-hand knowledge of the support worker role. In Manor, a patch-based system of care aided attempts by family and community services, and the health services, to develop a complementary and collaborative approach. At the frontline level, staff jointly operated the Elderly Mentally Ill (EMI) day centre and the bath run, and the physiotherapist contributed to training sessions. District nurses had begun to turn up to team meetings whenever possible, while a handful of support workers had, in turn, shadowed them out on the patch for a day.

But while support workers viewed members of the health team collectively as a 'good crowd' – friendly and approachable – they were, nevertheless, still seen, and, it was believed, saw themselves on a different level by dint of their professional training and expertise. Some support workers claimed that district nurses had understood collaboration to mean they could off-load a number of the routine practical aspects of care – bathing, in particular – onto their shoulders, freeing nurses to carry out medical tasks. Such misunderstandings were not helped by the fact that the health team was based at premises approximately half a mile from the NSU building.

Social workers were charged with having acted generally very defensively and jealously towards the development of the key worker component of the support worker role, while doctors generally needed far greater enlightenment. One GP practice on the Manor had kept abreast of changes, and consequently showed workers 'more respect' and 'credibility', but few hospital doctors had ever heard of the term 'support worker'.

Anthropology on the frontline

An anthropological approach to the topic of social care for older people has helped to provide me with a conceptual framework in which the core elements of care – identity and activity (Graham 1983) – can be fitted together in an everyday subjective experience of caring. It has increased the understanding of a sub-group – non-professional, formal carers – consideration of which is usually confined to the analysis of the cost and extent of service provision or to a straightforward description of duties.

The most important insight to emerge from my first study was that caring, in such a context, was not simply a 'vocational concern', but had to be understood in terms of a complex interplay of material and ideological factors. For home helps, a paradox was presented by the fact that their roles at home and at work were so closely related. The first qualified women to undertake the second. The second was constructed in terms of the first. Since they performed these roles simultaneously, women felt locked into a double bind: if they were devalued and found wanting as home helps then they themselves, as 'natural' housewives and carers, were found wanting.[5]

Payment did not automatically underplay the symbolic bonds that hold caring relationships together (Graham 1983: 19) but it did assume self-sacrifice as part of women's 'nature' (Porter 1983: 113). This is not to suggest that women did not enjoy or gain a sense of satisfaction from their job, particularly when treated as a confidant by users. However, work was described as both physically and emotionally very tiring and few felt able to treat the job as a 'nine-to-five'. Nevertheless, perhaps because it was cast as an 'obligatory' rather than an 'optional' role (Rossi 1972 quoted by Fransella and Frost 1977: 107), few workers articulated feelings of manipulation or exploitation: 'We do these things because we care. . . . We're home helps because we care.'

The NSU evaluation helped to confirm the pervasiveness of the familial model of care underpinning social care services for older people. From the perspective of frontline providers of care, NSUs had succeeded in achieving a more flexible and collaborative service which offered a comprehensive range of support, in a number of areas, beyond that outlined as necessary to constitute sufficient domiciliary care (Norton *et al.* 1986: 116). However, changing services involves not just new activities but new attitudes.

According to workers, the problem was that the 'outside was not educated'. Informing people by letter of the new aims of the Unit had not been enough, and support workers were left to deal, largely on their own, with 'a lot of aggro' from users. Indeed, some avoided confronting users' confusion or non-acceptance by continuing to refer to themselves as home helps. While it was thought that collaboration was increasing, albeit slowly, workers still encountered the defence of professional boundaries (Webb and Hobdell 1980; Wright *et al.* 1988; Meetham and Thompson 1992).

The issue of information was not just confined to users and other professionals, however. Once the Centre had opened, senior management personnel had 'never taken much notice' of the NSU scheme. The majority of support workers had received no more than the introductory two weeks' training provided prior to the Centre opening (if that) and that was described as 'squashed in', little different from that which they were given as home helps, and as failing to prepare them for the reality of being 'on district'. Effectively 'thrown in at the deep end' and without targeted follow-up training, it was not surprising that a number of workers reacted defensively to change: 'When you've been on . . . seventeen years you don't need no training. If you don't know now you will never know.'

USER-ORIENTED POLICY AND COMMUNITY CARE

The notion of user-oriented policy in community care has, perhaps, been more widely researched than has the work of frontline carers, despite their vital role in translating policy into practice. Yet although it is increasingly the focus of service reviews, the idea of user-oriented policy nevertheless remains a very vague and conceptually confused notion. Recent transformations, within health as well as social care systems, mean that greater prominence is now given to the 'consumption' alongside the 'production' of welfare (Barnes 1997). The service user as passive recipient is being replaced by the idea of an active co-producer of welfare (Walker 1987; Walker and Warren 1996). Indeed, empowerment has been declared the driving force within contemporary UK health and social services (DoH 1991). Yet such a sweeping claim hides important differences between various models of empowerment, not least those articulated by the users of social care services. From the idea that users could exercise a 'voice' about the services they receive (Mayer and Timms 1970), we have seen a shift in policy emphasis to the need to stimulate *choice* for service users (DoH 1989). In the ensuing period, commentators have employed other terms such as 'involvement', 'participation', 'partnership' and 'citizenship'. Not only is the concept of empowerment an 'elusive' one (Hollingberry 1994), it is also a 'contested' one (Means and Lart 1994b), charged with 'suggesting an equality which is rarely possible', or of drawing from frameworks, such as the consumerism debate (Walker 1989, 1991; Barnes and Wistow 1992; Barnes and Walker 1996), with which users, as well as professionals, do not necessarily agree (Stevenson and Parsloe 1993).

The account presented here – of NSUs and user involvement – demonstrates how an anthropological approach may combine a grasp of the structure and operations of social care systems with not only the fine-grained ethnography of interactions between officials and users, but also 'the analysis of the symbols, concepts and cultural processes that is needed for a critical evaluation of who is empowered by "empowerment"' (Wright 1994: 166).[6]

Answering questions of how differences between users and professionals are to be captured and, subsequently, to be taken into account in attempts to facilitate and encourage empowerment does not stop at the scrutiny of research. It also includes scrutinizing the role of the researcher (Warren forthcoming). Thus, the second part of this section begins a process of critical reflection, developed more fully in the concluding section, by considering to what extent researchers may play a part in the (dis)empowerment of the subjects of their study.

NSUs and user involvement

The notion of user-oriented policy first came under my scrutiny in the NSU evaluation, since the core aims of the NSUs were informed by the general trend towards more flexible and user-sensitive social services. Involvement and consultation were seen as working goals for service providers, based on the findings of a long series of research studies pointing to the divergence between the perceptions of need held by users and professional providers in the social services (Mayer and Timms 1970; Sainsbury 1980; Fisher 1989).

The wider objectives relating to involvement were invoked by senior staff pivotal to the day-to-day running of the scheme. As I have shown above, however, the manner in and extent to which support workers put key objectives into practice were constrained by a lack of resources and operational guidelines. Older people appeared to have very limited say in the organization of their individual support or care packages and believed that, ultimately, decision-making powers still lay in the hands of service providers.

What the case-study approach helped to underline was the crucial fact that the relationship between user involvement and service organization could not be fully appreciated without wider consideration of variations in need among older people and their understanding of the NSU initiative and its aims.

Older people have traditionally been assessed for and allocated social care on the basis of health and measurements of incapacity. A less structured exploration of need revealed a complex picture of often interlocking determinants based on individual perceptions of health, the nature and duration of illness or disability, and on how these factors fitted with varied personalities and life histories (Shanas *et al.* 1968; Wenger 1984; Warren 1988).

A number of very frail older people described their health as good, dissociating it from their physical fitness or taking pride in their longevity. In contrast, others indicated that particular events, which included withdrawal from long-term tranquillizer use and the experience of being burgled, were colouring their overall notion of well-being. Cases where people were terminally ill or suffering dementia required particularly close and frequent monitoring to obtain an accurate picture of need.

Some individuals, who stressed their independent nature, fought against increased reliance on support, accepting the minimum amount necessary to enable them to live at home. Others were judged by their informal carers to lean on them more heavily than was necessary. In three instances, older people were themselves looking after another person. All identified themselves primarily as carers and put the requirements of those to whom they gave support before their own.

Needs were also influenced by certain structural factors such as housing. A number of older people in upper-storey flats were effectively housebound by their fear of negotiating stairs on their own. Adaptations had been carried out in some cases, though the provision of alarms appeared of little use to highly confused older people who did not understand their purpose.

While the norm of family care was still very much alive, pressures on family members, typically relating to paid employment and to the responsibilities of caring for others, meant that the normatively approved hierarchical model of family care preferences (Qureshi and Walker 1989) was rarely realized straightforwardly or without stress. A number of carers relied on the telephone to check on the well-being of older people. In the absence of family care, neighbourly ties were activated, though support of this kind was generally not as substantial and was often provided by people who were themselves over sixty-five years of age.

Managers undoubtedly recognized the variation in user need. Why, then, was opinion divided on whether the NSU initiative had moved to being a more user-sensitive service? Reasons lay in two aspects of the scheme: the communication of aims and service organization.

Various channels were employed to convey the aims of the new Unit: public meetings, a coffee morning, pamphlets and letters, as well as verbal explanations to individual users. But the intensity of resistance and mistrust which greeted the changes suggested that not enough time or attention had been devoted to discussion with local people. Central goals, such as flexibility, were interpreted as support workers pleasing themselves.

Support workers' partial understanding of the new system, explained in the previous section, was compounded by a lack of guidelines for the managers of the NSUs. They were left to make decisions as they went along on such things as time-tabling of shifts, allocation of support and activities to be undertaken. Despite ongoing efforts to produce booklets and reports about the Manor Neighbourhood Centre, managers still believed that 'some kind of formal public relations programme' or 'outreach work' needed to be established which was targeted, not least, at 'deeply entrenched' professional attitudes towards the role of the social care workers.

Service organization issues also contributed to professional opinion about the NSU. Recognizing the movement towards models of case management and computerized information systems (Griffiths 1988), Family and Community Services made compulsory a new common assessment form during the course of the evaluation. In comparison with the NSU form, the common assessment form was much more detailed (see Walker and Warren 1996) and, in theory, should have elicited a more accurate picture of need, especially since users' and carers' contributions were 'an integral part of any assessment'. However, in practice, the forms were used in similar ways: the minimum of data was typically recorded, with very brief comments, and sections were often left incomplete. Indeed, responses to the new fifteen-page common assessment document suggested that (quality aside) quantity of information had an inverse relationship to the length of the form. Despite reduced caseloads, team leaders did not necessarily have the time to devote to paperwork due to the new demands of their roles, including running the day centres and supervising workers. The forms therefore tended to perpetuate the traditional culture of social care service organization, whereby considerable amounts of information about users were passed on verbally and staff operated on the basis of 'taken for granted' knowledge of older people.[7]

At the same time, there were no specific procedures or mechanisms to encourage or secure the involvement of potential users in assessment. Older people were described by senior staff as 'participating', and observation found team leaders to be very thorough in their consideration of people's circumstances, life-histories and informal support networks. Nevertheless, how people's views were recorded lay very much in the hands of individual team leaders rather than being a joint process.

A number of older people appeared to be unaware that they had been referred for help and/or to be confused about the purpose of the team leader's visit. Self-referrers included, few were active or assertive in setting out directly what they considered to be their needs. If they knew of the assessment forms, none made reference to the sections set aside for recording their own views. Statements about the importance of 'control', 'independence' and 'hav[ing] a say', were largely an expression of individual character. Otherwise, comments reflected the traditional passive user role: 'I'm simply grateful towards anybody who helps me.'

The language of senior staff was equally equivocal. While recognizing that 'different individuals have different needs', care managers also spoke of 'determining allocation by making comparisons with other service users'. Reference was made to people who were not capable of making decisions concerning receipt of help and could not be left at risk. For one senior manager, assessment rested on debate concerning 'the difference between quality of care and quality of life'. Older people might argue that cleaning was important to their quality of life, but to supply domestic help to all people defining their needs in this way would be to spread the jam of service provision too thinly, compromising the overall quality of the service. In sum, the power of decision regarding service allocation still lay firmly in the hands of staff whose actions continued to be shaped by a perception of finite resources.

Expansion in the scope of support worker activities, the allocation of key workers, and collaboration with the health care team were cited by senior staff as evidence of better provision, choice, packaging, and continuity of care. However, they also acknowledged that certain features of the wider care-giving culture compromised attempts to introduce change, especially the failure of senior staff to accept the necessity of 'prioritizing in a world which was far from ideal'.

In other situations, cost-effectiveness ruled the day: a twenty-four hour service was deemed too expensive to provide, the night-sitting service was restricted to terminally ill older people, and team leaders no longer staffed the Unit at the weekends but were on call instead.

Among the case-study sample, users reported feeling involved in the sense of participating in everyday outside or communal activities, and exercising choice in terms of remaining at home or continuing to care for significant others at home. Older people who had received home care prior to the introduction of the NSU highlighted the increase in 'personal attention'. However, satisfaction with services was also linked to the adequacy of help received. Here, some users believed that flexibility had compromised reliability or operated to the favour of workers. There was a clear sense that aspects of provision – especially with housework tasks – had been reduced, if not as a matter of policy, then as a matter of exigency. Support workers were looking after a wider range of users and were too stretched. Indeed, users appeared to be given little support of a motivational nature, especially when they were severely confused or frail.

There is a risk of explaining older people's lack of reference to areas of support lying outside current service provision solely in terms of the dominance of the traditional model of social care and, thereby, to play down the importance of adequate domestic help to their physical and emotional well-being. But, even among new referrals, the desire was expressed for more help with cleaning, though they did not feel in a position to make demands. Where choice was openly offered, it tended to be within boundaries. For example, older people determined the selection and ordering of a number of the day centre activities, but it was within a framework shaped by the availability of transport and a fixed lunch-hour.

Not only do users' circumstances change, with implications for their needs, but it is possible for older people to change their minds about the suitability of care. However, while the role of monitoring and evaluation was highlighted by senior staff, how the scoring of measures in assessment was translated into the particular services provided was not clear-cut and there was no obvious evidence of the standardized recording of unmet need, or the systematic collation of outcomes, over time.

Checks on the needs of 'routine clients' were very informal: '[The support worker] might just say "is there anything else?".' Two new referrals, who had required emergency cover following hospitalization, reported decreases in provision that reflected their recovery and had been made in consultation with themselves and their families. Elsewhere, evidence showed patterns of provision to be sensitive to developments in need among existing users, but largely on the basis of how staff perceived those changes. In respect of a terminally ill user who did not want to confront his imminent death, such an approach was understandable. Other users simply said that the support workers could be 'relied upon'. Yet situations still arose where users and/or their carers had to make requests because of the lack of response from service providers. The failure to find a stand-in for an auxiliary nurse on long-term sick leave was one example. And although it was the general expectation among older people and care staff alike that complaints would be settled at the local level by senior NSU staff, rather than by resort to the official, Family and Community Services, city-wide panel system, the expression of grievances was not made easy by limited contact between users and team leaders.[8]

User-group committees were set up with the aim of ensuring 'users' participation in the development and use of community facilities' (Building User Group Code of Practice: 1). However, meetings were often poorly attended or attended consistently by the same handful of individuals. The extent of members' participation in management decisions appeared to be concentrated chiefly on the use of the building and the minibus by people living locally, and on services run on site. Users who received support within their own homes, particularly those who were housebound and/or in the 75-and-over age range, were severely under-represented within the groups. Given that none of the case-study sample appeared to know of their existence or purpose, it seems fair to conclude that, as established, these groups were clearly not a route to ensure the effective involvement of older people in the organization of the NSUs.

The role of research and researchers in empowerment

The NSU initiative was borne on the springtide of the empowerment movement. A danger inherent in studies of areas where the development of policy is rapid is the ahistoric trap of judging innovations according to standards to which they were not designed to aspire. In the NSU study, anthropologically informed methods and perspectives helped to conceptualize empowerment as an 'evolving *process*' (Stevenson and Parsloe 1993) and to illustrate how and why, at given points in time, different actors may be involved in various ways and to various degrees in empowering processes. A pluralistic evaluation model (Smith and Cantley 1988), was fitting for the evaluation of a scheme which aimed to offer greater flexibility and user/carer involvement in service provision. At the same time, and ironically, what it helped to reveal as a central feature of the NSU initiative was the failure adequately to prepare people for change or to allow them time to adapt to new practices. It evidenced gaps between conceptions of reality construed in terms of varying professional and lay value systems (Grant 1992), and highlighted lived contradictions in policy and their effects on the lives of service users and providers.

Unfortunately, it is rarely the case that those deciding the research agenda are researchers alone. It may be shaped by a complex amalgam of funders, politicians, professionals and managers. Since the NSU evaluation, I have had experience of conducting small-scale, local level studies of user involvement funded by bodies with limited research monies and desirous of instant findings.

The resulting 'fast and dirty' research projects (Hudson and Warren 1993; Warren 1994a) may be held up as examples of the ways in which the need to approach empowerment as a process may be compromised by the lack of scope to do much more than provide a snapshot picture of the practical details of policy implementation (Warren forthcoming). Indeed, in a context where notions of accountability are particularly sharp, some service users have been deeply affected by the failure to consider their interests as stakeholders within the research process itself (Beresford 1992; Davis and Fleming 1992). Researchers working in the field of health and social care have thus begun to pursue models, echoing the classic bottom-up empowerment model supported by anthropologists, which allow for a far greater degree of user participation (cf. Barnes and Oliver 1995; Barnes *et al.* 1994; Cooper and Sidell 1994; for a review of such models, see also Haxby 1994; and Thornton and Tozer 1994).

REFLECTIONS

Amongst anthropologists trying to achieve a better understanding of their own society there has been a move towards a 'more subjective ("intuitive") and self-questioning position' (Jackson 1987: 9–10). Greater reflexivity is regarded as a general implication of anthropology at home (Strathern 1987a: 17). Feminism has, arguably, increased and 'accelerated the process' (Williams 1987: 101). The acknowledgement by feminist researchers of a complex interaction between the 'research phenomenon', 'feminist theory' and 'feminist consciousness', as well as more directly personal influences and effects (Stanley and Wise 1979: 359), has led them to making a case for the personal to be made political and for research accounts to be (more) reflexive (Stanley and Wise 1983).

Both stances, together and separately, have shaped and have significance for my own work on community care. My first account of the experiences of front-line workers caring for older people was written at a time when, through my teaching, I had become immersed in examining and discussing feminist theory (Warren 1990a). This is not to say that my studies up to this point were uninfluenced by feminist perspectives. For example, referring specifically to methodological issues, my desire to avoid creating a hierarchical relationship with interviewees (an essential consideration in an investigation of the very personal nature of caring for vulnerable people in their own homes) and my subsequent rejection of a structured research strategy were stimulated in large part by Ann Oakley's discussions of interviewing women (Oakley 1981). However, if initially I was simply aware of feminist perspectives in social research, now I had a strong preference for them on methodological and political grounds. If feminism had actually played only a part in my choice of research topic and fieldwork methods, it had become increasingly important in the interpretation of research results. In fact, as feminist perspectives helped my understanding of the experiences of home helps and older people (by placing them in relation to gender and age divisions within a context of oppression and subordination) so in a dialectical process my understanding of and commitment to feminism grew. Already aware of the well-established trend of self-reflection in anthropological ethnographies (cf. Whyte 1955), reflexivity became particularly important to me as a means of offering an understanding from the point of view of women's experiences of women's reality.

In my second opportunity to study frontline carers I had not dropped feminism, far from it as the analysis above shows, but the major imperative in this instance was to consider the impact of policy innovation on the lives of formal carers and the older people for whom they cared. Changing services involves not just new activities but new attitudes, and the focus was on the organizational culture of service provision, and its role and relative success in shifting views. The study was framed far more explicitly than my doctoral studies in an understanding of policy reform, specifically of the policy of care that has been adopted in all advanced societies, variously called community care, the promotion of independent living or 'ageing in place' (Walker 1982; Tinker 1995).

Placing the accounts side by side, it is clear that there is interplay between present and past which affects the deployment of particular past events and thoughts (Morgan 1987). As authors, we construct and reconstruct. What we produce each time is a version of many possible versions. It may be revision of previous papers. It may be based on those issues we did not or could not include in the last. If I had set my studies in a rural area, rather than in large, industrial urban areas, for example, I might have viewed community care from other angles. Cecil (1989) has shown how, in a small Northern Irish town and its rural hinterland, home helps' straddling of the boundary between formal and informal care is further complicated by the fact that they are commonly neighbours of the people for whom they care. In addition to the expectation that women's lives are largely domestic and family-centred, there is an ideal of neighbourliness which puts pressure on women to give their services willingly and without payment. Different again would be an account which concentrated on people from minority ethnic groups and their experiences of community care.

What, as researchers, we are funded (and personally motivated) to produce thus keeps open the question of the purpose of our analysis and communication: for whom we write (Strathern 1987a) and, indeed, for what occasion (Morgan 1987). We might also add to this the question of how we write. I am not, in this instance, implying the need for a critical appraisal of the written text, though this is an important phase of postmodernism (cf. Marcus and Cushman 1982; Clifford and Marcus 1986; Crick 1987; Strathern 1987b). What I am referring to instead, and particularly in the context of the empowerment movement, is the call to involve those who are typically the 'subjects' of research more fully in the production of accounts of their lives. This may go beyond the simple notion of jointly authored accounts. For users of services desirous of setting their own research agenda, this means finding ways of working *with* – or 'for' – groups, using our skills primarily in an advisory capacity to help individuals to set up their own proposals, secure funding, gather data and to decide on the format for its analysis and presentation. Indeed, if we are to make a claim for the role of anthropology in better understanding community care, we need to be open to the community reflecting on our own anthropological backyard and arrogant assumption of the academic as expert. To paraphrase Maiteny, by listening to some of the critiques directed at us by other[s] and even learning to use some of their methods and tools, we would improve our own effectiveness and empower ourselves' (1996: 47).

NOTES

1 BASAPP was renamed Anthropology in Action in December 1993, reflecting a shift from its British focus. The organization brings together people interested in anthropological approaches to current issues of policy or practice in the fields of health and social and community work as well as education, organizational change and overseas development. For a history of the organization, see Wright (1995).

2 The questionnaire survey was to involve the use of Manpower Services Commission sponsored researchers. The trade unions believed that this was work which should be carried out by the Department as a matter of course, by full-time staff on permanent establishment.

3 Interviews were also conducted with practitioners and frontline workers within the health team but the lack of resources meant that a detailed analysis of the health component of the project was not possible.

4 Individual users of services were allocated to a named support worker who was responsible for monitoring and reviewing care packages.

5 This was a problem pointed out by Poland (1986) in relation to mothers working as childminders, but it appears to me to apply equally to housewives and mothers working as home helps. Indeed, describing the intense pressures of the service for a home help and the huge burdens which she takes on, Bond concluded: 'to admit that she cannot meet all these demands with the resources available to her would strike at her good womanhood – at the very qualities for which the staff of the service are elected' (Bond 1980: 24).

6 Fuller discussions have included brief pen portraits of selected households to illustrate the kinds of circumstances, experiences and beliefs that had bearing on the process of user *and* carer involvement (Warren 1993; Walker and Warren 1996).

7 The new form was eventually abandoned by Family and Community Services and staff at the Manor Unit simply reverted to the tools used prior to its introduction.

8 While the recently introduced system of care management should in theory alter this situation, the creation of a new relationship between managers as purchasers and workers as frontline providers may remove the benefits of direct line-management.

BIBLIOGRAPHY

Allan, G. (1979) *A Sociology of Friendship and Kinship*, London: George Allen and Unwin.

Ballard, R. (1983) *Racial Inequality, Ethnic Diversity and Social Policy: Applied Anthropology in Urban Britain*, revised version of a paper presented at the 1983 Association of Social Anthropologists Conference, Cambridge.

Barnes, C. and Oliver, M. (1995) 'Disability rights: rhetoric and reality in the UK', *Disability and Society* 10, 1, 111–16.

Barnes, M. (1997) *Care, Communities and Citizens*, Harlow: Longman.

Barnes, M., Cormie, J. and Crichton, M. (1994) *Seeking Representative Views from Frail Older People*, Kirkcaldy: Age Concern Scotland.

Barnes, M. and Walker, A. (1996) 'Consumerism versus empowerment: a principled approach to the involvement of older service users', *Policy and Politics* 24, 4, 375–93.

Barnes, M. and Wistow, G. (1992) 'Consulting with carers: what do they think?', *Social Sciences Research* 1, 9–30.

Beresford, P. (1992) 'Researching citizen involvement: a collaborative or colonising exercise?', in M. Barnes and G. Wistow (eds) *Researching User Involvement*, Leeds: Nuffield Institute for Health, University of Leeds.

Bond, M. (1980) *Women's Work in a Women's World*, unpublished MA dissertation, Department of Applied Social Studies, University of Warwick.

Cecil, R. (1989) 'Care and the community in a Northern Irish town', in H. Donnan and G. McFarlane (eds) *Social Anthropology and Public Policy in Northern Ireland*, Aldershot: Avebury.

Clifford, J. and Marcus, G. E. (eds) (1986) *Writing Culture: The Poetics and Politics of Ethnography*, London: University of California Press.

Collins, J. (1992) 'The monolithic institution in social care systems', *Anthropology in Action* 13: 6–7.

Cooper, M. and Sidell, M. (1994) *Lewisham Older Women's Health Survey*, London: EdROP The City Lit.

Crick, M. R. (1987) 'Comments on paper by M. Strathern "Out of context"', *Current Anthropology* 28, 3, 270–1.

Davis, A. and Fleming, A. (1992) 'User-commissioned research – the shape of things to come?', *Social Services Research* 1, 50–3.

Department of Health [DoH] (1989) *Caring for People*, London: HMSO.

—— (1991) *Managers and Practitioners: Guide to Care Management and Assessment*, London: HMSO.

Dexter, M. and Harbert, W. (1983) *The Home Help Service*, London: Tavistock.

Douglas, M. and Nicod, M. (1974) 'Taking the biscuit: the structure of British meals', *New Society* 30, 744–7.

Egington, A. (1983) 'Knowing where to draw the line', *Community Care*, 2 June, 16–17.

Fisher, M. (ed.) (1989) *Client Studies*, Sheffield: JUSSR.

Fox, N. (1995) 'Postmodern perspectives on care: the vigil and the gift', *Critical Social Policy* 44/5, 107–125.

Fransella, F. and Frost, K. (1977) *On Being a Woman*, London: Tavistock.

Gearing, B. and Coleman, P. (1996) 'Biographical assessment in community care', in J. Birren, G. Kenyan, J.-E. Ruth, J. Schroots and T. Svensson (eds) *Aging and Biography: Explorations in Adult Development*, New York: Springer.

Gowler, D. and Clarke, G. (1983) 'The employment and training of British social anthropologists', paper given to the 1983 Association of Social Anthropologists Conference, Cambridge.

Graham, H. (1983) 'Caring: a labour of love', in J. Finch and D. Groves (eds) *A Labour of Love: Women, Work and Caring*, London: Routledge and Kegan Paul.

—— (1984) *Women, Health and the Family*, Brighton: Wheatsheaf.

Grant, G. (1992) 'Researching user and carer involvement in mental handicap services', in M. Barnes and G. Wistow (eds) *Researching User Involvement*.

Griffiths, R. (1988) *Community Care: An Agenda for Action*, London: HMSO.

Guba, E. G. and Lincoln, Y. S. (1987) *Effective Education*, (5th edn), London: Jossey-Bass.

Gubrium, J. F. and Silverman, D. (eds) (1989) *The Politics of Field Research: Sociology Beyond Enlightenment*, London: Sage.

Haxby, J. (1994) *Involving Older People in Planning and Evaluating Community Care: A Review of Initiatives*, York: SPRU, University of York.

Hollingberry, R. (1994) 'Elder power', in Counsel and Care (ed.) *More Power to Our Elders: Promoting Empowerment for Older People*, London: Counsel and Care.

Hudson, B. and Warren, L. (1993) *South West Durham Care Management Project: Evaluation Report*, Durham: Institute of Health Studies, University of Durham.

Jackson, A. (1987) 'Reflections on ethnography at home and the ASA', in A. Jackson (ed.) *Anthropology at Home*, London: Tavistock.

Maiteny, P. (1996) 'Empowering anthropology and the rhetoric of empowerment', *Anthropology in Action* 3, 1, 45–7.

Marcus, G. E. and Cushman, D. (1982) 'Ethnographies as texts', *Annual Review of Anthropology* 11, 25–69.

Mars, G. and Nicod, M. (1984) *World of Waiters*, London: George Allen and Unwin.

Mayer, J. and Timms, N. (1970) *The Client Speaks*, London: Routledge and Kegan Paul.

McCourt-Perring, C. (1992) 'The reproduction of institutional structures in the community', *Anthropology in Action* 13, 10–12.

—— (1993) *The Experience of Psychiatric Hospital Closure. An Anthropological Study*, Aldershot: Avebury Press.

—— (1994) 'Community care as de-institutionalisation? Continuity and change in the transition from hospital to community-based care', in S. Wright (ed.) *Anthropology of Organizations*, London: Routledge.

Means, R. and Lart, R. (1994a) 'Involving older people in community care planning', in Counsel and Care (ed.) *More Power to Our Elders: Promoting Empowerment for Older People*, London: Counsel and Care.

—— (1994b) 'User empowerment, older people and the UK reform of community care', in D. Challis, B. Davies and K. Traske (eds.) *Community Care: New Agendas and Challenges from the UK and Overseas*, Aldershot: Arena.

Meethan, K. and Thompson, C. (1992) 'Setting up the Scarcroft Project: the problem of joint working', *Caring for People* 9, 6–7.

Monks, J. (1992) 'Life stories and substantive issues: people with MS and their supporters', *Anthropology in Action* 13, 7–9.

Morgan, D. (1987) *'It Will Make a Man of You': Notes on National Service, Masculinity and Autobiography*, Studies in Sexual Politics, 17, Manchester: Department of Sociology, University of Manchester.

Norton, A., Stolen, B. and Taylor, H. (1986) *Councils of Care: Planning a Legal Government Strategy for Older People*, London: Centre for Policy on Ageing.

Oakley, A. (1974) *Housewife*, London: Allen Lane.

—— (1981) 'Interviewing women: a contradiction in terms', in H. Roberts (ed.) *Doing Feminist Research*, London: Kegan Paul.

Okely, J. (1983) *The Traveller Gypsies*, Cambridge: Cambridge University Press.

—— (1987) 'Fieldwork up the M1: policy and political aspects', in A. Jackson (ed.) *Anthropology at Home*, London: Tavistock.

Poland, F. (1986) 'Minding and mothering. The tension between "work" and "care"', in the Social and Research Seminar (ed.) *On Researching the Topic of 'Care'*, Studies in Sexual Politics, 11, Manchester: Department of Sociology, University of Manchester.

Porter, M. (1983) *Home, Work and Class Consciousness*, Manchester: Manchester University Press.

Qureshi, H. and Walker, A. (1989) *The Caring Relationship*, London: Macmillan.

Rossi, A. (1972) 'The roots of ambivalence in American women', in A. Rossi and J. Bardwick (eds) *Readings in the Psychology of Women*, New York: Harper and Row.

Sainsbury, E. (1980) 'Client need, social work method and agency function: a research perspective', *Social Work Service* 23, 9–15.

Shanas, E., Townsend, P., Wedderburn, D., Friis, H., Milhøj, P. and Stehouwer, J. (1968) *Old People in Three Industrial Societies*, London: Routledge and Kegan Paul.

Sixsmith, A. (1990) 'The meaning and experience of "home" in later life', in B. Bytheway and J. Johnson (eds) *Welfare and the Ageing Experience*, Aldershot: Avebury.

Smith, G. and Cantley, C. (1988) *Assessing Health Care: A Study in Organizational Evaluation*, Milton Keynes: Cambridge University Press.

Soloman, D. N. (1968) 'Sociological perspectives on occupations', in H. S. Becker, B. Geer, D. Riesman and R. S. Weiss (eds) *Institutions and the Person: Papers Presented to Everett C. Hughes*, Chicago: Aldine.

Stanley, L. (1986) 'A referral was made: behind the scenes during the creation of a social services department statistic', in the Social and Research Seminar (ed.) *On Researching the Topic of 'Care'*, Studies in Sexual Politics, 11, Manchester: Department of Sociology, University of Manchester.

Stanley, L. and Wise, S. (1979) 'Feminist research, feminist consciousness and experiences of sexism', *Women's Studies International Quarterly* 2, 359–74.

—— (1983) *Breaking Out: Feminist Consciousness and Feminist Research*, London: Routledge and Kegan Paul.

Stevenson, G. (1976) 'Social relations of production and consumption in the human service occupations', *Monthly Review* 28, 3, 78–87.

Stevenson, O. and Parsloe, P. (1993) *Community Care and Empowerment*, York: Joseph Rowntree Foundation.

Strathern, M. (1987a) 'The limits of auto-anthropology', in A. Jackson (ed.) *Anthropology at Home*, London: Tavistock.

—— (1987b) 'Out of context: the persuasive fictions of anthropology', *Current Anthropology* 28, 3, 251–81.

Strong, P. and Dingwall, R. (1989) 'Romantics and stoics', in J. F. Gubrium and D. Silverman (eds) *The Politics of Field Research: Sociology Beyond Enlightenment*, London: Sage.

Tambiah, S. J. (1985) 'An anthropologist's manifesto for the eighties', paper given to the 1985 Association of Social Anthropologists Conference, University of Keele.

Thornton, P. and Tozer, R. (1994) *Involving Older People in Planning and Evaluating Community Care: A Review of Initiatives*, York: SPRU, University of York.

Tinker, A. (1995) 'Housing and older people', in I. Allen and E. Perkins (eds) *The Future of Family Care for Older People*, London: HMSO.

Twigg, J. (1986) *The Interface Between NHS and SSD: Home Helps, District Nurses and the Issue of Personal Care*, Kent: University of Kent, PSSRU.

—— (1997) 'Deconstructing the "social bath": help with bathing at home for older and disabled people', *Journal of Social Policy* 26, 2, 211–32.

Ungerson, C. (1983) 'Women and caring: skills, tasks and taboos', in E. Gamarnikow, D. H. J. Morgan, J. Purvis, and D. Taylorson (eds) *The Public and the Private*, London: Heinemann.

Walker, A. (1982) 'Dependency and old age', *Social Policy and Administration* 16, 2, 115–35.

—— (1987) 'Enlarging the caring capacity of the community: informal support networks and the welfare state', *International Journal of Health Services* 17, 3, 369–86.

—— (1989) 'Community care', in M. McCarthy (ed.) *The New Politics of Welfare*, London: Macmillan.

—— (1991) 'No gain without pain', *Community Care*, 18 July, 14–16.

Walker, A. and Warren, L. (1996) *Changing Services for Older People: The Neighbourhood Support Units Innovation*, Buckingham: Open University Press.

Warren, L. (1988) *Home Care and Elderly People: The Experiences of Home Helps and Old People in Salford*, unpublished PhD thesis, University of Salford.

—— (1990a) *Doing, Being, Writing: Research on Home Care for Older People*, Feminist Praxis 31, Manchester: Department of Sociology, University of Manchester.

—— (1990b) '"We're home helps because we care": the experiences of home helps caring for elderly people', in P. Abbott and G. Payne (eds) *New Directions in the Sociology of Health*, Basingstoke: Falmer Press.

—— (1993) 'Community care and user participation', in P. Kaim-Caudle, J. Keithley and A. Mullender (eds) *Aspects of Ageing: A Celebration of the European Year of Older People and Solidarity between Generations*, London: Whiting and Birch.

—— (1994a) *Involving People in Social Services in Sunderland: A Case Study of People with Physical Disabilities*, Durham: Institute of Health Studies, University of Durham.

—— (1994b) 'Tradition and transition: the role of the support worker in community care in Sheffield', in D. Challis, B. Davies and K. Traske (eds) *Community Care: New Agendas and Challenges from the UK and Overseas*, London: Arena.

—— (forthcoming) 'Empowerment: the path to partnership?', in M. Barnes and L. Warren (eds) *Alliances and Participation in Empowerment*, Bristol: Policy Press.

Warren, L. and Walker, A. (1992) 'Neighbourhood Support Units: a new approach to the care of older people', in F. Laczko and C. Victor (eds) *Social Policy and Elderly People*, Aldershot: Avebury.

Webb, A. and Hobdell, M. (1980) 'Co-ordination in the health and personal social services', in S. Lonsdale, A. Webb and T. L. Briggs (eds) *Team Work in the Personal Social Services and Health Care*, London: Croom Helm.

Weiss, C. H. (1986) 'Research and policy-making: a limited partnership', in F. Heller (ed.) *The Use and Abuse of Social Science*, London: Sage.

Wenger, G. C. (1984) *The Supportive Network: Coping with Old Age*, London: Allen and Unwin.

Whyte, W. (1955) *Street Corner Society*, Chicago: University of Chicago Press.

Williams, A. (1987) 'Reading feminism in fieldnotes', in Feminist Research Seminar (ed.) *Feminist Research Process*, Manchester: Department of Sociology, University of Manchester.

Wright, J., Ball, C. and Coleman, P. (1988) *Collaboration in Care: An Examination of Health and Social Service Provision for Mentally Frail Old People*, London: Age Concern.

Wright, S. (1992) *Evaluation of the Unemployment Strategy*, Middlesborough: Cleveland County Council.

—— (1994) 'Part III: clients and empowerment. Introduction', in S. Wright (ed.) *Anthropology of Organizations*, London: Routledge.

—— (1995) 'Anthropology: still the uncomfortable discipline?', in A. Ahmed and C. Shore (eds) *The Future of Anthropology: Its Relevance to the Contemporary World*, London: Athlone.

Chapter 11

Treasures on Earth

Housing assets, public policy and older people in New Zealand[1]

Sally Keeling

INTRODUCTION

> Lay not up for yourselves treasures on earth, where moth and rust doth corrupt, and where thieves break through and steal; But lay up for yourselves treasures in heaven. For where your treasure is, there will your heart be also.
>
> (Matthew 6: 19–21)

By opening with a biblical quotation this discussion does not purport to preach a sermon, but to explore some connections between the cultural value expressed here, contemporary New Zealand public policy on 'user pays' in continuing care, and the views of some over-80-year-olds on 'treasures' – their tangible assets and less tangible values. These values and assets are ways in which the connections between older people and their communities of residence are made and maintained. They involve questions of belonging, identity, independence and autonomy, and express both through and beyond bricks and mortar, notions of roots in and ties with familial and community contexts.

For the purposes of this discussion, 'treasures' is used as shorthand for the idea that housing assets have both economic and financial meanings on the one hand, and symbolic social and personal meanings on the other. These dual meanings can be also represented by the use of the terms 'house' and 'home', each with their different connotations. For older people in New Zealand, the prospect of selling their house contains the prospect of losing their home.

AGEING, ANTHROPOLOGY AND COMMUNITY CARE IN NEW ZEALAND

Housing has been described as 'the essential element of community care' (Gurney and Means 1993: 123). Applying this to a New Zealand context, Thorns acknowledges the importance of the social relations and notions of independence and security which are enmeshed in physical structures, as areas needing research attention (Thorns 1993: 97). With Dupuis, Thorns has also gone on to present some of the meanings of home for older people with case extracts which echo strongly the material being presented here (Dupuis and Thorns 1996).

As an anthropologist working with older people in a New Zealand community, I have inherited from my discipline an array of concepts, theories and methods appropriate to this task. For instance, studies of reciprocity, and the exchange of goods and services in private, domestic and family domains, have a long history in anthropology (Goody 1983; Mauss 1922; Strathern 1992). In this work, the 'balance sheet' can exceed more than one generation, and 'repayments' are likely to be seen as deferred, but of equivalent type and value. So the caregiving one receives from one's parents is repaid by caring for them in later life, and the interdependency of generations is recognized throughout the life-cycle. Similarly, anthropologists have always treated questions of kinship, descent and inheritance as needing to be considered each in their own right, but also in relationship to each other: they are recognized as major conceptual and pragmatic building blocks of social structure. The theory is that, in a lineage-based society, one knows the line of gift and return will be continued.

In relation to housing, anthropology also offers a strong perspective on the range of social and symbolic meanings surrounding and embedded in culturally various settings of house, home and dwelling. The collection of cultural settings included in *About the House* (Carsten and Hugh-Jones 1995) reinforces a holistic focus on the house, and presents a view of houses 'in the round', on which this analysis of New Zealand issues around housing assets and older people very much depends.

Working in a medium-sized community located within a complex national structure, I needed to explore the possibility of local variations on national themes, so the prospect of looking at ideas about the complex values embedded in housing assets from both a national, media-based perspective, and with community-based informants, was both feasible and productive. The particular value of working with older people as informants was another process readily identifiable within my anthropological training. By virtue of their life histories and experience, older people impart a kind of knowledge about their community and their own roles within social contexts. I am something of an outsider to these, if only by virtue of the fact that in most cases, forty years separate our ages and lives.

PUBLIC POLICY CHANGES: HOUSING ASSETS

The public policy which has been at issue is that which requires housing assets to be spent down to a specified level before an older person qualifies for a residential care subsidy under Income Support Services. The current brochure prepared by the Income Support Service concerning the availability of the residential care subsidy asks and answers two key questions. The first is, 'What counts as assets?' The list specifies cash or savings, investments, shares or stocks, loans made to other people, house, chattels and car if the applicant lives alone, and gifts over the $5,000 per year to family members limit, in the five years prior to application. The second question is 'Who can get a subsidy?' In addition to specifying assessment and other qualifying criteria, the key point is that assets for single or widowed people must not exceed $6,500. In other words, all assets above this level, including the value of the family home, must be 'cashed up' and used to pay for care.

A brief presentation of public policy history helps to put perspective on the material that follows (cf. Blank 1994; Easton 1979). In essence, at the time of the major restructuring in New Zealand of service delivery for the elderly (on 1 July 1993), a four-part pattern of funding and provision of long-term care services for the elderly existed. Different regulations covered charging regimes in each of the four sectors of long-term care delivery: eligibility for state subsidy varied with the location of the service (in the public or private sector) and according to the level of care (represented as Rest Home or hospital care).

The effect of the 1993 changes was to extend the asset testing regulations, which had previously applied only in the private Rest Home sector, to both public and private hospital provision. Meanwhile, the public Rest Home sector was effectively closed down. This shift in resources was noted as being necessary to free up public funds for home support or community care services, which had previously been predominantly voluntary or fully 'userpays'. Full state or welfare funding had been limited to short-term services, such as Meals on Wheels, home helps and services on hospital discharge, and had not been widely available for long-term continuing care for older people in the community. Significant public reaction followed these changes.

MEDIA REVIEW OF ASSET TESTING DEBATE

Over the period January to April 1994, I monitored coverage of the asset testing debate in local newspapers while I was embarking on my anthropological field-work with older people in a local community. Two broad themes in the presentation of this issue were discerned. Moving from the sublime of the opening biblical quotation to the ridiculous, two cartoons by Garrick Tremain represent these themes (Figs 2 and 3). The first shows the political impact of the debate, in mobilizing older people as a political force opposing a key government policy. The second deals with the perceived social and family impact of the means-testing policies, here shown as impinging on inheritance patterns.

A sample of cuttings and headlines from this same period shows that the local and national media had no difficulty presenting this first area. For example: 'Govt "got it wrong" on asset testing' (*Otago Daily Times* 29 January 1994); 'Pensioner asset testing anger' (*Dominion* 11 January 1994); and 'Elderly vent anger at asset testing' (*Christchurch Press* 11 February 1994). Protest meetings were held throughout the country, where older people in significant numbers made their views public.

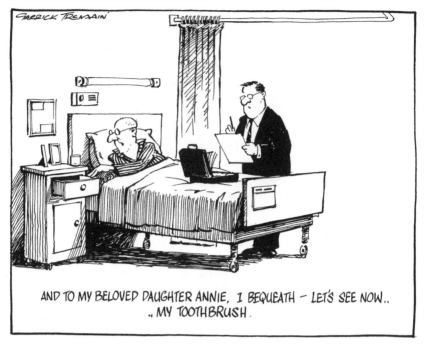

AND TO MY BELOVED DAUGHTER ANNIE, I BEQUEATH — LET'S SEE NOW..
.. MY TOOTHBRUSH.

Figure 2

Source: By Garrick Tremain

The second area received less focused coverage, and was generally based on a particular reported situation, where other social and family values were seen to be affected. For example: 'Asset, income testing "splitting family fabric"' (*Otago Daily Times* 22 February 1994); 'Asset rules put son's home at risk' (*Sunday Times* 27 February 1994); and 'Warning to elderly that divorce may end benefit' (*Otago Daily Times* 22 January 1994).

A new round of press coverage in August 1996 followed ongoing modification of the policy and practice of the asset testing scheme. It echoed coverage of thirty months previously: the political and personal issues had not been resolved, and the inconsistencies within the policy were becoming cumulative. There were now recorded cases of active resistance and legal challenges, such as the case reported in the *Otago Daily Times* (16 August 1996) under the headline 'Govt places caveats on homes of 1489 elderly'.

Since 1994, while this debate has continued, parallel issues, such as superannuation policies, in particular the tax surcharge (by which superannuitants pay a premium tax rate on private income), and income levels for over 65-year-olds, vied for media coverage and political supremacy. The superannuation and income issues have also received significant academic attention, particularly from

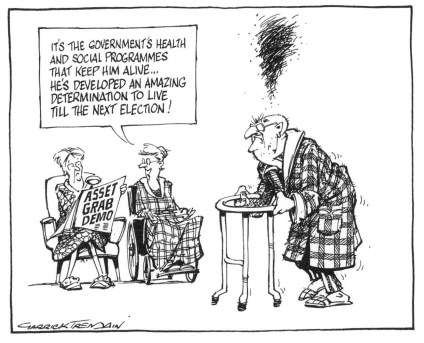

Figure 3
Source: By Garrick Tremain

economists (St John 1993) and historians (Thompson 1991). Both issues (surcharge and asset testing) resurfaced in June 1996, with submissions being called for by the Labour Select Committee on the Repeal of Asset Testing for Older People requiring Disability Support Services Bill. At the same time, a multi-party Superannuation Accord was reconsidering legislation to repeal the surcharge. Few reminders of the political potency of these issues were needed in an election year.

By the end of 1996, the outcome of New Zealand's first parliamentary election held under the mixed member proportional representation system was known, with a coalition being formed between the previously governing National Party and a newer party known as New Zealand First. In the coalition agreement released on 11 December 1996, key issues in the handling of the treasures of senior citizens were included: the abolition of the superannuation surcharge from 1 April 1998; the development of a home equity scheme to allow people solely reliant on superannuation to borrow up to 20 per cent of the value of their home, to be repaid with interest when their home is sold; the removal of income and asset testing for long-stay geriatric public hospital care, and asset testing for long-stay geriatric private hospital care; and the introduction of a significantly higher ($100,000) exemption on the family home for income and asset tests on Rest Home care by 1999/2000 (NZFVWO 1997: 13).

The government in New Zealand had proposed these funding policy shifts to develop a more 'seamless service', to remove anomalies and inequities which clearly existed, and to bring the public health sector into a competitive commercial environment (Health Matters 1993; Upton 1991). The concept of a continuum of care, where older people made choices as to the style and location of care, and appropriate services were to be matched to carefully assessed need, was, however, frequently disrupted by an 'all or nothing' choice. This choice involved either retaining home ownership, or obtaining publicly funded care; it jeopardized community residence and membership by being linked, at a policy level, with the choice of residential care.

OLDER PEOPLE AT HOME IN NEW ZEALAND

Thorns has documented a detailed housing history of cohorts of New Zealanders in the last fifty years, noting regional and ethnic variations. He concludes that, while the actual level of assets involved in housing owned by elderly people is modest, the debate on equity release in the period since 1991 has been seen by older New Zealanders as an 'attack on their status and on their past thrift' (Thorns 1993: 117). Thorns (1997) has continued tracing issues relating to house and home for older people in New Zealand during the period of recent change in policy and, following comparisons overseas, confirms that his research presents a strong New Zealand cultural tradition of home ownership and sense of belonging which is particularly evident amongst older people.

In the asset testing debate in New Zealand we see significant state intervention in family policy and action, as it regulates gifting, and the capacity to bequeath assets to family members or others. It is important also to note that home ownership is the predominant form of asset holding among New Zealand's population over the age of sixty-five. In 1991, 'more than three-quarters of the elderly lived in mortgage-free private dwellings' (Statistics NZ 1995: 55).

The homes of the older people I visited in the course of my research reflect in quite specific ways the general features of the meanings of 'home'. In New Zealand, 'home' has been identified as a place of shelter, a place of security, a place of shared memories and a potential store of wealth (Thorns 1993: 97). The disruption of leaving one's home to go to a Rest Home (the name by which an institution providing 24-hour residential care to frail elderly people is known in New Zealand) has not been masked by the continuous use of 'home' to describe the new setting, nor by the fact that the majority of such homes are in communities. Neighbourly and community relations are frequently cultivated within the Home. Many contemporary Rest Homes encourage their residents to bring familiar furniture and personal items upon their admission, to encourage a feeling of being 'at home' in their new surroundings. The implicit contrast is not between 'home' and 'community', but between 'home' and 'hospital', a setting where more clinical and nursing related features may be evident in both function and design. There is metaphorical ambiguity in the use of 'Rest' – does it allude to 'laid to rest', 'rest from . . . ' or 'the rest of one's days?'

The public and political debate over the appropriate use, by conversion into funds for care, of the housing assets of older people in New Zealand has raged over the last ten years. Over the same time period, there has been significant development in the practice of home care and the growth of owner-occupied retirement villages throughout the country (NACCH and DSS 1994; Statistics NZ: 1995). As Pool has argued cogently (in relation particularly to superannuation) 'in conceptualizing policy, any dichotomy between social and economic is misleading' (Pool 1991: 173).

It is in the area of linking public policy to the family context of older people that there is a great deal more by way of assumption and contradiction than validated knowledge. The brunt of the asset testing policy is currently affecting those assessed as needing long-term residential care; a standard figure of 6 per cent of those over sixty-five is frequently quoted, with the proportion of those over eighty-five years much higher (see Koopman-Boyden 1993). The more detailed figures for residential care rates in 1991 are given by Statistics NZ (1995: 54, 81) as 1 per cent of people aged sixty-five years and over, rising to 22 per cent of those aged eighty-five years and over, and 65 per cent of those aged ninety-five years and over.

There are also increasing intrusions of the means testing policy into the 'domestic sphere' and the more private economy of the household – in the area of policies relating to older couples, where one partner needs residential care, and through income assessments for those being offered publicly funded, home-based services. Charlotte Paul has recently foreshadowed the similar overflow effect of these policies in the funding and quality of services for the long-term needs of the chronically ill, whether old or younger (Paul 1996).

Current research brings us much closer to this more private familial setting, the setting in which public policies are acted out, as older people make decisions in the light of the law, policies, regulations and (dis)incentives, as well as their own values, about the use and disposal of their 'treasures'. A 1977 anthropology thesis from Auckland marks one end of the trail (Johnson 1977). Johnson links anthropological work on gift-giving and financial aid within families, with his informants' notions of closeness or emotional proximity. More recently, Opie (1992) has focused New Zealand caregiver research by presenting the experiences of family members caring for confused elderly people at home, interpreting both the intensely demanding daily patterns of care, and the gendered provision of care. In addition, implicit in the presentation by some of her caregiver respondents of eventual residential placement as a decision of 'last resort', the emotionally charged aspect of this decision, let alone any consideration of its financial consequences, is accentuated.

New Zealanders have rather taken for granted a cultural tradition of the quarter-acre paradise (Mitchell 1972) and freeholding one's home as the predominant arena for asset accumulation over a lifetime. This intensifies the heat of the debate in this country. Add to this the clear pattern for women to outlive their husbands, and for the earnings of women over their lifetime to have been less in dollar terms than their husband's, and the value of the family home as the last major asset available to women is raised yet further.

Some members of parliament have recently espoused the cause of raising the exempt asset level closer to the value of a 'family home equivalent'. Going further than this, the full repeal of asset testing was argued with a complex rationale (Bills Digest 1996) including age discrimination, advantaging the wealthy and those able to avoid the means test through early establishment of family trusts, and contradictions between this policy and other aspects of retirement income policies. The coalition government's proposals outlined earlier reflect the state of play at the time of writing.

UNITED KINGDOM AND AUSTRALIAN EXPERIENCE

There is a significant body of overseas academic literature which considers the complex relationship between the state, older people and their families, and the private sector. Such studies are valuable for the comparative perspective they offer on the problems faced by the elderly in New Zealand. In the United Kingdom, Walker's 'welfare triangle' shows the mix of private/market, public/state and informal family care (Walker 1995: 202–5). The 'taken for grantedness' of family care for older people has been explored from a variety of perspectives: negotiation of family responsibilities (Finch and Mason 1993), caregiver burden (Baines et al. 1991), exploitation and elder abuse (Phillipson et al. 1995), public policy, economic and service provision (Allen and Perkins 1995), and inheritance patterns and issues around legacy (Kane 1996).

It was in the 1980s that studies began to explore the relationship between family support and public assistance. Qureshi and Walker (1989) set out to explore the implicit assumptions they saw in public policy in the United Kingdom at the time: that family support for ageing relatives was an underutilized resource available to the state, and that as the state pulled back from meeting the increasing needs of frail older people, families would fill the gap. Their series of reports based on this work challenged these assumptions, and made certain other broad features of the patterns of family support in this situation quite clear. While public policy statements refer to 'family', the reality of both work and commitment falls on women (Finch and Groves 1983). Further, while the partners in this relationship (the older people and their family caregivers) value independent living over residential services, there is still a gap between the availability and provision of family and state resources.

Allen and Perkins (1995) begin to make predictions based on existing knowledge about the future of family care. Baldwin (1995), Groves (1995) and Hamnett (1995) each turn their attention to economic aspects of the policy of drawing further on family resources in order to protect the state's resources for the most needy. They consider that the advanced state of research in investigating the internal workings of extended families, following in the tradition of Finch and Mason (1993), allows them to extrapolate policy impacts on individual families in such areas as costs to caregivers, pensioners' own financial resources, and housing equity release and inheritance. Hamnett describes the fluctuations in the housing market in the United Kingdom over the last twenty years, and the rapidly rising ratio of owner-occupiers to tenants, with its implications for the passage of wealth from one generation to another.

In the United Kingdom, Oldman has reviewed closely what is known in that context about older people's capacity to use home equity to fund care, together with a consideration of their willingness and current practice in doing so. She traces UK Age Concern's acknowledgement in 1988 that 'community care reforms involve shifting care services', and that particularly in relation to 'long term care . . . the goal posts have moved' (Oldman 1991: 184). In that same year, she notes Sir Roy Griffiths' recommendations to government based on the finding that the elderly represented a group who were 'asset rich but often cash poor' (*ibid.*: 185). She concludes 'policy development in the area of using housing equity in old age is hampered by large gaps in knowledge', and that 'the Government has not developed a coherent or consistent policy towards home equity and its conversion' (*ibid.*: 196–7). Henwood (1996) notes that the recent shift in exempted asset level in the United Kingdom has been made because of its likely political impact.

In Australia, about ten years ahead of New Zealand in terms of paying research attention to the social and personal side of the policy framework designed for an ageing society, Kendig and his team mounted a major multidisciplinary study of ageing in Sydney (Kendig 1986). Of particular interest from this team project is the work of Alice Day (1985), which goes beyond present patterns of family and community support for over-75-year-olds to consider 'contingency planning'. She classifies the responses of the older people interviewed according to four basic orientations, which she labels on a scale from a 'high' to a 'low' belief in the efficacy of planning: the four are described as planners, procrastinators, fatalists, counters on family support.

Day claims that there is growing evidence that 'the ethos of self-help among the aged is related to their perception of their capacity to reciprocate in the exchange of help', and raises the question of whether the deterioration in the power to *give* might affect older people's receptivity to *receive* (*ibid.*: 99). This notion gives tangible expression to the language of dependency which is still prevalent in the literature on ageing (Wilkin 1990).

In Day's full discussion of support between family members, there is no reference to 'deferred payments' or inheritance; the participants in this Sydney study are apparently focused on the here and now. More recently, Australian interest in these issues has been pursued further by Davison *et al.* in *'It's My Place'* (1993). They begin by talking with older people about their *housing* then progress to more symbolic levels of meaning around *home*. They trace the policy importance of 'ageing in place', and support the need for flexible and integrated policies across a continuum, stressing that roles and responsibilities across the range of services for older people (from acute health care and residential care to home and community care) need to be considered together (Davison *et al.* 1993: 10).

THE MOSGIEL STUDY: AGEING IN A LOCAL COMMUNITY

The research and case material presented here illustrate some of the practical and semantic issues confronting older people as they make decisions about where and how they live. The community in which the interviews took place represents a case study of 'ageing in place', as the study outline follows the changes in personal health, social networks and social support over a six-year period of residence in the town.

Mosgiel is in the province of Otago, in the South Island of New Zealand. It is situated on the outskirts of Dunedin city, which had a population of 119,000 in 1996. Mosgiel itself has a population of 13,500 and, since the project began, it has strengthened its reputation as a retirement township with the development of two major retirement villages, which have drawn residents from throughout the province. At the edge of the Taieri Plains its flat residential land, sheltered aspect and ready access to services are seen as attractive to older people. In its general demographic outline, Mosgiel represents many of the features of the South Island generally: outmigration of younger people leaves an older and more rapidly ageing population pattern (Statistics NZ 1995: 39).

The study population within the project comprised all those in Mosgiel who were aged seventy or over at a given date in 1988, and those still living in the community were re-interviewed six years later. The original group at baseline numbered 794, and at the six-year follow-up, 313 were re-interviewed. More extensive and open-ended interviews were taped with twenty of those over eighty years of age at the six-year follow-up.

The taped interviews were all conducted in the homes of the older people in the sample group, although my first meeting with them was at the health centre, during the research interview process. In some cases, I was asked and was able to drive them 'back home' after their health centre interview. As the follow-up interview was arranged, it was clear that its preferred location for all concerned was in their own homes. None expressed any discomfort with this location, and most were genuinely welcoming and in a full sense 'at home' during the interview. In what follows, names have been changed to protect anonymity.

The assumption 'that families, can, will and should do more' for their ageing parents and relatives fuelled the urgency of research interest in addressing some related questions in a local context. These found a fruitful channel for enquiry in the current Mosgiel project, from which the following case material derives. What is the picture now, in Mosgiel, of social networks and social support for those aged seventy and over? How has the pattern changed over the last ten years? Is there a particular pattern for the 'old old', those in the eighty- to ninety-year age group, still living in the community? What are the relative contributions of family, friends and professionals (the blend of informal and formal care, in Walker's terms)? How varied are roles within and between families?

It is important to remember that the answers to these and all the questions posed by the Mosgiel study are phrased in terms of the views and experiences of the older people themselves. In contrast to many other social network studies, and to research with caregivers, it is hoped that, by giving centrality to the older people themselves, we will get a clearer focus on the nub of the wheel, the centre of the web, or the heart of the issue. For if public policy is contradicting the deeply held beliefs of 80-year-olds, for example by denying them control over their assets at the end of their lives, and requiring them to accept a position of dependency on either the state or their families, without reciprocity, it may be denying them what it claims to offer – independence, dignity, security.

The interviews with people in the eighty- to ninety-year age group in Mosgiel were carried out during 1995 and 1996. The living situation of the approximately 300 involved in the follow-up study shows that just over half live alone, with a further 23 per cent sharing their home with a spouse; just over 10 per cent live with a son, daughter or other relative in the house. Residence in a Rest Home or in a long-term hospital situation each accounts for 7 per cent of this population at follow-up, although these people were not included in the sub-group participating in the taped interviews. From the twenty interviewed in this sub-group of people who have continued to live in their own homes over the period of the longitudinal study, a variety of ways of handling housing and asset-use decisions could be discerned.

DESCRIPTION

The following description is based on an amalgam of fieldnotes made at the time of the interviews, and is intended to paint an archetypal picture of the physical setting in which these interviews were conducted. A typical address I was given was '12B Side St.', reflecting the pattern of flats and units which have been built in the last twenty or so years in Mosgiel, often in pairs, or groups of four. Such ownership flats have a relatively standard design in these situations, being finished externally in low-maintenance permanent materials. The garden and access path to 12B is clearly labelled, and has its own letterbox in a group, and might commonly have visual separation from the adjoining units, such as a trellis or garden edging.

While waiting in the porch or entranceway for the door to be opened on my arrival, I could see from the pot plants and tub gardens that a small-scale interest in garden maintenance was well within the capacity of this resident. An opening conversational gambit, commenting on the quality of the peony bush, or the deep and unusual colour of this particular geranium, was often all that was required to generate numerous cues to follow, should there be any risk of the conversation drying up on tape.

Once past the entranceway, and through the front door, I would find myself in the sitting room of a cosy unit – the indoor temperature was often visibly boosted by a bar heater, although one or two people had woodburners, which would be glowing at a low level, even in the mornings. In this case, I could follow up in the interview whether any assistance was required with wood supply and clearing of a heat source which is acknowledged as entailing hard work.

Even without additional heating, the sitting rooms of these units tended to share also in solar gain, as they have generally been well placed to catch the sun, and might also use net curtains for some sun protection and privacy. Furniture in the sitting room would typically include a settee, and a couple of easy chairs, one with all the signs of being the favourite of the regular user. It would perhaps have a side table at hand, with the day's paper (often folded open at the TV programmes for the day), reading glasses, the TV remote control, a book, and a knitting or sewing bag. Many of the sitting rooms gave an initial impression of crowdedness. A complex array of framed photographs, prints, dried and artificial flowers, indoor house plants, ornaments and tapestries covered the TV set, shelving, window ledges and mantlepiece, as well as available wall space.

Crowdedness does not imply untidiness, but rather an intensely used and appreciated space. Glassware and china would sparkle in the sunlight from clean windows, and polished wood would gleam if its surface were exposed, rather than covered with a lace or embroidered cloth. Handcrafts of a wide variety of types would be evident, particularly in textiles, with crochet blankets draped over armchairs, and individual cushion covers each telling a personal story.

This style of interior decor in the sitting room, or lounge, includes rich and complex colour combinations, in carpet and drapes, and is in striking contrast to the style in the bedroom area, which is more likely to use pastel tones and more 'frilly' fittings. The homes of the men I visited for these interviews did have fewer of the softer and floral elements which were so evident in the women's homes, and also tended to have a more limited colour range of greens and browns. They were markedly more dusty, almost on the dingy side, and I also found their rooms colder in a literal sense.

The kitchen area of a unit or flat of this type would often be separated by a bar or dividing unit from the sitting room, or located in the short end of an L-shaped space in an open-plan layout. Kitchen fittings would tend to be older style, in terms of the age of the stove, toaster, kitchen clock and kettle, etc., and bench-top small ovens would be visible, with by no means everyone having a microwave. Bench surfaces would also be older style, but always clear and clean. Depending on the time of the interview, subtle cooking smells might be evident, and could well become a point of comment with some pride.

Those whom I interviewed who were still in the house in which they had spent a much longer period of their lives offered an even stronger sense of belonging in their space. They would generally have a larger living area, and additional bedrooms beyond the one they occupied, but in most other ways, their style of living was similar to those in a smaller unit, who might have lived there mostly on their own for perhaps the last eight years.

Even in this description it is difficult to separate the physical and functional aspects of the home setting from the more personal and symbolic. These people have clearly all claimed their flat or unit as their own, made their personal mark upon it with the choice of decor and personal memorabilia.

In a variety of ways, people talk in the interviews about the often implicit connection between values and policy, irrespective of whether the 'treasures' they refer to are more specifically seen as assets, income, or resources such as money and time. All would be appropriately described as 'asset rich and income poor' in the sense that the majority have basic pension incomes and do not currently pay the surtax; the majority own their own homes. In the four cases which follow, they describe several different ways in which they manage their own resources – assets, space, health – in the maintenance of a style of independence appropriate to their situation.

CASE STUDIES

Mrs Lachlan

Mrs Lachlan was born in 1913, grew up in the region, married a local small businessman, and was widowed over twenty-five years ago. She lives alone with regular daily visits from her son, who took over the family business at a young age, on his father's death. Two other daughters live locally. Her attitudes to continuing to live independently in the family home are quite explicit, although her judgement in relation to her own situation differs from how she sees her friend's needs.

MRS LACHLAN: My family have been close, and have been good to me. And I want to share what I've got. I don't want it to get eaten up in a Home five and six hundred dollars a week . . . if I went . . . into a Home and you lived ten years. You wouldn't be – you'd eat up your house, all the money you had in your house, too. Your family would get nothing. There's that way of looking at it too. You do them out of their inheritance. . . . Yes, well my friend lost her husband, and she's lost – she worries me, because she's got stairs, in the house down there . . . and she says, I'm not moving out of my house into any Home, but I'm worried about her eyes. Because she's really lost her sight, she's got to get right up here with a magnifying glass, and she counts the stairs, but I'm afraid that one of these times, she'll miscalculate, and have an accident. She wants to do something about that – get out of the house, and get herself a little flat here, if she wants to be on her own. Stairs are no good when you get old.

Mr Wilson

Mr Wilson was born in the district in 1912, and has been married for fifty-six years. He lives with his wife and only son, who has never married or left 'home'. Under asset testing rules, this house would be exempt if either or both parents were to need long-term care, and in his own way, Mr Wilson recognizes this continuity.

MR WILSON: Oh, well, we have thought that we'd like to see him married, and settle down with a family of his own, but that's not likely to happen now, he's forty-five, or forty-six very shortly, and you couldn't get a happier man . . . mind you . . . we look forward to him coming home every night from work. He makes – our life would be a long way different. . . . Well, I think we would be . . . more self-centred if we hadn't had him at all. We would just be thinking of ourselves, whereas now, he comes into it, we're thinking of him, more than we are of ourselves, quite often.

In response to questioning about household management, he describes a subtle transfer of 'ownership':

MR WILSON: Well, I have been the boss of the outside. We always said that May looked after the inside, I looked after the outside, sort of style.
SALLY KEELING: And where does your son fit in that?
MR WILSON: Well, he didn't fit in as far as the garden went, until I had a big operation, and then he took on the lawns – he does all the lawns, now. . . . Well he did a bit of lawn there – but, no, I don't think we needed to ask when he saw that I wasn't fit enough to do it, at that time. And we were surprised that – he'd taken no interest in the lawns up till then, and now, he calls them 'my' lawns – he says that they're his lawns now! So, that pleased me very much.

Mrs Rongen

Mrs Rongen was born in 1910, and has been widowed since 1975. She has one adopted daughter who lives locally. Two years ago, she moved to an ownership unit in a retirement village, a decision she described as being made without support from her daughter.

MRS RONGEN: Oh, no, my daughter was very much . . . very much against me coming here. . . . Well, what I mean, it was, she wouldn't admit, but you know . . . um . . . well, she says, that she'd have looked after me. She says, I'd have given up work and looked after you. But, goodness me, I know quite well, that she wouldn't have been happy doing that. And, ah, she'd have . . . I'd have been sitting in the home, whether she came to my home, or I went to her home, and I'd have been on my own. Look, it wouldn't have worked. But, she – I don't know whether she just didn't want me to go out of my home, or whether she thought that this was costing too much, and what I mean, I wouldn't have the same money to leave her . . . I don't know. . . . I don't know really why. . . . I had said all along, I had a very nice comfortable home, and I said I'm never shifting from here. Just shows you how you say these things. I'm never shifting from here. . . . I'll be carried out of here. . . . I'm not going to go into a Rest Home, and I'm not going to this, that and the next thing.

There followed a discussion about how it was the experience of a friend which prompted Mrs Rongen to make her move, assisted and advised by a Public Trust Manager. Mrs Rongen concludes:

MRS RONGEN: Oh, yes, she knows it's a relief for me to be here. Oh, yes. Oh, I think I've done the right thing all right, but it did worry me.

Mrs Rongen has an unmarried sister in a church-run hospital in Dunedin, and clearly asserts her right to use her assets in terms of her own values; she describes her sister as still wishing to make financial gifts to the church, rather than accepting that she is paying them for her care.

MRS RONGEN: Yes, well, I've a niece in Dunedin that really takes responsibility for my older sister, which is good, because I used to be fit to do things for her, but you see, now I'm not fit. I've got to have people do things for me. And it is frustrating, terribly frustrating. . . . Yes, well our niece is very kind. And she tends to my sister's – sees to buying her clothes, and that sort of thing, and her finances, her banking, and that kind of thing. But I feel sorry for that sister, because she was in [church] work all her life, and lived very frugally, and she had lots of things that she was very interested in, and saved money, so as she'd be able to leave them something, but you see now, it's all dwindling away. It's nine hundred dollars a week, that it's costing for her. So her bit of capital that she had, it's dwindling away. And she said, last night, must see my niece, and just see what money I have got. I haven't given anything to the Church for a long while. And of course, she was very interested in the Church work, and I haven't given anything, she's given regularly. Well, you see, you can't tell her not to do that. There's no need for her to worry about that. And she'll do without herself, for the sake of giving to other people. So it's rather sad.

Mrs MacDonald

Mrs MacDonald was born in Scotland in 1909, and migrated to New Zealand after World War II, with her husband and only daughter. Her husband died fourteen years ago, following a period when both lived with the daughter and her family in a country town about four hours from Dunedin. Mrs MacDonald has several major health problems, and has had increasing sight problems in recent years, and at the time of the interview was receiving a range of home-based services (Meals On Wheels, day programmes and home help). In the first interview, she clearly expressed a desire to 'hold on' in her flat, despite her 'pretty hopeless' ability to manage on her own; her main concern is to be able to leave her flat to her daughter. She had previously taken a mortgage out on the flat she owned to pay for private hip treatment.

MRS MACDONALD: Well, I don't often have treatment – I had my hip done, I had to get that, a loan out of my flat, you know – I cried here for a week, to think I'd bought everything, never owed anything, and I had to take this money, a loan out, and that cost me . . . it's terrible, what was it? Three hundred dollars to get to – transfer the title deeds, a copy of the title deeds to the bank. And then I had to pay to take it out. My daughter took me last week, and I paid it off. She said, 'Mum, I'm proud of you – we were ready to step in, give you some money towards it anyway', she said, 'we'd be able to sell some – shares we had', and I said to her, 'I'm glad you didn't'. I said 'I want to be independent'. So . . . that Scotch instinct! I'm so independent. I still don't want to go into a home, unless I'm pretty bad. That's – it's the eyes that are the problem now – I can't . . . I can't make your face out at all.

SALLY KEELING: Do you think that you and your daughter see that differently?

MRS MACDONALD: Well . . . we could have an argument like that, and I – she doesn't realise it, but that's not good for me. And I know, she wants me to go up there for the winter. . . . Well, she said, 'I'll come down. And I'll stay a couple of days with you.' So of course, she wants me to go back with her – this is the story, but . . . I . . . just have a feeling, we'd be better . . . we're friendlier apart – that sounds terrible, because I do love her, and she loves me in her own way – but she's a – she's a one – She's just – you know, she just lives for her husband.

Six weeks later, in attempting to make my final return visit to Mrs MacDonald, I found the phone disconnected, and learnt through a project contact person that she had in fact gone to live with her daughter. In this way, she had apparently conceded her personal independence in order to retain her financial independence, by being able to continue owning the flat to be able to leave it to her daughter.

CONCLUSION

This chapter has explored some aspects of the interface between private and personal values and public policy concerning assets. It raises questions about ownership and stewardship of assets, and whether it is possible to separate the economic and personal value of the family home, in the present New Zealand cultural setting.

The Bible clearly refers to tangible treasures, those that 'moth and dust corrupt', and rates them as less valuable than intangible treasures (treasures in heaven, those of the heart). It casts those who 'rob' those assets as thieves, whether in the guise of the state, family or other potential beneficiaries. The message, both from the Bible and the means-testing policy, is that it is better to spend, share, give and consume assets than to save and protect them. Over the previous seventy years, people have been encouraged to save 'for their old age', yet when that day comes, they are reluctant to use those resources, on the grounds (in part) that these savings were also intended for the next generations, and in particular, that they are entrusted via the 'family home' to maintain those values across the generations.

There is also a sense in which any share in the 'family home' coming from the death and legacy of a parent in their mid-eighties and going to sons or daughters themselves in their sixties remains just that: a protection against the vagaries of health and dependency for those with very limited ability to vary their earning power. As a corollary to this, any benefits to the state are short term. Without the cushioning effect of a share in the family home passing on to today's 60-year-olds, they in turn will qualify for state subsidy sooner – and under present demographic trends, there will be more of them, and they are likely to cost more for longer (Pool 1991; Koopman-Boyden 1993).

It would seem that the most recent political compromise in New Zealand goes some way towards restoring some balance in this debate. The proposed policy which exempts the family home from asset testing at the level of $100,000 recognizes that New Zealanders value their homes as treasures, in both biblical senses. It recognizes more equally both the tangible (individual user pays) and intangible (family continuity of assets), and accepts the dual value of both house and home.

NOTE

1   An earlier version of this work was presented at the 1996 meeting of New Zealand Association of Social Anthropologists, Palmerston North. Acknowledgement is due to the Health Research Council of New Zealand for the award of a postgraduate scholarship for the period 1996–7.

BIBLIOGRAPHY

Allen, I. and Perkins, E. (eds) (1995) *The Future of Family Care for Older People*, London: HMSO.

Baines, C., Evans, P. M., and Neysmith, S. (eds) (1991) *Women's Caring: Feminist Perspectives on Social Welfare*, Toronto: McClelland and Stewart.

Baldwin, S. (1995) 'Love and money: the financial consequences of caring for an older relative', in I. Allen and E. Perkins (eds) *The Future of Family Care for Older People*, London: HMSO.

Bills Digest (1996) Bills Digest no.192, 21 May, Wellington: New Zealand Parliamentary Library.

Blank, R. H. (1994) *New Zealand Health Policy: A Comparative Study*, Auckland: Oxford University Press.

Carsten, J. and Hugh-Jones, S. (eds) (1995) *About the House: Lévi-Strauss and Beyond*, Cambridge: Cambridge University Press.

Davison, B., Kendig, H., Stephens F. and Merrill, V. (1993) *'It's My Place': Older People Talk About their Homes*, Canberra: Australian Government Publishing Service.

Day, A. T. (1985) *'We Can Manage': Expectations about Care and Varieties of Family Support among People 75 Years and Over*, Monograph no. 5, Melbourne: Institute of Family Studies.

Dupuis, A. and Thorns, D. C. (1996) 'Meanings of home for older home owners', *Housing Studies*, 11, 4, 485–501.

Easton, B. (1979) *Social Policy and the Welfare State in New Zealand*, Auckland: George Allen and Unwin.

Finch, J. and Groves, D. (eds) (1983) *A Labour of Love: Women, Work and Caring*, London: Routledge and Kegan Paul.

Finch, J. and Mason, J. (eds) (1993) *Negotiating Family Responsibilities*, London: Tavistock/Routledge.

Goody, J. (1983) *The Development of the Family and Marriage in Europe*, Cambridge: Cambridge University Press.

Groves, D. (1995) 'Costing a fortune? Pensioners' financial resources in the context of community care', in I. Allen and E. Perkins (eds) *The Future of Family Care for Older People*.

Gurney, C. and Means, R. (1993) 'The meaning of home in later life', in S. Arber and M. Evandrou (eds) *Ageing, Independence and the Life Course*, London: Jessica Kingsley.

Hamnett, C. (1995) 'Housing equity release and inheritance', in I. Allen and E. Perkins (eds) *The Future of Family Care for Older People*.

Henwood, M. (1996) 'The future of long term care', in *Health Crisis – What Crisis?*, proceedings of the Fabian/Socialist Health Association New Year Conference, Fabian Society Pamphlet, no. 574.

Johnson, P. (1977) 'Perceptions of ageing among the middle-aged: a contribution to the ethnography of adult life', unpublished MA thesis, Department of Anthropology, Auckland University.

Kane, R. (1996) 'From generation to generation: thoughts on legacy', *Generations*, Fall.

Kendig, H. L. (ed.) (1986) *Ageing and Families: A Social Networks Perspective*, Sydney: Allen and Unwin.

Koopman-Boyden, P. (ed.) (1993) *New Zealand's Ageing Society: The Implications*, Wellington: Daphne Brassell Associates.

Mauss, M. [1922] (1970) *The Gift: Forms and Functions of Exchange in Archaic Societies*, translated by I. Cunnison, London: Routledge and Kegan Paul.

Mitchell, A. (1972) *The Half-Gallon Quarter-Acre Pavlova Paradise*, Christchurch: Whitcombe and Tombs.

NACCH and DSS (1994) *Living at Home: consensus development conference report*, Wellington: National Advisory Committee on Core Health and Disability Support Services.

NZFVWO (1997) *Dialogue*, the newsletter of the New Zealand Federation of Voluntary Welfare Organisations, no. 93, 12–13.

Oldman, C. (1991) 'Using housing to fund care', in F. Laczko and C. Victor (eds) *Community Care and Elderly People in the 1990s*, Aldershot, Avebury.

Opie, A. (1992) *There's Nobody There: Community Care of Confused Older People*, Auckland: Oxford University Press.

Paul, C. (1996) 'Chronically ill: is there deliberate neglect?', *Otago Daily Times*, 13 July, 8.

Phillipson, C., Biggs, S. and Kingston, P. (eds) (1995) *Elder Abuse in Perspective*, Buckingham: Open University Press.

Pool, I. (1991) 'The demographic transition of the New Zealand family: a key determinant of major policy needs and responses', in Population Association of

NZ/NZ Planning Council *Population Change and Social and Economic Policy in the 1990s: Proceedings of a Conference*, Population Association of NZ: Wellington.

Qureshi, H. and Walker, A. (1989) *The Caring Relationship: Elderly People and their Families*, Philadelphia: Temple University Press.

St John, S. (1993) 'Income support for an ageing society', in P. Koopman-Boyden (ed.) *New Zealand's Ageing Society: the Implications*.

Statistics NZ (1995) *New Zealand Now: 65 Plus*, Wellington: Statistics New Zealand.

Strathern, M. (1992) *After Nature: English Kinship in the Late Twentieth Century*, Cambridge: Cambridge University Press.

Thompson, D. (1991) *Selfish Generations? The Ageing of New Zealand's Welfare State*, Wellington: Bridget Williams.

Thorns, D. (1993) 'Tenure and wealth accumulation: implications for housing policy', in P. Koopman-Boyden (ed.) *New Zealand's Ageing Society: the Implications*.

—— (1997) 'Intergenerational conflicts: impacts upon policies and the experiences of the elderly', unpublished paper presented at the International Conference on 'Living Environment, Health and Wellbeing for the Elderly', Tokyo.

Upton, S. (1991) *Your Health and the Public Health, A Statement of Government Policy*, Wellington: New Zealand Department of Health.

Walker, A. (1995) 'Integrating the family into a mixed economy of care', in I. Allen and E. Perkins (eds) *The Future of Family Care for Older People*.

Wilkin, A. (1990) 'Dependency', in Peace, S. (ed.) *Researching Social Gerontology: Concepts, Methods And Issues*, London: Sage.

Chapter 12

Residents' participation in the management of retirement housing in the UK

Peter Lloyd

INTRODUCTION

Community care: the two words carry such a positive resonance. Community implies shared interests and loyalties and, indeed, care. The community is caring. But the words are ambiguous too; the very breadth of their meaning enables each of us to find in them what we seek. Care *in* the community signals the discharge of persons from the allegedly impersonal long-stay geriatric wards or mental institutions into smaller domestic-like units; it connotes the moves to enable frail people to remain in their homes rather than be transferred into institutional care. Care *by* the community signals the support by a network of friends, neighbours and voluntary organizations; though in practice, as so many have argued, it is by the family. As the resources of the welfare state are increasingly stretched, they are targeted on those in most acute need. Preventative care is left to 'the community', even though a modest state expenditure here could obviate the much more costly treatment of crises.

Complementing the rhetoric of community care is that of consumer choice. Care delivered to the user should constitute a package to meet individual needs. The user should be able to choose what services are needed and by whom they are delivered. Service delivery should be co-ordinated – a 'seamless service' from 'the one-stop-shop'.[1] Citizens' charters, in a wide variety of spheres from hospital waiting lists to train punctuality, spell out what we should expect in service delivery.

However, in this environment of increasing participation older people are usually absent or left out; they are silent and ineffective. 'The voices of older people who use or need community care are rarely heard directly' state Thornton and Tozer (1995: 4) in their study of the many ways in which older people might have a say in issues that effect them (see too Lloyd 1991; Thornton and Tozer 1994).

Well over half a million people live in sheltered – or retirement, as it is increasingly termed – housing; that is more than the combined total of those in residential care and nursing homes. These people are living independently in their own homes; the independence fostered by retirement housing schemes contrasts with the dependency so often created in residential care and nursing homes. They are living *in* the community. But the retirement housing scheme is itself a little community – at very least in the physical sense. How far it constitutes a community in the social sense is a matter for investigation; those living in such a scheme might be as unaware of their neighbours as are residents in a typical block of flats – or they might interact as intensely as members of a commune.

In this chapter I shall examine the degree to which residents of retirement housing schemes are actively involved in the management and social life of their schemes, the reasons for the present lack of such activity and measures currently being promoted to increase involvement.

This chapter is based on nearly ten years' study of retirement/sheltered housing – an interest which grew out of earlier studies of community action in Third World shanty towns, via a subsequent interest in neighbourhood action, especially as it affected older people, in Brighton. During this period I have visited scores of schemes to talk with residents and scheme managers, maintaining contact with many over a number of years, though never engaging in a lengthy period of intensive participant-observation – true social anthropological fieldwork! The Sussex Gerontology Network's Sheltered Housing Group which I convene has, since November 1991, held fifteen workshops which uniquely bring together those who live in, and those who manage, retirement housing. Throughout these workshops two themes have predominated: first, the potential of retirement housing to cater for residents who grow increasingly frail, enabling them to live independent lives rather than be obliged to move into increased dependency in residential care and nursing homes; and, second, the potential for residents to manifest their activity and independence in taking an active role in the management of their own schemes.

As social anthropologists move from academia into spheres of practice and policy they often feel that it is inappropriate to justify explicitly their thinking in terms of the canon of their discipline. It is only when, apparently doing what comes naturally to them, they discover that the 'common-sense' of others is somewhat different, that they reflect upon the basic premises of their own thinking.

My initial interest in retirement housing focused on the degree to which residents in a scheme constituted a community (see Cohen 1989), linked through an intricate pattern of relationships with cohesion maintained through patterned ties, symbols and rituals. As I visited various schemes, I realized that each managing agency – local authority, housing association or private company – had its own organizational culture (see Wright 1994: Ch. 1). As my concern with participation developed I realized that residents' empowerment lay not in response to questionnaires and management-set agenda, but in expressing their own views of retirement housing, what it meant to them and what they wanted from it, in their own words.

WHAT IS RETIREMENT HOUSING?

Retirement (or sheltered) housing schemes are typically blocks of between twenty and sixty flats – or more rarely bungalows or maisonettes.[2] They are constructed and managed by local authority housing departments, registered housing associations and private companies. Most are in the rental sector; access is here by application sometimes involving assessment of need and restriction to those already living locally. In others, the leasehold of units may be purchased – either in full or through equity-sharing schemes. In all schemes there is minimum age of entry – usually sixty years (applicable to the elder member of a couple). But the average age of entry has, in recent years, been rising: in many schemes it is now in the late seventies as residents delay moving until they become unable to manage their home, or because they have had difficulty in selling it. Changes in state benefits have led some who would otherwise have entered a residential care home to explore the viability of retirement housing. The average age of current residents is thus in the eighties, with some still quite active whilst others are becoming frail. In the 1970s sheltered housing was often seen as a staging post; but the prospect of a sequence of traumatic moves in the last decades of one's life is now anathema to residents: they hope to remain in their scheme until the end of their life.

Units in the retirement housing schemes tend to be small. Many schemes built in the 1970s and 1980s consisted of bed-sitting rooms with shared toilet facilities. These are unpopular and many such schemes are now designated hard-to-let. The consequent claim that there is an over-provision of retirement housing is countered by the waiting lists for more recently built schemes. These tend to have separate sitting and bedrooms with en suite facilities and there is increasing demand for two bedrooms. Older schemes, albeit ostensibly constructed for older people, have many design deficiencies which are now being addressed. Location factors too are recognized – one does not site schemes on steep hills, far from shops, amenities and public transport.

In the past schemes have been classified, in the official nomenclature, as Categories One, Two and, less officially, Two-and-a-half. The Category One scheme has few communal facilities and probably a non-resident or peripatetic scheme manager/warden. The typical scheme is Category Two – having a communal lounge with kitchenette, laundry and guest room. The scheme's manager lives on-site and, although 'off duty', is available to meet emergencies out of work hours. As the population of retirement housing schemes ages and frailty increases, more schemes are being designed or developed to meet their needs; these are sometimes termed Category Two-and-half (to distinguish them from residential care homes, termed Category Three) or very sheltered housing, extra care sheltered housing, etc. These tend to have more facilities – one or two assisted baths, a treatment room, provision of lunch – together with 24-hour duty cover by staff.

Concomitantly the role of the erstwhile wardens – now scheme, resident or estate managers (the term 'scheme manager' will be used hereafter) – is changing from that of an amateur 'good neighbour' to a professional role encompassing both property management and facilitation of care provision.[3] An 'extra care' scheme is likely to have a care team located on site managed either directly by the scheme manager or independently by an outside agency.

The design of the retirement housing scheme with its communal lounge implies a minimal level of common social activity; the job description of the scheme manager usually includes the facilitation of such activity. Thus most schemes have a weekly coffee morning, the occasional lunch or supper, bingo or card games, and outings. These are arranged variously by scheme manager and residents – with the former often taking the more active role.

With their physical proximity as close neighbours, and with such social activity, one might legitimately ask 'how far do the residents constitute a community?' In this chapter I am concerned primarily with residents' involvement in the management of their scheme – in its daily running and the over-arching policies of the managing agency, be it local authority, housing association or private company. What say do the residents have in these vital aspects of their lives? What influence or control do they want to have?

WHAT IS PARTICIPATION?

Participation is one of today's buzzwords – acceptable to almost everybody because of the wide range of meanings embraced. Many scales of participation have been devised – these are here reduced to three levels (see Richardson 1983).

Information underlies all involvement: unless they know what is going on people cannot play any part in active decision making. Managing agencies are required by legislation and codes of practice to supply their residents with information packs outlining policies and practices, with annual financial statements and performance indicators. But the giving of information often implies little or no response; channels of communication are not clearly indicated. This is not participation as generally understood. Consultation with residents, too, is advocated in codes of practice. But the initiative usually lies with the managing agency which decides how and when to consult residents, and sets the agenda. There is no guarantee that residents' views will be accepted; and indeed, residents often feel that they are consulted after a decision has already been taken. This constitutes minimal participation.

Actual participation occurs when residents are included on decision making bodies where they may determine, or at least influence, policy. Such decision making bodies exist at several levels. Most obvious are the residents' groups or associations, informal or formal, which exist within the individual scheme. Residents *may* be involved in a very wide range of issues: the selection, appointment, job description and daily routine of the scheme manager; house rules – security, smoking areas, keeping of pets, use of the lounge; finance rents and service charge – the use of 'spare' money to provide improvements; repairs maintenance and service charges; the use of the scheme's communal areas by outsiders; allocation policy and procedures; the delivery of care and support to frail residents; the possible transfer of management to another agency. The amount of power devolved to residents must be negotiated with the managing agency.

At the other end of the scale managing agencies have allowed residents to occupy up to one-third of the places on their higher boards or committees of management. Such representatives are frequently co-opted from among residents who so express an interest, are nominated by line managers and are deemed suitable by the managing agency. Such representatives are not elected by residents and so cannot be mandated to speak on their behalf. In as much as the remaining two-thirds of these boards comprise the managing agency's senior executives who have agreed a common strategy and policy before coming to any meeting, the resident representatives would seem to have little or no opportunity to alter agency policy.

In between are the regional area forums established by many managing agencies. In their initial stages one or two informally selected residents from each scheme are invited to attend; the meetings are consultative, rather than decision making. These forums differ in the extent to which they are led by the managing agency or the residents. A logical development here is for the resident representatives to be elected within their schemes and for the forum to elect the resident members of the top policy making boards. But until this process is completed there exists a disjunction between scheme residents' associations and the managing agencies' policy making bodies.

None of these participatory structures would seem to tax one's comprehension – all look quite straightforward – so why have they not been more widely adopted?

MODES OF PARTICIPATION

As Hester Blewitt (1992) noted, 'participation in sheltered housing ranges from highly developed schemes, where tenants and owners have legal responsibilities for managing, to situations where professionals appear to be running elderly people's lives for them'. The former remain a small minority, the latter the vast majority.

Active participation in retirement housing schemes seems to arise in three situations. First, some local authority housing departments have fostered participation among their tenants through a small team of tenant participation officers. Their efforts have extended to retirement housing schemes where tenant associations have been formed. Representatives of these associations then meet either with those from other retirement housing schemes or from neighbouring general needs housing estates to constitute an area committee. This feeds into higher committees in a pyramid structure which influences the local authority's housing committee of elected councillors.

Second, one private company – Retirement Security Ltd (RSL), founded by Robert Bessell, a former Director of Warwickshire Social Services – now operates almost twenty extra care or very sheltered schemes. It decrees that each owner contributes one share to form a management company which elects a board of directors. RSL is appointed as managing agency by this board, and can be removed. The board exercises a very strong control over the day-to-day management of the scheme.

In both of these situations, the impetus for resident participation has come from above, from agencies with a culture of participation. In a third situation it comes from below, from the residents themselves. A crisis arises and the residents feel that their complaints are not being addressed by the managing agency. They create a formal residents' association in order to give weight to their representations. In one scheme known to me, a scheme manager still had not been appointed several weeks after the first residents had moved in; they then decided that they did not really need a scheme manager and that one of them, a relatively young and active resident, would act as 'volunteer warden' for a small honorarium. She now has a team of ten 'deputy volunteer wardens' which effectively runs the scheme, under the direction of the residents' association and with the services of a managing agent who collects the service charges, draws up contracts and executes such formal business. This arrangement has now been working well for several years. (For a more detailed description of these and similar cases, see Lloyd and Wilcox 1997.)

It is sometimes suggested that levels of participation are related to social status: the middle classes are more active and accustomed to committee work, the working classes are more passive and dependent. It may certainly happen that older people with fixed incomes, and who are annually dipping into savings, will be more concerned to challenge their rent and service levels, than will those reliant on state benefits where any increase in these outgoings is compensated by benefit increase. But tenants in local authority retirement housing may well have been active, in their earlier years, in tenant movements, in trades unions and the like. We are still left asking why there should be such differences in activity level.

WHY PARTICIPATE?

There is widespread support for the idea that residents *ought* to participate:

> Policies that encourage tenants to participate in setting rules and influencing decisions contribute to increased tenant satisfaction and a sense of pride among elderly tenants. Structures such as active tenant organizations and meaningful social programming build a sense of community among elderly tenants and increase social interaction. Finally, management policies help to give tenants a sense of direction, set realistic boundaries concerning the rights and responsibilities of

elderly tenants, increase mutual support among tenants, and reduce the likelihood of interpersonal conflicts.

(Sheehan 1992: 95)

Residents have a citizen's right to share in the control of their environment and control of all that affects their daily lives. Furthermore it is argued, though it would be difficult to prove conclusively, that such activity promotes health and longevity; sickness and death will come most quickly to those who sit and wait for it. Participation too may lead to more cost-effective management; as managing agents attempt to cut costs, removing layers of line management and allocating extra duties to scheme managers (already facing increased tasks as their role is professionalized), any devolvement of tasks to the residents is likely to be beneficial. Finally, as they co-operate in the tasks of management, residents will become more aware of each other's personal situations and needs, and will be better able to offer informal support. The potential for self help among residents increases in importance as the resources of statutory agencies are targeted to those in most acute need and withdrawn from many preventative care services (which would delay or remove the onset of crises).

So why have these challenges not been met? Factors operate from above and below. Ageist assumptions, common within society, are frequently articulated by managing agency staff and shared by older people themselves. Older people, it is asserted, want a quiet life, free from conflict or hassle. Retirement is seen as a signal for withdrawal – from unwelcome tasks, unnecessary relationships. Such themes were prominent in the psychological literature of recent decades. One of the frequently cited advantages of a move into retirement housing is that major issues of property maintenance, such as tiles falling off the roof, and blocked drains, fall to the scheme manager.

Again, it is said that older people do not want 'responsibility'. For those becoming forgetful, the collection and recording of money – for an outing perhaps – can provoke anxiety. One hesitates to promise a regular performance, such as making breakfast for a neighbour, when one's own health and ability is uncertain. But used thus, 'responsibility' differs from 'taking responsibility', making decisions about one's environment, making one's view known.

The line management of local authority housing departments and housing associations are almost all professionals trained in housing law, finance and construction; they have little or no personal experience of life in retirement housing or the concerns of older people. Their daily discourse, replete with its jargon and technicalities, is alien to the residents. Only where a line manager is specifically responsible for care in retirement schemes might he/she have a social service or health background. Scheme managers are apt to claim that they know the views of their more frail residents and should be the ones to speak on their behalf; for it is they who see them every day, not the neighbours who meet only those who actively move within the scheme, attending the coffee mornings and group events.

In keeping with retirement housing's stress on independence, the rights of the *individual* are continually stressed. In the codes of practice, scheme and line managers are abjured to respect individual rights and the individuality of each resident. The collectivity is obscured. In their own documentation many managing agencies state, in as many words, that whilst residents have every right to set up a residents' association (when the agency will provide them with guidance, a draft constitution, etc.) they do not have to do so; furthermore nobody can be obliged to participate if they do not wish to.

In general, managing agencies have done little to encourage participation, though there are some noteworthy exceptions. Often advocacy of participation appears hypocritical – 'you may organize if you wish, but we would be happier if you didn't'. The message is not lost on the residents. Even where a management agency adopts a 'culture of participation' – providing copious information packs, employing tenant participation officers, etc. – it finds it difficult always to follow it in practice. As one senior manager said 'we reach decisions here in the office and then we remember "Oops! We ought to have consulted the tenants first."'

A mere expression of support for formal residents' associations falls well short of positive action – the appointment of resident participation staff, the provision of resources for the association (office space, typing and photocopying facilities, etc.), training for officers and reimbursement of out-of-pocket expenses in attending meetings.

In 1993–4 Hanover HA carried out a survey of resident opinion, obtaining a 59 per cent response rate. To the question 'Do you feel that Resident Participation could give you more of a say in how your estate is run?', slightly more than one-half said no; almost all the 'no's' said they 'were happy to leave Hanover to manage the estate'. 'Would you get involved in a residents' association on your estate?' attracted 81 per cent negative answers, though only 42 per cent thought that residents' associations were not a good idea. Faced with such a response, countering its own wish to promote participation, it is understandable that Hanover HA should focus on resident membership of top-level boards and the establishment of area forums:

> From the results it seems that there will not be a sudden increase in the number of Residents' Associations at Hanover – we respect your views on this subject, as setting up Residents' Associations is entirely your decision. But we would like to see a gradual expansion and are working to assist you, should you want to set one up. For those of you who are interested in getting involved in Residents' Associations, we feel that an alternative approach could be considered. One such approach is the setting up of Regional Residents' Forums through which residents would be elected to Regional Committees, and ultimately main Committee. To be democratic, elections would be required. This concept represents a shift away from using Residents' Associations as the principle vehicle for Resident Participation and instead directly

elects representatives from all the estates. Once established, Residents' Forums could be involved in a variety of policy and service issues from a very early stage in the process.

(Hanover Property Management Ltd 1994)

But not all surveys point in the same direction. In an independent survey on behalf of the Anchor Trust, Moyra Riseborough (1996) found an overwhelming majority of respondents felt it either important or very important that they should have a say in the way in which their schemes were run; salient issues were rent and service charge increases, scheme security and the redecoration or refurbishment of communal areas.

Why should there be such a difference in response? One possible answer is that an in-house survey is likely to provoke responses of gratitude rather than opposition, although the Anchor respondents seemed no less pleased with the service which they were receiving. Another is the manner in which the question is posed – or at least, interpreted by residents: 'do you want to participate in the management of your scheme?' provokes the response 'no, we pay the scheme manager to do it'. 'Do you want to have a say in how the scheme is run?' provokes a more positive response. Furthermore Riseborough's lengthy questionnaire, probing a wide variety of attitudes to retirement housing, probably provides a more rounded picture of residents' views then Hanover's three management-oriented questions. Many managing agencies poll their residents in what might be termed consumer satisfaction surveys; at best these can indicate shortcomings; at worst they are little more than invitations to express gratitude to the agency. In general there is a dearth of studies which explore the residents' views of the little world in which they live, or, in social anthropological parlance 'to grasp the native's point of view, his relation to life, to realise *his* vision of *his* world' (Malinowski 1922: 25). However, ongoing research through unstructured interviews by Dilys Page and Sheila Cunnison is exploring residents' attitudes towards scheme managers.[4]

THE SCHEME MANAGER'S ROLE

The role of the scheme manager is crucial. Some, because of their personal convictions or of their management agencies' policies, have striven to promote resident participation. More have been antipathetic, and one even hears stories of scheme managers who have advised residents against attending area forums. In conferences of scheme managers a talk on resident participation usually provokes a negative response. The scheme manager's job is quite attractive: it is a caring role, and it encourages creativity in providing a congenial atmosphere and social events. The scheme manager is a gatekeeper between management and residents, and control can be exercised through 'divide and rule'. Codes of practice insist that all residents be treated identically, but inevitably the scheme manager helps some – for example, by making a cup of tea or collecting a prescription – more than others. These acts are seen by residents as favours, to be withdrawn from 'difficult' or non-compliant residents. Residents frequently believe (and not without cause) that their scheme manager will play a major part in decisions about their ability to cope within retirement housing rather than be moved on to residential care or nursing homes; they fear, in common with so many older people, that any criticism of services provided will lead to their withdrawal, the complainants being labelled as 'trouble makers'. In most, but certainly not all, schemes, the manager is seen by the residents as a 'most wonderful person – kind, caring, supportive, etc.'. And almost invariably it is believed to be the scheme manager who creates the difference between a 'good' and a 'bad' scheme.

The scheme manager has considerable independence; a line manager visits perhaps monthly. Indeed, the most frequent complaint of scheme managers is lack of support when things go wrong; they seek more understanding from their line managers, a greater opportunity to share their problems with their peers.

In this situation the last thing that a scheme manager wants is residents, either individually or collectively, looking over their shoulder all the time, questioning, challenging or seeking justification for every act, because this could make their job intolerable. Such a situation is aggravated when, as is still often the case, the scheme manager is an 'old-style warden', the 'good neighbour', the relatively poorly paid post resulting in holders with little education, and few professional qualifications, who are of lower social status than most of the residents and in consequence feel threatened by them.

Issues of resident participation hit scheme managers at a time when their role is already threatened by other changes. In order to cut costs, many managing agencies are removing a level of line management and devolving duties upon scheme managers; others talk of making scheme managers non-resident but responsible for two or more schemes. Their role as facilitators of care packages is stressed. The rapid professionalization of the role (see n. 3) taxes the skills of many scheme managers.

The scheme manager is expected to facilitate the development of participatory structures. But when a residents' association is established, what is their role in it? Residents may demand their exclusion or allow attendance by invitation only. The residents' association may communicate directly with the line manager, thus marginalizing the scheme manager who is used to 'running' the scheme. How can they work if they do not know what the residents are deciding?

Scheme managers must be given support and training for such changing roles. Managers in one local authority admitted that, in their enthusiasm for working with their tenants, they had neglected to carry their scheme managers with them and were surprised by their obstructionist stance.

THE RESIDENTS' ROLE

Not all the fault lies with the managing agency or scheme managers; the residents themselves rarely initiate participatory activity. Most residents select a retirement housing scheme on the basis of its location, amenities and cost. Few have any appreciation of the structure of the managing agency, let alone its culture.

Before the first residents move into a new scheme a scheme manager will have been appointed, a job description agreed. The management structure is already in place. Advice is frequently given that one should move into retirement housing whilst still active and thus able to make the adjustments necessary to a new mode of life. But very many enter in a state of trauma, after a serious illness or loss of a partner has rendered them incapable or unwilling to continue to live in their former home. Often the scheme has been chosen by children anxious to have mum/dad living nearby but not with them. For some older persons first sight of the scheme is on moving-in day. Moving house is traumatic for most people, but even more so when one has had to lose many personal possessions, items of furniture with their memories, in squeezing into a much smaller space. On moving day the scheme manager will introduce her/himself and outline her/his role in the scheme; it is likely to go in one ear and out of the other. In the following weeks the new entrant will be trying to adjust to the new circumstances – not to alter the environment to meet their own needs. Routines become established and each successive new entrant in turn seeks to adjust, to fit in with the existing company of residents. Such routines become difficult to break. When two politically active residents moved into a scheme which for fifteen years had enjoyed no communal activity (in spite of having two spacious lounges), they faced great opposition to the establishment of a weekly coffee morning. Over the years their perseverance has resulted in a much greater activity level – but it has been hard work.

Rarely is it suggested by the scheme or line manager that residents ought to express an opinion on issues such as those listed above. So often residents are presented with a fait accompli: the first they hear about the redecoration of their lounge is with the arrival of the painters! In one scheme, the manager and line manager considered the tenders for maintaining the gardens. Their choice was announced at the following day's coffee morning. The residents did not demur but it became apparent that several were keen gardeners and had personal knowledge of the contractors; they could have made a valuable input into the decision.

In spite of the large number of people living in retirement housing, they do not constitute a recognizable constituency in the sense that pensioners, or members of the various disability groups, such as stroke, Alzheimer's or diabetes, or their carers do. It is difficult to obtain comprehensive lists of schemes within any area. Residents are unaware of other schemes close by. In one part of Brighton eleven schemes (managed by eight agencies) are sited within half-a-mile of each other, yet few of their residents are probably aware of this. Even scheme managers are unaware of the nearby schemes of other agencies. Many housing associations provide quarterly newsletters for their own schemes' residents – sometimes containing useful information about rents or service charges, but more often with chatty accounts and photographs of eighty-fifth birthday parties. Outings may be arranged to other schemes within the same agency.

Managing agencies could try to act collaboratively within a locality. For example, they could co-operate in providing training for their scheme managers. But all is arranged in-house and, although they have common interests, they are in effect competing with each other to provide a product that best satisfies the customer.

PROMOTING PARTICIPATION

How, then, does one break this deadlock, created by the apathy towards participation still fostered by many managing agencies and the absence of collective identification among the residents and their passive acceptance of the status quo?

It is not that participation does not work – there are too many examples to the contrary (see the case studies in Lloyd and Wilcox 1997). But most remain unrecognized in the wider society. The management practices of the Retirement Security Ltd schemes, with nearly 1,000 residents, seem completely unknown outside the company. There exists no forum in which comparisons can be made and debated. Few monographs have been written on the social structures within retirement housing, least of all in Britain. Two of the best examples (Carlin and Mansberg 1994; Keith-Ross 1977) refer to the USA and France respectively; the latter author is a social anthropologist. In each scheme the residents are active participants in management; in the latter it was rivalry between those attached to communist and non-communist trade unions which generated action. But those books are unknown to those who manage or live in retirement housing.

Again, little attention has been paid to residents' participation in the training of scheme managers. *Effective Sheltered Housing* (Parry and Thompson 1993), an excellent text book widely used in courses leading to the National Warden's Certificate and similar professional courses, devotes less than one of its 180 pages to 'The importance of tenant participation'. Both authors are known to support participation; their explanation of their brevity was that the subject is not in the Chartered Institute of Housing syllabus (personal communication)! So one must move to higher circles of decision making. Nevertheless, many individual tutors of these courses are known to include a session on resident participation.

As we have already noted, participation is being stressed increasingly in the directives of funding bodies and in codes of practice. Thus the Housing Corporation decrees (in the Tenants Guarantee 1994) that 'opportunities should be given to exercise genuine influence over the service they receive'. The

Association of Retirement Housing Managers supports participatory activity in its code of practice. But these bodies are speaking to managing agencies, not residents; the latter body is composed of managing agencies. One suspects that in both cases their formulations reflect a lowest common denominator to which all can subscribe. Information-giving is prescribed, consultation is advocated; real collective action, decision making by residents, is ignored. One knows that within each managing agency there are a few individuals who are, from personal conviction, promoting residents' participation. However, on boards and committees they are matched by others who will budge only as far as the threat of negative sanctions demands. The Centre for Sheltered Housing Studies, which as its name implies is one of the few organizations concerned specifically with retirement housing, has as its primary function the provision of training for scheme managers; it has little contact with residents.

There is an abundant literature on tenant participation, in general; much of this is provided by the Tenant Participation Advisory Service (TPAS), a most effective organization which holds frequent conferences, and provides support and advice. But this is restricted to tenants – it does not service leaseholders or owners. The residents of retirement housing are thus divided into two distinct and separate legal categories, obscuring the many interests which they hold in common. The content of TPAS' and other organizations' activities focuses on issues of property maintenance and the legal rights of tenants – issues which predominate in general needs housing estates. Here an adversarial approach is most usual, such as 'how can one force the council to effect repairs in time?', 'how can one counter threats of eviction?' These issues are of course relevant to residents in retirement housing, but do not embrace the many others which arise, for instance, around their communal activities and the role of the scheme manager. A small voluntary organization, Federation of Residents Associations in Sheltered Housing (FRASH), has recently been established to promote the interests of residents in leasehold schemes, liaising with managing agencies and campaigning on relevant issues. Advice Information and Mediation Service for Retirement Housing (AIMS), in association with Age Concern England, provides advice on legal issues and offers a conciliation service to residents and managers. Such organizations do not provide a basis for collective action among retirement housing residents.

There seemed, therefore, to be a need for a guide to participation which would focus specifically on older residents of retirement housing schemes, both tenants and leaseholders. In writing *Get Involved!* (Lloyd and Wilcox 1997), we were guided by oft-repeated issues raised within practice and policy; we were not consciously trying to introduce social anthropological concepts.[5] Yet the differences between this guide and earlier literature do reflect the basic premises cited earlier – a concern with community and culture. The guide is addressed not to residents alone but also to managing agencies and scheme managers. It covers, in a different format, the issues raised in this chapter: reasons for participation, modes of participation, spheres in which residents ought to become involved, selecting the method by which one becomes involved, and making involvement work. The guide includes case studies illustrating both good practice and some of the problems which nevertheless arise. It neither advocates an adversarial approach nor does it prescribe any single structure of participation, but invites instead the three parties cited to *negotiate* among themselves.[6] This seemed, to the authors and their steering committee, to be the proper approach; it seemed appropriate too given the difficulties in reaching an audience of residents other than through their managing agencies and the necessity of winning the support of the managing agencies in fostering participation.

Negotiation implies equality between those involved. Each party must have similar rights to draw up agenda, and each must try to understand the discourse of the other. When not meeting face to face appropriate channels of communication must be established. Residents should feel that they are being empowered, and that the balance of power is tilting towards them.

MAKING PARTICIPATION WORK

Even when all parties – managing agency, scheme manager and residents – express themselves as fully committed to participation, one hears the ultimate deterrent – 'it's fine and we've tried it, but it doesn't work'.

Sometimes the cause of failure can be attributed to lack of management support: the managing agency has failed to provide information upon which residents might act and residents feel that their views are ignored by management. Their frustration results in apathy in place of struggle, and the scheme manager is unco-operative. But often the causes lie in the dynamics of community living.[7]

The residents of a scheme *are* a community in many respects. They are linked by cross-cutting ties and multiplex relationships, the latter defined by Gluckman (1955: 19) as 'relationships which serve many interests'. Close friendships exist: some residents discover that their new neighbours are schoolmates of six or seven decades earlier. Others play cards together or collaborate in organizing social events while some rely on the help of others to do shopping. These ties are valuable. It is said that older people find it hard to make new friends. In moving into retirement housing one loses many old friends and needs new ones.

Formal decision making creates divisions: some will vote for, others against. These divisions threaten existing relationships. Some issues may be sufficiently trivial to be managed. Others may go deeper. More affluent residents may seek increased services and a raised rent or service charge whilst poor residents fear that they might be forced out of the scheme. Divisions can be obscured by attempting to reach an informal consensus whereby matters are discussed but no decisions are taken by the residents, as the scheme manager takes them instead. In one recent case, a residents' group had gone far in setting up a formal residents' association. On the day that a training session was arranged it apparently had cold feet and decided to proceed informally instead, in effect reasserting the *status quo ante*. The scheme manager is a convenient scapegoat for decisions which are, or become, unpopular and which would otherwise threaten the status of individual residents.

It is frequently claimed that it is hard to find leaders among retirement housing residents. Indeed, many are too frail to assume the levels of performance necessary. But almost every organization finds it difficult to recruit leaders, and retirement housing schemes seem no exception. Ageing, however, does raise some particular issues. Loss of authoritative work roles through retirement creates in some a need to create an alternative role; they are people who want to be in charge. But furthermore ageing also leads to mental impairment, to aggression resulting from fear of illness or dementia, and to consequent personality change.

In many schemes the manager will complain about the 'self-selected leader' who is continually 'troublesome'. Often there exist no formal channels through which residents might express opinions so vociferous protest is the only avenue available. Sometimes other residents are supportive but remain silent lest they spoil their relationship with the scheme manager. Sometimes the protests lead to the creation of a formal residents' association, and in the secret ballot for officers their 'leader' receives only his/her own vote.

Many leaders of formal associations fulfil their roles well. Perhaps through experience they manage meetings effectively or they are punctilious in giving all an opportunity to speak and in making them feel that their opinions are valued. Information on which to base decisions and subsequent actions is adequately provided.

But other leaders may not have these skills, and the managing agency does nothing to promote training. So one hears, usually from scheme and line managers, stories of leaders, albeit elected, who become highly autocratic even to the extreme of brow-beating other residents into supporting them. Other residents are likely to express their dissatisfaction by withdrawal; a formal challenge, a motion of no-confidence would probably create too much disharmony for the community to manage. Autocratic leaders, themselves being active older people, may in fact represent the views of the active residents, to the exclusion of the frail who remain invisible, absent from coffee mornings and scheme events, and sometimes discriminated against. Here the scheme manager may feel obliged to represent the frail residents in opposition to the elected resident leaders of the scheme.

Such situations place the scheme managers in an invidious position. Their job descriptions may state that they should promote and facilitate resident participation, yet they may be admitted only by invitation to resident association meetings. Should they try to stimulate opposition to the autocratic leader? Should they 'blow the whistle', and report events to their line manager? What action can a line manager take against such a leader who appears to be democratically elected and to hold quarterly meetings at which decisions are taken?[8] Such extreme cases are rare, but every line manager seems to have one in their repertoire of 'problem issues'.

CONCLUSION

It is time to return to our opening question: why, in the context of community care, do older people have so little voice and influence? We have looked at this with regard to the involvement of residents in the management of retirement housing schemes.

There are sufficient, albeit few, examples, covering a wide variety of situations, to support the assertion that there is clearly nothing inherent in the ageing process that inhibits participation. Obviously some residents are so frail that their contribution to activities must be limited, but others with severe physical impairments can be very alert mentally. We have seen that the mode of entry into retirement housing promotes acquiescence. The network of ties between residents may impel them towards informal consensus rather than formal division of opinion. Poor leadership may result in withdrawal from active participation.

However, a major handicap to participation lies with the managing agency and its staff, since residents can only participate when management accepts. Rhetorical support for participation becomes meaningless if management fail to provide residents with information, listen to their views, provide resources and training for elected representatives, and training and support for their own staff too.

Negotiation implies the setting of boundaries. Residents may express demands and opinions of any kind. But scheme managers are entitled to career prospects and better conditions of work. Managing agencies must respect their duties to manage properly, and may be constrained by mission statements, legally binding covenants and the like. This is a game where all cards lie face upwards on the table, not one in which, shielding one's own hand, one attempts to trump one's opponent.

There is a good case for employing development workers to stimulate activity amongst residents. However, this can only be effective if managing agencies provide and support the appropriate participatory structures.

NOTES

1 Although community care rhetoric, and the several reports of the Audit Commission in the UK, stress the need for collaboration between housing and social services, resource restriction encourages budgetary division. In the UK the notorious 'Ealing judgement' decreed that local authority housing revenue money should not be used to pay for the social care provided by scheme managers; more recently it has been suggested that housing benefit should cover only the property element of any rent or service charge and not the care element. Initiatives to create a 'seamless' service are bedevilled by such bureaucratic constraints.

2 Age Concern (1995) *The Buyers' Guide to Retirement Housing*, in advising prospective residents what to look for, gives a good overview of the range of facilities and services available.

3 A consortium of nearly forty housing associations and similar organizations has recently produced a leaflet, 'Sheltered housing is changing: the emerging role of the warden', for distribution to staff in social and health services across the country. It

stresses the professionalism of the scheme managers' role and urges other professionals to collaborate with them.

4   Cunnison was, in fact, one of the founder members of the Manchester shop-floor studies group in the 1950s and 1960s (see Wright 1994: 10–14).

5   *Get Involved!* was funded by the Housing Associations Charitable Trust with a matched contribution from six major housing associations. The project was administered and the guide published by TPAS.

6   The concept of negotiation of meanings has a significant place in social anthropological theory. An early attempt to conceptualize organizations as a continuous process of organizing and negotiating meaning is Strauss *et al.*'s (1963) treatment of a hospital as a 'negotiated order'. They show the aim of the hospital, to 'turn patients out in better shape', was adhered to by all, but masked discrepancies on how to achieve it. Formal rules were minimal and not widely known. A sense of order was achieved by the different professionals, lay staff and patients daily negotiating agreements over individual patient care. These became patterned understandings between staff who worked together for any length of time but were continually susceptible to change. When these negotiations broke down a crisis was solved by a committee making a formal decision which became a 'rule' until it was forgotten. Similarly, informal ward rules would be forgotten 'until another crisis elicited their innovation all over again' (1963: 306). Both formal and informal spheres were part of a daily round of negotiating order. This action-oriented or transactional analysis locates 'culture' – the process of continuously organizing and negotiating order – in the surface of everyday activities (from Wright 1994: 20).

7   Much of Tom Douglas' (1986) description of interaction between residents of residential care homes is relevant to retirement housing.

8   Gluckman's (1955) study of the situation of the African village head can easily be transposed. The village head is not only a political leader but may also be relative, in-law, landlord, etc. to members of his village; he is situated in a difficult intercalary position between his obligation to his community and to the colonial administration.

BIBLIOGRAPHY

Age Concern (1995) *The Buyers' Guide to Retirement Housing*, London: Age Concern England and the National Housing and Town Planning Council.

Blewitt, H. (1992) 'Participation in sheltered housing', *TPAS News* 5.

Carlin, V. F. and Mansberg, R. (1994) *If I live to be a 100*, Princeton: Princeton Book Company.

Cohen, A. P. (1989) *The Symbolic Construction of Community*, London: Routledge.

Douglas, T. (1986) *Group Living: The Application of Group Dynamics in a Residential Setting*, London: Tavistock.

Gluckman, M. (1955) *The Judicial Process among the Barotse of Northern Rhodesia*, Manchester: Manchester University Press.

Hanover Property Management (1994) *Hanover (Retirement Housing) News Special Edition*, Hemel Hempstead: Hanover Property Management.

Keith-Ross, J. (1977) *Older People, New Lives*, Chicago: University of Chicago Press.

Lloyd, P. (1991) 'The empowerment of elderly people', *Journal of Aging Studies* 5, 2, 125–35.

Lloyd, P. and Wilcox, D. (1997) *Get Involved! Resident Participation in the Management of Retirement/Sheltered Housing*, Salford: Tenant Participation Advisory Service.

Malinowski, B. (1992) *Argonauts of the Western Pacific*, London: Routledge.

Parry, I. and Thompson, L. (1993) *Effective Sheltered Housing: A Handbook*, Harlow: Longman.

Richardson, A. (1983) *Participation*, London: Routledge and Kegan Paul.

Riseborough, M. (1996) *Listening to and Involving Older Tenants*, Oxford: Anchor Trust.

Sheehan, N. W. (1992) *Successful Administration of Senior Housing: Working with Elderly Residents*, Newbury Park CA: Sage Publications.

Strauss, A., Schatzman, L., Ehrilich, D., Bucher, R. and Sabshin, M. (1963) 'The hospital and its negotiated order', in E. Friedson (ed.) *The Hospital in Modern Society*, New York: Macmillan.

Thornton, P. and Tozer, R. (1994) *Involving Older People in Planning and Evaluating Community Care: A Review of Initiatives*, York: Social Policy Research Unit, University of York.

—— (1995) *Having a Say in Change: Older People and Community Care*, York: Joseph Rowntree Foundation.

Wright, S. (ed.) (1994) *Anthropology of Organizations*, London: Routledge.

Chapter 13

Using experiential research methods

The potential contribution of humanistic groupwork methods to anthropology and welfare research

Iain R. Edgar

INTRODUCTION

The chapters in this book mainly examine the contribution that social anthropology can make to the development of social welfare policy and practice. However, I think that the general field of welfare practice, and humanistic groupwork methods in particular, have a significant contribution to make to the development of research methodology in the social sciences. Social anthropology in particular stands to benefit from this engagement. As some of the other chapters in this volume show, social anthropology still relies significantly upon participant-observation as its main and discipline-defining research method. Such a method seeks access to the implicit world-view of the individuals and groups studied. This method does not rely solely upon what people say but rather seeks to evaluate their action and interaction. Social anthropology aims then to elicit both the spoken and unspoken perspectives of those studied.

Some of the methods used by welfare practitioners, derived principally from humanistic groupwork practice, can be used to access such perspectives. The methods I consider are artwork, sculpting, imagework, dreamwork, gestalt and psychodrama. These methods are most used in the UK state welfare sector by family therapists working in clinical settings, whether from a medical, psychological or social work discipline. They are also widely used in the independent group-based therapy sector. However, these techniques have been little used and theorized by social science researchers.

The study of the actual and potential use of some of these methods from the social welfare/therapy field will be the focus of this chapter. The *Handbook of Qualitative Research* (Denzin and Lincoln 1994) makes almost no mention of these methods, even though photography is a well-established method of artwork (Harper 1994), as are the 'personal experience methods' of journals, diaries, annals, storytelling, etc. (Clandinin and Connelly 1994). My hypothesis is that using such 'therapeutic' methods can enhance research data by eliciting implicit perspectives and identities of respondents.

The chapter will combine the introduction of the above methods with a review of their contemporary use as research methods. I shall use Bourdieu's concept of 'habitus' (1977), a sociological theory which articulates the 'taken-for-granted' nature of our implicit knowledge of self, others and social interaction. I continue by giving examples of the use of some of these methods, such as imagework, gestalt, and dreamwork, from my own research practice. Finally I consider briefly some of the methodological, ethical and epistemological implications of these methods for potential research practitioners.

SCULPTING

Sculpting involves a group member using some of the other group members to physically represent past or present relationships in his/her current family, family of origin or a significant group such as a work group. The person doing the sculpt arranges the key people to display how he/she feels about, or would like to represent, the group or family in question. So the sculpt may display the whole gamut of feelings in relationships whether they be togetherness, security, conflict, anger or hurt. Alliances and hostilities in a group can easily be shown by using 'typical' motifs such as the 'clenched fist' or 'hugging', and the spatial representation of people through closeness and distance is a powerful way to express feelings. The 'sculptor' may be very surprised by how he/she places significant people in his/her life such as siblings or parents. The 'knowledge' that he/she represents in the sculpt may be surprising, and show feelings and perceptions that have remained unacknowledged. The evocation of such unacknowledged perceptions through the use of techniques such as sculpting, if utilized by the researcher, may allow the opportunity for the researcher to access profounder perceptions than the interview or questionnaire normally allows. Perceptions barely conscious to the respondent could then become conscious.

An example of the possible use of sculpting might be the intention to research family members' views on 'health in the family'. A sculpt involving each family member physically positioning family members in relation to each other and in relation to the question 'how do you see health in your family?' is very likely to generate, through evoked experience and subsequent discussion, significant insights into individual and family lifestyles, communication patterns within the family, and data as to how the issue of 'health' itself is perceived. For instance family members, I have found, may be much more orientated to psychological rather than physical definitions of health.

ARTWORK

Artwork is an established, though infrequently used, method in social science research. Bendelow (1992), in her own study of the gendered dimensions of the perceptions of pain, has used artwork as a way to access respondents' perceptions. Her study used paired sets of reproduced artwork to trigger respondents' expression of 'beliefs about pain'. The responses were subsequently analysed for gender distinctions. James (1993) used children's artwork as both an interviewing trigger and as a way of accessing their perceptions of 'significant others' in the school setting. Artwork can express the felt and intuited aspects of life experience in a way that logic and language often cannot (Benson 1987).

I have used artwork to seek respondents' view of their personal life history or more particularly their view of their experience of health. In both examples I asked respondents to draw a sequence of pictures on a large A1 or A3 sheet of paper to represent the 'felt' experiences of their lives, or their experiences of health during their life-course. We then made a wall gallery of their results and each respondent had a few minutes to talk to the group about their 'picture of health' in as confidential a form as they wished. No artistic ability was needed and the variety of imagery was immense. Respondents might choose to present their life as a road map, a slow ascent, descent or circular journey, or even as a helter-skelter! What was noteworthy in this case was how broad a range of experiences people considered relevant to their experience of health. Typically, I found older respondents had a more holistic ideology of health than younger respondents, who tended to focus on a more medical view of health and so emphasized the broken bones of living more than the acute sufferings of interpersonal life events. In these examples we can see the possible benefits of using such approaches to reveal and disclose that of which the respondent is only implicitly, or dimly, aware.

IMAGEWORK

Imagework has variously been called 'active imagination', 'visualization' and 'guided fantasy'. Imagework is also a powerful therapeutic method as described by Glouberman (1989) and Achterberg (1985). Imagework has developed from the active imagination technique of Jung, and the theory and practice of psychosynthesis developed by Assagioli (1975). Jung's (1959: 42) concept of the 'collective unconscious' underpins imagework. The concept of the 'collective unconscious' represented Jung's perception that the human psyche contained impersonal and archaic contents that manifested themselves in the myths, dreams and images of humans. Jung's idea that all humans contained a common and universal storehouse of psychic contents, which he called 'archetypes', is the core model of the unconscious that enables imagework practitioners (e.g. Glouberman 1989: 25) to consider the spontaneous image as being potentially a creative and emergent aspect of the self. More recently transpersonal psychotherapy has integrated the work of Assagioli and Jung to form an imaginatively based approach to therapy. Rowan's definition of active imagination suggests that:

> In active imagination we fix upon a particular point, mood, picture or event, and then allow a fantasy to develop in which certain images

become concrete or even personified. Thereafter the images have a life of their own and develop according to their own logic.

(Rowan 1993: 51)

The imagework method is an active process in which the person 'actively imagining' lets go of the mind's normal train of thoughts and images, and goes with a sequence of imagery that arises spontaneously from the unconscious. It is the quality of spontaneity and unexpectedness that are the hallmarks of this process.

The method of imagework could be considered as a version of projective testing which has a long history in anthropology (e.g. DeVos and Wagatsuma 1961; Edgerton 1971). Imagework and projective testing both certainly share a common concern with articulating 'aspects of the personality . . . not susceptible to direct verbalisation by the informant' (Johnson 1978: 127).

There are significant differences between the various kinds of projective tests, such as Thematic Apperception Tests (TAT) and the Rorschach Inkblot Test, widely used by anthropologists in the 1950s and 1960s. TAT tests offer the respondent an ambiguous image of a social situation, such as an incomplete picture of a family group, for the respondent to imagine and define as an actual scene or story. The ambiguity of the portrayed scene allows the respondent a range of possible interpretations of what is pictured. Rorschach inkblot tests offer an abstract image, as in an inkblot, from which the respondent can describe 'what they see' and in so doing usually create images and patterns which reflect their own 'idiosyncratic way of interpreting themselves and their relationship to the world around them' (Mead and Wolfenstein 1955).

TAT tests suffer from being highly prestructured in comparison to imagework. They do not fully facilitate the imaginative resources of the respondent and considerably prefocus him/her on the imaginative task required. The Rorschach inkblot tests are too open and unspecific. Rorschach tests are very difficult to interpret in a culturally unbiased way and are now hardly used (Johnson 1978). Imagework is both less structured than TAT tests and less open than Rorschach tests.

Imagework does however clearly involve some prestructuring, as in guiding the imagination in the various forms of imagework. Whilst personal and social imagery evoked through imagework is undoubtedly culture-specific, in principle it is applicable for use in non-western cultures in a way which has been found highly problematic with projective tests such as the Rorschach and TAT tests (Johnson 1978: 127–33).

Imagework exercises could be used in Third World settings and particularly in development work. It could be used to facilitate respondents' unarticulated views. For instance, with respect to eliciting villagers' views of a prospective new road development, the researcher could ask a group of respondents to imagine the present day's activity without a road. Then the researcher could ask the group to imagine how a road would change their daily pattern of activity. Instead perhaps of a long walk each day to fetch water, villagers would be able to travel quicker, thereby spending more time on other pursuits but needing to gain money for bus fares. The daily water collection might be seen as a time for singing and discussion, when women had time for themselves. The hypothesis informing my advocacy of the imagework method is that facilitating a group imaginatively to make such journeys would provide richer data, and empower muted groups such as children and women to be able to express their latent perceptions and feelings.

Another difference and advantage of imagework is that most uses of imagework articulate not just a 'single frame' image such as may happen in projective tests, but rather an entire inner, visual, often felt and certainly subjectively experienced, drama. I use imagework to evaluate a course programme and facilitate respondents/students remembering how they felt at the beginning and end of the programme and imaginatively to picture key moments of personal, academic and professional change. This often evokes a stream of significant images which have a narrative and felt component, sequence and plot, and implicitly contain issues of self and personhood, cultural context and the genesis of personal and social change. Thus imagework avoids many of the in-built weaknesses of projective tests with respect to their cross-cultural usage and limited, evocative potential.

The imagework method is particularly effective in accessing participants' implicit awareness of such areas as personal and cultural identity formation and change; interpersonal dynamics; organizational culture; and individual and collective vision development. Imagework has to date been little used in social science research though recently Stuhlmiller and Thorsen (1997: 140–9) have reported on their use of imagework, which they call 'narrative picturing'. Whilst the application of the imagework method may be considered relatively innovative, the principles and practices governing the organization and analysis of data derived from this method remain firmly within the established qualitative domain.

DREAMWORK

The dreamwork movement itself began in the USA in the 1970s as an offshoot of the human potential or personal growth movement. At this time the publication of works by authors such as Garfield (1974), and Ullman and Zimmerman (1979) both popularized and guided groups and individuals into ways of working with their dreams. The dreamwork movement values dream imagery as being of potential benefit to the dreamer and the 'meaning' of such imagery as being accessible and understandable to the interested person (Hillman 1989). Dreamwork groups are relatively commonplace in the USA but are less frequent in the UK (for which, see Edgar 1995).

Most dreams are initially seen as incomprehensible to the dreamer. However, the group members who work on their dreams are often able to derive some insight into an aspect of themselves that is currently preoccupying them. The action methods of gestalt, psychodrama, sculpting and artwork can be used as ways of getting further in touch with the latent perceptions of the dreamer. Examples of this process and its sociological rather than therapeutic outcome will be offered later in the chapter. While sociology's interest in dreaming has been largely dormant since the work of Bastide (1966), social anthropology has continued its tradition of interest in this field, which is seen as of considerable value in the exploration of world-view and particularly the mythological aspects of a society. Whilst Bastide viewed dreams as both expressing and trying to resolve the conflicts of each society, anthropologists such as Tedlock (1987) have developed an innovative 'communicative theory' of dreaming. This considers not only the dreams themselves but the dream narration as a communicative event involving the act and creation of narration, the psychodynamics of narration and the dreamer's interpretive framework. This theory of dreamwork considers dream analysis as more than a hermeneutically based textual analysis. Instead, it is a social and cultural process or activity that has both expressive and instrumental outcomes.

The 1980s also saw more use of researchers' and respondents' dreams for ethnographic research purposes. Levine (1981) analysed the dreams of three of her informants for transference material concerning her relationship with them. She was able to gain an increased awareness of issues such as power, asymmetry between herself and informants, poverty and dependence, and about the degree of gender support she was offering to one of her informants who had marital difficulties. Hillman (1989: 137) has also recently suggested that dreams can provide the ethnographer with important insights into emotional and conflictual aspects of the fieldwork situation. Goulet (1994: 22) found that 'knowing how to dream' was essential for his study of Guajiro (South America) culture. Kohn (1995) writes about the value of the dreams of her principal informant during the time when this informant, Kamala, visited her in England. Coming from a remote hill village in Nepal, Kamala's awareness of cultural change seemed heightened by her experience of travel and, unusually, she shared several dreams of her homeland with Kohn. Kohn relates how 'ideas about the cosmos which many hours of taped interviews had not uncovered in the field' (1995: 48) were shared through the dialogue about Kamala's dreams in Durham, UK.

Recently two very interesting chapters have appeared dispelling the silence around ethnographers' dreams. Ewing (1994) describes and discusses a dream experience and the recounting of her dream and its impact on her belief system. While studying Sufism in Pakistan she had the experience of a Sufi, regarded as a saint by his followers, having foreknowledge of both her dream and its meaning for her. This experience of the Saint's foreknowledge led her to question the anthropological tradition of observational scepticism with regard to data collection in the field. Based on this experience she began to value the possibility of belief in aspects of her informants' world-view co-existing with rigorous anthropological enquiry.

The fear of being labelled as 'going native' by the anthropological community initially kept undisclosed George's (1995) similar experience of dreaming during fieldwork amongst the Barok of Papua New Guinea. That her informants manifestly 'knew' the content of her dreams on several occasions profoundly shook her cultural preconceptions about the dichotomy between public and private experience. One time (1995: 23) she had a divinatory dream which indicated where to dig to find the remains of a sought-after clan house. She experienced an informant having apparent prior knowledge of the content of this dream. Another dream George recounts is of herself giving birth, followed, most unexpectedly and coincidentally, by the reality of a woman giving birth in the canoe that she was in. I have tried (Edgar 1996) to relate dreams experienced during my fieldwork to eventual analytic themes developed in my PhD thesis. Whether the anthropological study of the 'other' will necessarily one day embrace the researcher's own unconscious has yet to be seen, though Caplan has suggested, in her discussion of 'engendering knowledge', that:

> the time has come for us all, male and female, to recognise that the sense of self which has sustained the practice of ethnography for so long is irrelevant and that as the French poet Rimbaud put it 'Je suis un autre'.
>
> (Caplan 1988: 17)

These examples demonstrate the validity of conceptualizing dreams as a significant field for social scientists to consider. Just as 'anthropology at home' is now well accepted within the discipline (Jackson 1987), so it is appropriate to assert the value of dream analysis and narration (both one's own and of one's informants) as a potentially valuable part of the fieldwork and ethnographic process.

ADVANCED TECHNIQUES: GESTALT AND PSYCHODRAMA

Gestalt and psychodrama are experiential methods which require considerable competence before a researcher embarks upon using them. Gestalt techniques, derived from the innovative work of Perls (1969), offer similar opportunities. Gestalt therapy focuses on the 'here and now' of people's felt consciousness. Perls moved away from the idea of the unconscious and instead developed an integrative model of the self in which the 'therapeutic task' was to reclaim buried and incomplete aspects of the self through a form of directed roleplay. In gestalt the person working on an issue 'becomes' the person they wish to dialogue with and this is often symbolized and made more powerful by the person changing seats when in the role of their mother, daughter or boss. Through this process of spatial change and emotional disclosure the person is expected to 'get in touch' with suppressed and repressed parts of themselves. In, for instance, the context of dreamwork, from which examples will later be presented, Perls considers that each part of the dream represents a part of the self and the process of working with dreams involves this imaginative identification with different images from a particular dream.

Psychodrama is a dramatic re-enactment of some past, present or future situation. Whilst gestalt typically involves the client mainly in *dialogue* with him/herself and the therapist, psychodrama involves a directed and changing *drama* involving the group participants as well as the client. Such a dramatic recreation of past or possible events is a group-based psychotherapeutic activity initiated by Moreno (1946). The group members are used in the drama to act out the different roles of a particular situation concerning one of their members. Since a 'typical' psychodrama evokes strong emotions concerning basic human experiences such as loss, love and fear, the feelings of the rest of the members of the group will be evoked. Facilitating respondents to do a psychodrama in a therapeutic situation may allow the respondents to either rehearse or occasionally to experience a form of catharsis about an unfinished aspect of their personal life. Such a process of involvement may and often does generate new insight and some form of reformulation of the self-concept. Psychodramas can be constructed from participants' dreams and then the dream 'events' are 'acted out' in the group. This dramatic process and its subsequent discussion can evoke fresh perspectives for participants on personal and social issues. The benefit for the researcher is that views are expressed about many things which would not usually emerge using the more 'traditional' research methods of questionnaire and interview.

THE SOCIOLOGICAL ENCOUNTER

Such novel encounters with aspects of the self potentially offer a serious criticism of the nature of personal and social data provided by the more orthodox research methods, such as focus groups, interviewing or social surveys. The limitations of more orthodox methods are well documented (Bernard 1994; McNeill 1985), but usually the critique is limited to the truthfulness of the respondent and issues of procedural reactivity and the implicit biases that can enter the interview process by way of race, gender, age and class dimensions. What more experiential research methods, such as those outlined above, offer is the opportunity to reach levels and forms of knowledge not immediately apprehensible by the respondent in interview or through his/her participation in a focus group. The researcher, of course, is also involved in the production of experience as well as its recording and analysis. Using these methods as a researcher gives a new meaning to the term participant-observer!

All these powerful techniques from humanistic psychology have as a common theme the intended arousal of neglected and avoided aspects, experiences and emotions contained within the self. Often the body itself is held to represent suppressed emotion and a gestalt therapist, for instance, will often point out the difference between the verbal and non-verbal expression of the self.

The 'new' methodologies so far presented offer the opportunity for researchers to further encounter the psyche of the respondent, and occasionally of ourselves, to obtain material suppressed and repressed by the conscious mind. That we carry and contain forms of implicit knowledge, even values, within us is not a novel concept in the social sciences. Bourdieu (1977) has shown how social values are retained and contained in the posture, gait and gaze of its members. It is no accident, according to Bourdieu, that totalitarian institutions, like British boarding schools with their emphasis on 'good manners', spend so long inculcating cultural forms. The body is then 'treated as a memory' and

> The principles em-bodied in this way are placed beyond the grasp of consciousness, and hence cannot even be made explicit; nothing seems more ineffable, more incommunicable, more inimitable, and, therefore, more precious, than the values given body, *made* body by the transubstantiation achieved by the hidden persuasion of an implicit pedagogy, capable of instilling a whole cosmology, an ethic, a metaphysic, a political philosophy, through injunctions as insignificant as 'stand up straight' or 'don't hold your knife in your left hand'.
>
> (Bourdieu 1977: 94 [emphasis in original])

Bourdieu's concepts of habitus and body, explaining how the social is written into all aspects of our lives, provide a conceptual link between the 'worlds' of humanistic groupwork methodology and the social sciences. Bourdieu's explanation of how social knowledge is unknowingly acquired and internalized by individuals uses a similar notion of the 'body' as the humanistic psychologies described. Both view people as containing within an idea of the body, that includes the mind, all manner of dispositions and orderings of experience that are capable of becoming conscious. However, normally these would remain unconscious and unknown in some form without intervention from others, either in the form of therapy or in long-term social analysis such as participant-observation. Given the unconscious nature of both personal and social knowledge, we can begin to answer and later offer examples of the reclamation of this knowledge of self and society. However I would now like to illustrate, through examples from my own fieldwork, the possible scope and anthropological/sociological value of using approaches derived from dreamwork, imagework and gestalt.

DREAMWORK

I will now present an example of dreamwork drawn from research with recent dreamwork groups that I co-facilitated with a colleague, a female freelance groupworker, in Newcastle in 1989–90. The overall research aim was to analyse how group members made, through the group process, cultural and personal 'sense' out of the phantasmagoric 'nonsense' of dream imagery. The example I give shows the generation of a feminist 'sense'.

These dreamwork groups consisted of three ten-week groups of approximately two to two-and-a-half hours duration. Recruitment was by local advertising, word of mouth and through a local independent training agency. The groups were held on that agency's premises. Group size was between six and twelve. All the group members were white; there was a majority of female members and most members were employed, many in social work or counselling or teaching settings. The group started the evening by each person saying how they felt in general and whether they had a dream to share. During the evening typically two or three dreams would be selected to be 'worked on'. Having a dream 'worked on' meant telling the dream and any real life context and references that the dreamer was aware of; thereafter group members discussed possible ways of understanding the dreams; often dream images were imaginatively identified with, as in gestalt practice, or dramatized, as in psychodrama; sometimes they were painted or became the basis for a separate imaginative journey (imagework). For example, when two members had both dreamt of a door that they had been frightened of going through, we developed an imagework exercise in which members imagined that they went through a door. Dreams were prioritized for being 'worked on' if they were repetitive, felt urgent or particularly powerful as with a nightmare, or if the dreamer had not 'worked on' a dream for a while. All such 'working on' was, of course, voluntary.

The chosen dream reflected a woman's concern with her current job situation and an impending interview. The dream in summary concerned this woman going for interview in a bookshop. She was carrying a large loaf of bread in her arms. There was icing on top of the bread which suddenly started to drip off. Her ex-partner and his girlfriend were also there.

The unpacking of meanings from this dream imagery was long and complex and involved the member reflecting on her present job situation, and feelings about current and past key relationships. The dreamer identified the linking of the bread, the icing and the interview, with her concern about maintaining her physical attractiveness and avoiding her male partner's rejection if she became overweight. The group on this occasion focused on affirming the innate attractiveness of the dreamer, without reference to male expectation, and the ability of the dreamer to define herself – to become 'her own loaf'! Overall the dream reflected her anxiety and fear of assessment linked to a present fragility of self-image in the domestic sphere. The dreamer made a gestalt identification with the icing on the bread in which she imagined that she actually 'was' the icing on the bread. Through this exercise she got in contact with very basic feelings and perceptions about her mother and her mother's expectations of her. Throughout the discussion and exercise a powerful theme for the group was the spontaneous discovery of the various metaphors of bread embedded in ordinary language use such as 'using your loaf', being 'kneaded', being 'proved', 'being good enough to eat', a 'bun in the oven' and 'loafing about'. These became both humorous asides and also powerful metaphorical summaries, via the puns, for example, on 'being kneaded' and 'being proved', of the dreamer's self-state and current self-image. She, during this session, developed an identification with the bread which became a multi-vocal symbol of the self capable of many different amplifications of meaning.

Such meanings were derived from the dialogue between self (dreamer), and group. They were elicited in the group by reflecting on how we derive our dream imagery from our culture, and then in turn understanding and developing the imagery of this particular dream by considering the use of and playing with metaphor in everyday language.

The group in this session focused on assisting the dream narrator and playing with these 'bread' metaphors. However, the issues arising from the discussion reflect structural aspects of culture, in this case patriarchy. It is unlikely that a social scientist investigating the gendered nature of self-identity would have encountered or evoked such a depth of feeling in either an unstructured interview or in a focus group. Gestalt-based dreamwork practice, as in this example, aims to evoke buried, disowned or avoided feelings and also to support the integration of these 'lost parts of the self'. The groupworker/researcher is then co-producing novel insight and emotion. The results can be both therapeutic and richly informative.

IMAGEWORK

The first example of the use of imagework is at an 'introductory level'. This 'introductory level' imagework is designed to facilitate a group in sharing and analysing how participants are feeling about a certain situation. Such a method can be used as a part of interviewing or in group-based interviews and in focus groups. The technique simply consists of asking respondents to imagine an image that reflects the situation being considered. It is as easy as that! In a recent example, the situation was a two-session study of personal and professional identity change amongst students on a vocational master's program in social work at a UK university.

What was immediately striking about the student feedback was first, that all of the twenty students were able to relate an image that they had pictured and second, how 'discontented' their images were. Students particularly described 'seeing' pictures of train scenarios such as 'being in a siding', 'being derailed', 'in a tunnel' and 'I thought I was on a modern train but it's not!' Apart from the surprising amount of train imagery apparent, other notable imagery presented included feeling 'in a fog', being 'up against a brick wall' and 'climbing up a mountain without enough footholds'! I later realized that students had previously been attending a staff-student meeting about the course, and that individual and group morale at that point was low.

However, the whole point about imagework is to facilitate the movement from 'seen' inner image to articulated theme through a process of 'reading' the imagery much as one might 'read' a picture in an art gallery; and indeed further 'readings' can be obtained by asking the respondents to make a simple external picture of their imagery and then displaying their results on the wall for further individual and group discussion. Each respondent then speaks to their picture in turn before the researcher/facilitator possibly develops a group-based analysis of pertinent themes based on comparing the individual narratives that have emerged. Further amplification of meaning from such imagery can be made by doing a sculpt which in the above case would have consisted of inviting the group to first design and create a train station and railway line, using chairs and tables as props. Then each person would have been asked to position themselves in a pose that represented their feeling state about their position on the course (e.g. 'being stuck in a tunnel' or 'derailed' etc.) This can be jolly, is not difficult to facilitate (see Jennings 1986 for details), and as people talk from their positions and poses in the sculpt, new levels of insight and implicit knowledge can be revealed. It is also enhancing of group cohesion and identity, and that in itself can facilitate richer levels of discussion, of disclosure and group analysis.

So we can articulate a research process that starts with imagework and then can move on into artwork, sculpting and possibly drama. Yet at whatever point the 'experiential' process stops, public analysis by each respondent needs to begin. Themes need to be drawn out and 'read' from the imagery and, as respondents talk about their imagery, they engage the intuitive and affective dimensions of the self in ways unlikely to be achieved solely through a cognitive engagement with an interviewer/researcher. Using the binary opposition model of the brain, Markham (1989) suggests imagework connects many people to the right-hand side of their brain, the centre for creative, intuitive and lateral thinking, whilst the left-hand side brain hemisphere is known to control cognitive and intellectual processes. So imagework is particularly powerful as a tool in accessing the unarticulated views of individuals and groups in the research process.

What imagework and related 'experiential' research methods can achieve is the articulation of respondents' as yet dimly perceived aspects of self and world. So, for instance, in the postgraduate masters programme evaluation presented above, students speaking of their imagework articulated through this process their feelings about the nature, content and structure of the course, and their individual and group progress on it. Furthermore, they accessed their original hopes and fears for 'the course' and how their imagery reflected their intuited and existential predicament concerning 'the course' and their life in the 'here and now'. Not only did they reflect their immediate felt concern but, through further experiential techniques, such as the use of art and sculpting, the process gave respondents the opportunity of 'working with' and changing their existential predicaments. When I asked respondents at the end of the session as to whose 'images' had changed during the course of the session, three respondents replied affirmatively. The one who had thought she was 'on a modern train but wasn't', felt she was now on an 'express train'! Another felt there was less 'fog' around her and another felt there were more 'footholds' on her mountain!

Thus imagework and its amplification (artwork, sculpting and drama etc.) can evoke both significant insights into psycho-social situations, and even change personal and group orientations, so becoming applicable in action-research settings. For instance, in this last example respondents had almost no idea that fellow respondents/students felt so similarly about the course experience. Using imagework, even at this most simple and introductory level, can evoke rich levels of personal and group insight, and facilitate enhanced self-disclosure and group analysis. Moreover, I find groups can be easily encouraged to develop their own meta-analysis of imagery presented; asking respondents to 'identify common themes and significant differences' usually provides very useful analysis as respondents, if reasonably facilitated, are 'warmed up' by their personal and group encounter with the affective and intuitive aspects of themselves, something still relatively rarely encountered in contemporary western lifestyles.

Imagework can be used as part of an oral history approach. The method consists of leading participants through their early biographical memories as a way of picturing forgotten or little-considered aspects of their childhood awareness. Remembering and (re)picturing one's first experiences of a child of another race and/or gender to oneself can be powerful triggers for recollecting the earliest experience of culturally formed and/or stereotypical thinking. This pilot session involved a group of twelve anthropologists as guinea pigs. The session involved, after a suitable relaxation exercise, a guided journey forwards in 'imaginative time' starting with participants' early memories/pictures of home, school and play experiences. Following the exercise, discussion and analysis took place as to how early concepts of race, gender, ability and other differences were constructed. Participants' awareness came through recollecting others' bodily characteristics and social customs, such as table manners and joking behaviours, and their implications for the formation of self-concept and peer group formation.

Another exercise consisted of facilitating a group of forty participants to visualize early memories in order to assist an analysis of their implicit awareness of class. They were guided to remember their thoughts and feelings around, for example, dress, food, play, humour and significant moral advice received. The material retrieved was effectively a raw psycho-ethnography that could then be subject, through paired and small group discussion, to an analysis of the development of personal and cultural identity, in this case with a focus towards class position and understanding. I was particularly interested in excavating their unarticulated awareness, yet embodied mastery, of the values and practices of a culturally specific class position.

The 'reading' of imagework, referred to earlier in this section, can have up to four levels: first, the descriptive level wherein respondents 'tell their story'; second, analysis by participants of the personal meaning of their experience of symbols used; third, analysis of the models and perspectives used to inform their imagery; fourth, the comparative stage when respondents compare their imagework with that of others in the group. Each of these levels needs facilitation and is promoted through the amplification of the imagework into art and drama.

ETHICAL CONSIDERATIONS

This chapter has intended to show how experiential methods derived from humanistic psychology can be usefully appropriated in pure and applied social science research. These methods have particular value when the aim is to access the implicit knowledge of the respondents and is a powerful way of doing this. Such techniques may yet be widely used in such diverse fields as the social sciences, health and social care, development and even business and marketing. Yet it is evident that they may have particular value in researching repressed areas of feeling, such as when focusing on possible sexual abuse involving children and adults. However, their use in such sensitive research areas would demand effective strategies for their ethical use and appropriate clinical training.

Clearly the use of the more advanced of these techniques requires considerable familiarity with their use, and skill in their application, though arguably a researcher could observe a groupwork practitioner using such techniques, rather than using them his/herself. Basic counselling ability, or the availability of a counsellor, may be appropriate. The concern with careful use is particularly important since, as we have seen, these techniques tend to reveal latent feelings and unrealized intuitions that are often only partially conscious or are possibly even repressed. On the other hand, the use of sculpting, artwork, dreamwork and some levels of imagework are not difficult to learn to use sensitively.

The ethics of using such approaches is important. Some researchers may feel that these methods are unacceptably intrusive, provocative, and raise power issues that are very problematic. However, these methods have, as their intention, the gathering of more profound data. I would argue that any data collection method involves intrusion and can provoke problematic self-disclosure. Even a simple interview can suddenly trigger a sensitive area for the respondent and leave the researcher with ethical considerations in terms of how to handle supportively the resulting situation. The methods I have outlined will often be a catalyst for various degrees of disclosure, yet the negative aspects of disclosure can be largely prevented by the sensitive explanation of the task and technique to participants beforehand, and by similar aftercare. Having more than one group leader/researcher is recommended, as leadership, support and research roles can be negotiated and shared. Having leaders of different gender, race and age can be important in balancing possible implicit leader bias in the group process.

In using these experiential methods it is also important to realize that, whilst they incorporate non-verbal activities such as artwork, they all finally elicit a verbal communication into which the respondents' interpretation is incorporated. Therefore, a respondent explaining a piece of artwork or sculpt will typically explain to the group, including the researcher, why they have chosen their particular artistic symbols and physical positions to reflect their previous personal experience. Imagination and behaviour become, using these methods, a form of verbal communication capable of transcription and thus a 'field text' (Clandinin and Connelly 1994) for the researcher.

CONCLUSION

This chapter has shown, through suggestion and example, how experiential research methods, using humanistic groupwork-based techniques, offer researchers the means of accessing the latent knowledge and unexpressed feelings of respondents. Bourdieu's concept of the body helps us to conceptualize how our bodies contain implicit forms of understanding through which we categorize and make sense of experience. Geertz (1983) has described this as 'cultural commonsense'. Experiential methods can elicit basic assumptions of the self and society, even though outcome in research terms remains verbal transcription. The way is open, however, for further studies using these methods, perhaps in controlled studies that would compare the value of such experiential methods against the use of more traditional research practices.

BIBLIOGRAPHY

Achterberg, J. (1985) *Imagery in Healing*, Boston: Shambhala.
Assagioli, R. (1975) *Psychosynthesis*, London: Wildwood House.
Bastide, R. (1966) 'Sociology of the dream', in V. Grunebaum and R. Caillois (eds) *The Dream and Human Societies*, Berkeley: University of California Press.
Bendelow, G. (1992) 'Using visual imagery to explore gendered notions of pain', in R. Lew and C. Renzetti (eds) *Researching Sensitive Issues*, London: Sage.
Benson, J. (1987) *Working More Creatively with Groups*, London: Tavistock.
Bernard, H. (1994) *Research Methods in Anthropology*, London: Sage.
Bourdieu, P. (1977) *Outline of a Theory of Practice* [originally published in French by Librairie Droz: Switzerland, 1972] Cambridge: Cambridge University Press.
Caplan, P. (1988) 'Engendering knowledge: the politics of ethnography', Part 2, in *Anthropology Today* 4, 6, 14–17.
Clandinin, D. and Connelly, F. (1994) 'Personal experience methods', in N. Denzin and Y. Lincoln (eds) *Handbook of Qualitative Research*, London: Sage.
DeVos, G. and Wagatsuma, H. (1961) 'Value attitudes towards role behaviour of women in two Japanese villages', *American Anthropologist* 63, 1204–30.
Denzin, N. and Lincoln, Y. (eds) (1994) *Handbook of Qualitative Research*, London: Sage.
Edgar, I. (1995) *Dreamwork, Anthropology and the Caring Professions: A Cultural Approach to Dreamwork*, Aldershot: Avebury.
—— (1996) 'Dreaming as ethnography', paper given at the Society for the Anthropology of Consciousness 1996 conference in Los Angeles.
Edgerton, R. (1971) *The Individual in Cultural Adaptation*, Berkeley: University of California Press.
Ewing, K. (1994) 'Dreams from a saint: anthropological atheism and the temptation to believe', *American Anthropologist* 96, 3.
Garfield, P. (1974) *Creative Dreaming*, New York: Ballantine Books.
Geertz, C. (1983) 'Common sense as a cultural system', in C. Geertz *Local Knowledge: Further Essays in Interpretive Anthropology*, New York: Basic Books.
George, M. (1995) 'Dreams, reality, and the desire and intent of dreamers as experienced by a fieldworker', *Anthropology of Consciousness* 6, 3.

Glouberman, D. (1989) *Life Choices and Life Changes through Imagework*, London: Unwin.

Goulet, J.-G. (1994) 'Introduction', in J.-G. Goulet and D. Young (eds) *Being Changed by Cross-Cultural Experiences*, London: Routledge.

Harper, D. (1994) 'On the authority of the image: visual methods at the crossroads', in N. Denzin and Y. Lincoln (eds) *Handbook of Qualitative Research*.

Hillman, D. (1989) 'Dreamwork and fieldwork: linking cultural anthropology and the current dreamwork movement', in M. Ullman and C. Limmer (eds) *The Variety of Dream Experience*, Wellingborough: The Aquarian Press.

Jackson, A. (1987) *Anthropology at Home*, London: Tavistock.

James, A. (1993) *Childhood Identities: Self and Social Relationships in the Experiences of the Child*, Edinburgh: Edinburgh University Press.

Jennings, S. (1986) *Creative Drama in Groupwork*, Bicester: Winslow Press.

Johnson, A. (1978) *Research Methods in Social Anthropology*, London: Edward Arnold.

Jung, C. G. (1959) 'Archetypes of the collective unconscious', in C. G. Jung *Collected Works of C. G. Jung*, vol. 9, part 1, London: Routledge and Kegan Paul.

Kohn, T. (1995) 'She came out of the field and into my home: reflections, dreams and a search for consciousness in anthropological method', in A. Cohen and N. Rapport (eds) *Questions of Consciousness*, London: Routledge.

Levine, S. (1981) 'Dreams of the informant about the researcher: some difficulties inherent in the research relationship', *Ethos* 9, 276–93.

Markham, U. (1989) *The Elements of Visualisation*, Shaftesbury: Element Books.

McNeill, P. (1985) *Research Methods*, London: Routledge.

Mead, M. and Wolfenstein, M. (1955) 'Introduction to Part 5', in M. Mead and M. Wolfenstein (eds) *Childhood in Contemporary Cultures*, Chicago: University of Chicago Press.

Moreno, J. (1946) *Psychodrama*, Vol.1, Beacon House: New York.

Perls, F. (1969) *Gestalt Therapy Verbatim*, Lafayette CA: Real People Press.

Rowan, J. (1993) *The Transpersonal: Psychotherapy and Counselling*, London: Routledge.

Stuhlmiller, C. and Thorsen, R. (1997) 'Narrative picturing: a new strategy for qualitative data collection', *Qualitative Health Research* 7, 1.

Tedlock, B. (1987) 'Dreaming and dream research', in B. Tedlock (ed.) *Dreaming: Anthropological and Psychological Interpretations*, Cambridge: Cambridge University Press.

Ullman, M. and Zimmerman, N. (1979) *Working with Dreams*, Wellingborough: Aquarian Press.

Index

Abraham, C. 122
Achterberg, J. 248
active imagination 248–9
Adler, G. 157
Advice Information and Mediation Service for Retirement Housing (AIMS) 240
Age Concern 240, 243
agricultural community: anthropology of welfare in 18–19; care in 18–19, 23–6; as family orientated 27–9; female depression in 28–9; gender expectations in 27; occupational identities in 19–23; stoical attitude in 27–8, 29–31
Alasewski, A. 36
AIMS *see* Advice Information and Mediation Service for Retirement Housing; Association for the Improvement of Maternity Services
Allan, G. 190, 191
Allen, I. 216
Allensbach, 81
Allison, J. 34, 42
All-Wales Strategy 123, 124, 129
American Psychiatric Association 146
Anderson, B. 2, 103
Anthony, W. A. 139
anthropology 1; applied 183–4; and categories 4; and collaboration 97–8; and concept of negotiation 244; contribution of to social welfare policy 246; and ethnic minorities 4; and the exotic 3, 4; role of in community care 183–4, 186, 204; simple/complex societies 2; and social care for the elderly 195–6
anthropology of welfare: in an agricultural community 18–19; application of 11–12; concerns of 3–5; development of 1–3; representation and reflexivity 5; *see also* welfare
Arney, W. 35
Association for the Improvement of Maternity Services (AIMS) 34
Association of Radical Midwives 34

Association of Retirement Housing Managers 240
Audit Commission 53, 98–9, 243

Baines, C. 216
Baldwin, D. M. 138
Baldwin, S. 216
Ballard, R. 183
Banton, M. 12
Barke, M. 180
Barnes, C. 202
Barnes, J. A. 7, 121
Barnes, M. 17, 196, 202
BASAPP *see* British Association for Social Anthropology in Policy and Practice
Bastide, R. 251
Batley, R. 3
Bayerisches Landesamt für Statistik und Datenverarbeitung 81
Beard, J. H. 139, 140
Bendelow, G. 247
Benn, S. I. 98
Benson, J. 248
Beresford, P. 202
Bernard, H. 253
Blank, R. H. 211
Blewitt, H. 232
Bloor, M. J. 140
Bond, M. 204
Booth, T. 121
borderline personality disorder (BPD) 11, 138, 146–8, 149–51, 152–3, 156, 157
Borneman, J. 78, 91
Bott, E. 7, 102
Bourdieu, P. 6, 17, 31, 247, 254
BPD *see* borderline personality disorder
Bridenthal, R. 91
British Association for Social Anthropology in Policy and Practice (BASAPP) 184
Brooks, D. H. M. 7
Brown, G. W. 137

Brown, H. 121, 129
Brown, P. 145, 156, 157
Bulmer, M. 7, 122
Bundesministerium für Familie und Senioren 93

Calloway, H. 5
Cambridge, C. 13
Campbell, R. 34
Cannan, C. 3
Cantley, C. 201
carers as resources model 17
Carlin, V. F. 236
Carr, W. 76
Carrithers, M. 181
Carroli, G. 47
Carsten, J. 210
Cecil, R. 186, 203
Central Council for Education and Training in
    Social Work (CCETSW) 5
Centre for Sheltered Housing Studies 240
Chacko, R. C. 137
Chamberlayne, P. 91, 92
Chambers, E. 12
Changing Childbirth (DoH) 38–9, 51, 52
Chartered Institute of Housing 239
child care 10, 11; conflict in 57–8, 67–8; family
    vs institutional model 60–1, 67, 70–1;
    options for 79–80; Portuguese welfare debate
    on 67–71; and setting up of mothers' centre
    83–7; *see also* The Lar
Christchurch Press 211
Christenson, P. 22, 28, 31
Churchill, N. 6
Clandinin, D. 246
Clarke, G. 183–4
Clifford, J. 5, 203
Clubhouse model 139, 140–2; and client
    heterogeneity 155–6; contradictions within
    143–4; diagnosis in 145–54; *see also* Harbor
    House; Treatment model
Coffield, F. 180
Cohen, A. P. 12
Coleman, A. 167
collaboration 97–8; and culture 102–3; defined
    102; HIV world 104–8, 114–17; Swedish
    model 104–18; in the UK 104
collaboration/co-operation model 109–10; case
    studies 112–14; and the HIV network
    114–17; and social inclusion 108, 117–18;
    with the 'third sector' 110–11
collective unconscious 248
Collins, J. 100, 184
Comas d'Argemir, D. 70
Commission of the European Communities 78
community 2, 7–8, 17, 19, 108–9; and culture
    9–11, 240; learning disabled in 120–1,

134–5; and neighbourly surveillance 28; and
    retirement housing 241
community care 3, 16–17, 69; in and by 228; as
    consensus model/arena for competing
    interests 50–2, 53; defined 97, 100; for the
    elderly *see* retirement housing; feminist
    perspective 121, 202–3; and frontline
    workers 186–95; and full family support
    23–5; and grid/group analysis 100–3; and
    the learning disabled 120–1, 122, 124–35;
    midwifery in the twentieth century 33–6;
    models and practice 98–100; and partial
    family support 25–6; and
    personal/communal identities 16, 29–30,
    31–2; as popular option 120; and progress
    99; and reflections on maternity care 48;
    responsive research into 185, 186; results of
    120–1; rhetoric and practice of 17; and role
    of anthropology in 183–4, 186, 204; and
    role of the hospital 36–7; and user-oriented
    policy 196–202
Community Care Act (1990) 99
Community Mental Health Centers Act (1963)
    137
Confusion Group 151
Connelly, F. 246
Cooper, M. 202
co-operation *see* collaboration/co-operation
    model
Crick, M. R. 203
Cushman, D. 203
Cutileiro, J. 61, 65, 66, 70

Dahrendorf, R. 93
Dalley, G. 22, 120, 121, 134
Damer, S. 161, 170, 173
D'Andrade, R. G. 3
Dasey, R. 90
Davies, C. A. 135
Davis, A. 202
Davis-Floyd, R. 37, 47
Davison, B. 217–18
Day, A. T. 217
Dean's estate 161; action research in 162–3;
    contexting narratives concerning 164,
    170–1; as dump for problem families 10, 12,
    171, 172, 174–5; and grading of tenants
    177–8; influence of location/design on
    167–70; and interaction with the local
    authority 171–2, 173, 174–9; myths
    concerning 164, 170–1; origins of 164–6;
    outside interventions in 180–1; residents as
    Pioneers, Settlers, Refugees 172, 173; and
    self 179–80; social situation in 170–9;
    treatment of new arrivals on 172–3; and use
    of horror stories 172, 173–4, 175
Delamney, C. 76

Delvechio Good, M. 138
Denzin, N. K. 170, 246
Department of Health (DoH) 34, 36, 38, 50, 52, 196
DeVos, G. 249
Dexter, M. 191
DGB-Bundesvorstand 82
diffusionism 99
Dincin, J. 139, 140
Dingwall, R. 185
Dixon, J. 3
Dominelli, L. 5
Dominion 211
Douglas, M. 98, 100–1, 190
Douglas, T. 244
Dumont, L. 89–90
Dunne, J. 179
Dupuis, A. 209–10
Durkheim, E. 1, 4

Easton, B. 211
Economic and Social Research Council (ESRC) 184
Eddy, E. 12
Edgar, I. 250, 252
Edgerton, R. B. 120, 249
Egington, A. 189
elderly people: ageist assumptions concerning 234; assessment of 197–8; and asset testing debate 211–14; case studies 221–4; and costs of caring for 199–200; and decisions on how/where to live 218–19; descriptions of at home 219–21; domiciliary services for 185, 186; empowerment of 229; and the family 195, 198, 210, 216–19, 221–4, 225; and home helps 188–91; housing for *see* retirement housing; impact of neighbourhood support units on 185, 187, 198; and Income Support Service 210–11; involvement of 199–201; Mosgiel study 218–24; needs of 198–9, 200–1; New Zealand experience 214–16; personal networks of 121–2; and problem of information 195–6; and support workers 191–5, 198, 200–1; UK and Australian experience 216–18; and value of inheritance 210, 224–5
empowerment 4, 51–2; of the elderly 229; role of research and researchers in 196, 201–2, 203, 204; *see also* power
Esping-Anderson, G. 77, 80
ESRC *see* Economic and Social Research Council
evolutionism 98–9
Ewing, K. 251
experiential methods 6–7, 246–7; artwork 247–8; dreamwork 250–2, 254–6; ethical considerations 259–60; Gestalt techniques 252–3, 256; imagework 248–50, 256–8; psychodrama 252–3; sculpting 247; sociological encounter 253–4

Fabrega, H. 156
family 17; and child care 8, 66, 67, 70–1; and the elderly 195, 198, 210, 216–19, 221–4, 225; and the learning disabled 124–35; normative concepts of 10; position of women in 80, 88, 90–2; and self 17; solidarity of 68; support of 18–19, 23–6, 106, 217
Federation of Residents Associations in Sheltered Housing (FRASH) 240
Feuchtwang, S. 13
Filstead, W. J. 140
Finch, J. 17, 22, 216, 217
Fisher, M. 197
Fiske, S. 12
Fleming, A. 202
Flynn, M. 121
Focus 79, 92
Foley, H. A. 137
Foner, N. 8
Forder, A. 72
Foucault, M. 36, 98
Fountain House 139, 140
Fox, N. 184
Frankenburg, R. 43, 138
Fransella, F. 195
Fraser, G. 55
FRASH *see* Federation of Residents Associations in Sheltered Housing
Frazer, E. 121
Freidson, E. 52
frontline workers 186–7, 203; anthropological approach to 195–6; home helps 188–91; support workers 191–5, 197, 198, 200–1
Frost, K. 195

Gaines, A. D. 138, 145, 157
Garcia, S. 70
Gardiner, A. 92
Garfield, P. 250
Garfinkel, H. 47
Gateway Club 133
Gaynor, C. 5
Geertz, C. 6, 9, 260
George, M. 252
Gerbert, F. 92
Gergen, M. M. 180
Ginsburg, N. 3
Glaser, B. 105
Glasser, I. 2
Glastonbury, B. 98
Glouberman, D. 248

Gluckman, M. 241, 244
Goffman, E. 36, 47, 98, 137
Goffman, I. 179
Good, B. J. 138
Goody, J. 210
Goulet, J.-G. 251
Gowler, D. 183–4
Graham, H. 190, 191, 195
Grant, G. 186, 201
Green, J. 46, 53
grid and group analysis 100–3
Griffiths Report (1988) 97, 99, 217
Groves, D. 17, 22, 216
Gruenberg, E. M. 137
Guardian 179
Guba, E. G. 185
Gubrium, J. F. 184
Gunderson, J. G. 140
Gurney, C. 209

Habermas, J. 93
habitus 6, 10, 17, 31, 247, 254
Hahn, R. A. 138
Hamnett, C. 216, 217
Hanover HA 235–6
Harbert, W. 191
Harbor House 137, 139, 141, 142–3; and client heterogeneity 155–6; and contradictions within the Clubhouse 143–4; dual diagnosis and diagnostic uncertainty in 153–4; setting, staff and clients 143; staff beliefs about treatment 148; staff evaluations/treatment of BPD clients 149–51; staff evaluations/treatment of schizophrenic clients 151–3; staff understandings of client diagnoses 145–8; structure/explanatory models in 155; and the therapeutic imperative 144–5, 149; treatment and rehabilitation in 154–5; *see also* Clubhouse model; Treatment model
Harper, D. 246
Haxby, J. 202
Health Matters 214
Heidenheimer, A. J. 3
Helman, C. G. 145
Henwood, M. 217
Herskovits, E. 29, 32
Higgins, J. M. 3
Hill, M. 3
Hillman, D. 251
HIV world 10–11; case studies 112–14; key components 114–17; and philosophy of the *kurators* 106–8; project 104–5; research methods 105–6; roles of the *kurators* 111–12
Hobdell, M. 196
Hockey, J. 8–9
Hodnett, E. 41

Hollingberry, R. 196
home, meaning of 210–11, 214–16, 225
House of Commons (HoC) 52
Housing Corporation 239
housing for the elderly *see* elderly people
housing estate research *see* Dean's estate
Huby, G. 4
Hudson, B. 99, 202
Hugh-Jones, S. 210
Humphries, B. 180
Hunt, S. 34, 43
Hyatt, S. 11

identity: female 21–3; occupational 19–23; personal/communal 16, 29–30, 31–2
institutions: culture of 9; and family *vs* professional/carers 9; formal/informal 8; ritual/symbolic practices in 8–9

Jackson, A. 183, 202, 252
Jacobs, J. 167
James, A. 5, 71, 248
Janicke, C. 78
Jeffrey, W. D. 140, 157
Jenkins, R. 13, 135
Jennings, S. 257
Johnson, A. 249
Johnson, P. 215
Jones, C. 5
Jones, M. 139, 140, 157
Jordan, B. 1, 36, 37, 41, 53
Jung, C. G. 248

Kahn, A. 78, 79
Kakar, S. 17
Kamerman, S. 78, 79
Kane, R. 216
Karasu, T. B. 140
Kaye, G. 100
Keith-Ross, J. 236
Kendig, H. L. 217
Kessen, F. S. 71
Kirkham, M. 35, 43
Kitzinger, S. 47
Kleinman, A. 138
Kohn, T. 251
Koonz, C. 91
Koopman-Boyden, P. 215, 225
Krumrey, H. 92

Lacey, N. 121
La Fontaine, J. 13
Lar, The: children in 59–60; and definitions of childhood 65; family *vs* institutional model in 60–1; origins 58–9; politics in 62–3; public/private aspects in 66–7; sex in 65–6;

spatial layout of 61–2; staff 59; tensions in 63–5; treatment of property in 62
Lart, R. 196
Lather, P. 181
Layder, D. 161, 163, 167, 179
Lazarus, E. S. 138
Leap, N. 42
learning disabled: adjustment of 120–1; and concerns of the parents 124–35; and employment 130–3; experiences of 128–30; in group homes 120–1, 125; perspectives on 124–8; research methods 122–4; and social networks 130–3
Leinhardt, G. 98
Lewis, J. 73
Light, D. 145
Lincoln, Y. 185, 246
Lloyd, P. 228, 233, 239, 240
Lock, M. 145
Lorenz, W. 3

McCourt, C. 41
McCourt Perring, C. 50, 121, 184, 188
Macfarlane, A. 34
McKeown, T. 42
McLeod, E. 5
McNeill, P. 253
Main, T. 139
Maines, D. R. 163–4
Maiteny, P. 204
Malinowski, B. 236
Mansberg, R. 236
Marcus, G. E. 203
Markham, U. 257
Mars, G. 190
Mason, J. 216, 217
maternity care: in the community 48, 52–3; development of policy for 36–8; from midwifery to obstetrics 33–6; and one-to-one midwifery 38–9, 40, 42–5, 52, 53, 54; policy as consensus model/arena for competing interests 50–2, 53; responses to research into 49–50, 52; status/role of women as patients/users 47–8, 54; women's responses to 39–40, 45–6
Mauss, M. 69, 210
Mayer, J. 196, 197
Mead, M. 249
Means, R. 120, 121, 196, 209
Meetham, K. 196
mental illness: Clubhouse and Treatment models 140–2, 143–56; research methods 142–3; therapeutic community and psychosocial rehabilitation 138–40, 144–5; treatment programmes 137–8
Messerschmidt, D. 12
Methven, E. 43

midwives see maternity care
Midwives Act (1902) 34
Ministry of Health 34
Mitchell, A. 216
Mitchell, C. 7
Mitchell, J. C. 121
Modica, L. C. 6
Moeller, R. G. 78, 91
Monks, J. 184
Moore, H. 76
Moreno, J. 253
Morgan, D. 203
Morgan, L. M. 138
Morgan, W. J. 138
Morsy, S. 138
mothers' centre 10, 12; as community of families 88; and environmental awareness 88–9; as informal, non-hierarchical and flexible 87; leadership structure of 85–6; location of 85; membership of 86–7; setting up of 83–5
Müller, U. 74, 79
Munday, E. 61, 71

Nader, L. 9
National Advisory Committee on Core Health and Disability Support Services (NACCH) and NSS 215
National Board of Health and Welfare (Sweden) 103
Nations, M. K. 138
neighbourhood support units (NSUs) 185, 187, 197–201
Nemec, P. B. 139
Nettleton, S. 16, 22
network analysis 7–8, 105–6
network conferences 113–14
New Zealand Federation of Voluntary Welfare Organisations (NZFVWO) 214
Newman, O. 167
Nicod, M. 190
Noah's Ark: Bavaria 89; Sweden 110, 114, 116
Norton, A. 195
NSUs see neighbourhood support units
Nuckolls, C. W. 138, 156
Nunes, J. A. 69

Oakley, A. 38, 41, 46, 191, 202
Okely, J. 5, 183, 184
Oldman, C. 217
Oliver, M. 202
Opie, A. 215
Orme, J. 98
Ortner, S. B. 138
Osmond, H. 142
Ostner, I. 77, 78, 91
Otago Daily Times 211, 212

Page, L. 41
Pankhurst, F. 54
Pappas, G. 138
Pardes, H. 157
Parry, I. 236
Parsloe, P. 196, 201
Parsons, T. 47
participation *see* retirement housing
Partridge, W. 12
Patch programmes 122, 123, 124, 125, 129–30,
   134
Paterson, W. 90
Paul, C. 215
Payne, M. 99
Perkins, E. 216
Perls, F. 252
Pfau-Effinger, B. 81
Phillipson, C. 216
Pill, R. 145
Pina-Cabral, J. 65
Pithouse, A. 5
Pizzini, F. 37, 42, 53
Poland, F. 204
Pool, I. 215, 225
Porter, M. 195
postmodernism 184
power: in clinical relationships 138, 154; local
   161, 172, 174; and place 10; *see also*
   empowerment
Price, D. 165, 166, 167
Prout, A. 71
psychiatry 137–8
psychosocial rehabilitation 139–40

Quataert, J. 90
Qureshi, H. 197, 204, 216

Rapoport, R. N. 140
Rapoport, R. S. 140
RCOG *see* Royal College of Gynaecologists
retirement housing 228–9, 243; defined 230–1;
   making participation work in 241–2; modes
   of participation 232–3; participation in
   231–2; promoting participation in 239–41;
   reasons for participation 233–6; residents'
   role in 238–9; and scheme manager's role
   236–7
Retirement Security Ltd (RSL) 233, 239
Reyer, J. 74, 79
Rhodes, L. A. 142, 154
Richardson, A. 126, 231
Riseborough, M. 236
Ritchie, J. 126
Robinson, F. 176
Rojek, C. 5
Roosens, E. 138
Rorschach Inkblot Test 249

Rossi, A. 195
Rossi, J. J. 140
Rothman, D. J. 138
Rowan, J. 249
Royal College of Gynaecologists (RCOG) 35
RSL *see* Retirement Security Ltd
Runge, B. 74, 83
Ryan, J. 120
Ryle, G. 170

Sainsbury, D. 73
Sainsbury, E. 197
St John, S. 213
Santos, B. de S. 57, 69
Savage, W. 35
Scharf, T. C. 3
Scheper-Hughes, N. 68, 138
Scheurell, R. 3
Schiewe, K. 77, 82
Schimmel, P. 140
schizophrenia 11, 138, 146, 147, 148, 151–3,
   155, 156
Scott, 105
Seed, P. 100
Sgritta, G. 80
Shanas, E. 197
Sharfstein, S. S. 137
Sheehan, N. W. 234
sheltered housing *see* retirement housing
Shweder, R. 17
Sibley, D. 167, 177
Sidell, M. 202
Siegel, A. W. 71
Siegler, M. 142
Silverman, D. 184
Singer, M. 138
Sixsmith, A. 193
Smith, G. 201
Smith, H. 121, 129
Smith, M. K. 140
Smith, R. 120, 121
social organization analysis 7–9; context 163–6;
   self 179–80; settings 167–70; situated
   activity 170–9
sociology 183
Spicer, P. 6
Spiegel, Der 93
Stanley, L. 185, 202
Statistics NZ 214, 218
Statistische Jahrbuch Deutschland 79–81
Stebbins, R. 179
Stein, H. F. 145
Stephens, S. 72
Stern, F. 90
Stevenson, G. 188
Stevenson, O. 196, 201
Stoker, G. 3

Strathern, M. 202, 203, 210
Strauss, A. 105, 244
Strong, P. 185
Stuhlmiller, C. 250
Sunday Times 212
Sussex Gerontology Network, Sheltered
    Housing Group 229
Symonds, M. 34, 43

Talbott, J. A. 137
Tambiah, S. J. 184, 185, 186
TAT *see* Thematic Apperception Tests
Taylor, A. 7
Tedlock, B. 251
Tenant Participation Advisory Service (TPAS)
    240
Tew, M. 34
Thematic Apperception Tests (TAT) 249
therapeutic community 138–40
Thomas, F. 12
Thomas, H. 37
Thompson, C. 196
Thompson, D. 213
Thompson, J. W. 137
Thompson L. 236
Thompson, N. 180
Thorns, D. 209–10, 214
Thornton, P. 202, 228
Thorsen, R. 250
Timms, N. 196, 197
Tinker, A. 203
Titmuss, R. M. 1, 70
Tomlinson, D. 2
Tozer, R. 202, 228
TPAS *see* Tenant Participation Advisory Service
Treatment model 140–2, 144, 145, 155, 156; *see
    also* Clubhouse model; Harbor House
Trevillion, S. 7, 99, 104, 121, 122
Truman, C. 180
Turnbull, G. 180
Twigg, J. 17, 184, 189, 190

Ullman, M. 250
Ungerson, C. 193
Upton, S. 214

van Putten, T. 157
van Velsen, J. 138

Wagatsuma, H. 249

Wagner, G. 98, 100
Walker, A. 161, 187, 191, 194, 196, 197, 203,
    204, 216
Wallman, S. 13
Walter, E. V. 170, 171
Warren, L. 186, 187, 188, 189, 191, 194, 196,
    197, 202, 204
Watson, J. 13
Webb, A. 196
Weiss, C. H. 186
welfare 184; consequences of assumptions in
    social policy 78–83; contribution of social
    anthropology to 246; culture of 9–11;
    experience of 6–7; gender
    needs/assumptions 73–5, 77–8, 92–4; as
    ideology and system of stratification 75–6;
    languages of 2; methods *see* experiential
    methods; social organisation of 7–9;
    German social policy 77–8; *see also*
    anthropology of welfare
welfare state/society difference 57, 69–70
Wenger, C. 3, 7, 121
Wenger, G. C. 197
Whyte, W. F. 7, 203
Wilcox, D. 233, 239, 240
Wilkin, A. 217
Williams, A. 202
Willigen, J. 12
Wing, J. K. 137
Wise, S. 202
Wistow, G. 196
Wolfenstein, M. 249
women: in agricultural community 21–3;
    depression in 28–9; educational expectations
    of 27; and employment 80–3; maternal
    identity of 88–90; position of in the family
    80, 88, 90–2, 93; response to maternity care
    39–40, 45–6; and setting up of mothers'
    centre 83–7; status/role of as maternity
    patients/users 47–8; and welfare
    needs/assumptions 73–5, 77–8, 93
Woodside, H. 140
Wright, A. L. 138
Wright, J. 196
Wright, S. 9, 188, 197, 204, 229, 244
Wulff, R. 12

Yanagisako, S. 76
Young, I. M. 121

Zimmerman, N. 250